Language Disorders in Children

*An Introductory
Clinical
Perspective*

Language Disorders in Children

An Introductory Clinical Perspective

Barbara Ann Johnson
Ph.D., CCC-SLP
Director and Associate Professor
Communication Disorders
University of Texas–Pan American
Edinburg, Texas

Delmar Publishers

I(T)P An International Thomson Publishing Company

Albany • Bonn • Boston • Cincinnati • Detroit • London • Madrid • Melbourne
Mexico City • New York • Pacific Grove • Paris • San Francisco • Singapore • Tokyo
Toronto • Washington

NOTICE TO THE READER

Cover Design: Sergio Sericolo

Delmar Staff
Acquisitions Editor: Kimberly Davies   Production Coordinator: John Mickelbank
Project Editor: Eugenia L. Orlandi

COPYRIGHT © 1996
By Delmar Publishers
a division of International Thomson Publishing Inc.

The ITP logo is a trademark under license

Printed in the United States of America

For more information contact:

Delmar Publishers
3 Columbia Circle, Box 15015
Albany, New York 12212-5015

International Thomson Publishing Europe
Berkshire House 168 - 173
High Holborn
London WC1V 7AA
England

Thomas Nelson Australia
102 Dodds Street
South Melbourne, 3205
Victoria, Australia

Nelson Canada
1120 Birchmount Road
Scarborough, Ontario
Canada M1K 5G4

International Thomson Editores
Campos Eliseos 385, Piso 7
Col Polanco
11560 Mexico D F Mexico

International Thomson Publishing GmbH
Königswinterer Strasse 418
53227 Bonn
Germany

International Thomson Publishing Asia
221 Henderson Road
#05 - 10 Henderson Building
Singapore 0315

International Thomson Publishing - Japan
Hirakawacho Kyowa Building, 3F
2-2-1 Hirakawacho
Chiyoda-ku, Tokyo 102
Japan

1 2 3 4 5 6 7 8 9 10 XXX 01 00 99 98 97 96 95

Library of Congress Cataloging-in-Publication Data
Johnson, Barbara Ann.
    Language disorders in children : an introductory clinical
perspective / Barbara Ann Johnson.
        p.   cm.
    Includes bibliographical references and index.
    ISBN 0-8273-5533-5
    1. Language disorders in children.   I. Title.
    [DNLM: 1. Language Disorders—in infancy & childhood.   WL340   J66L   1996]
RJ496.L35J635   1996
618.92'855—dc20
DNLM/DLC
for Library of Congress   94-36579
                                                                              CIP

Contents

Chapter 6
Introduction to Multicultural Issues:
Identifying, Assessing, and Treating
Children of Various Cultural Backgrounds   *265*
by Barbara Ann Johnson
and Teri Mata-Pistokache

Appendices

List of Illustrations

List of Tables

Dedication

*To my wonderful family
Bill and Alyssa Ann
Love and many thanks*

Foreword

It was the beginning of a long-term friendship. I think it was in the summer of 1976 that Barbara Johnson, then Barbara Matthews, a master's-level graduate student in my Department of Communication Disorders, came into my office and said very confidently: "I want to do a thesis. I want to do some research. I like to write, and I want to work with you"—and she did. I cannot remember the exact order of delivery of her comments, but I do know that everything she said was spoken in the same cadence as the Latin proverb, *"Veni, Vidi, Vici:* I came, I saw, I conquered." Almost 19 years later, I recall that she had the same air of confidence when I approached her about writing a book in the area of child language disorders. Her response was very similar: "I want to write a book. I have done research in the area of child language disorders. I like to write and, yes, I would like to work with you [again]." Influenced by the same confident composure she had shown in 1976, I enthusiastically recommended Barbara as an author to Delmar Publishers, Inc. As a result of this collaboration, Barbara has written *Language Disorders in Children: An Introductory Clinical Perspective,* a book that most readers will regard as a long-term friend.

It is not easy to write a book about language disorders in children because there is so much material to cover. Indeed, it is a challenge for an author to determine how to select information from this widespread discipline that best meets the need of the reader. Even more challenging is to write a book at the introductory level, because the nature of the topic is complex, controversial, and transdisciplinary. In order to cover the topic of language disorders in children in a comprehensive, efficient way, one not only has to have a clear understanding of the important issues involved in this area, but also a grasp of other, related disciplines such as linguistics, psychology, sociology, and education, and their impact on language behavior as well.

Barbara Johnson has confronted all these literary challenges and succeeded. She has adroitly written a first-rate piece of work about language disorders in children. The chapters about family-centered clinical procedures, Chapter 5, and multicultural issues, Chapter 6, help to distinguish this book from other books in the same field. These chapters, in particular, also provide readers with important information that will prepare them for the reality of future service delivery with language-disordered children.

This text is designed for courses related to language disorders in children. It is very suitable for students who are taking their first course about language disorders and need a comprehensive, basic introduction to the topic. Johnson has done an excellent job of establishing a relationship between basic processes and clinical information. The text is up-to-date and written in a manner that accommodates a deductive teaching process. The inclusion of definitions, learning objectives, and an extensive study guide in each chapter make the book student-friendly. The custom-designed materials provide the reader with many helpful and interesting learning tools. Barbara Johnson's book will provide a strong introductory foundation about language and language disorders. Anyone who reads this book will find it to be an invaluable practical resource.

With pride,
Charlena M. Seymour, Ph.D., 1994

Preface

The available knowledge on the subject of childhood language disorders is enormous and growing rapidly, yet undergraduate majors in speech-language pathology are faced with establishing a comprehensive knowledge base comprising the topic's most consequential issues. It is on this foundation that students add subsequent knowledge and experience in order to achieve the goal of becoming independent, competent speech-language pathologists. Therefore, this volume summarizes the basics of language and normal language acquisition and then proceeds to present a cohesive exposition on the fundamentals of language disorders and related clinical issues. In combination with appropriate course work, it not only provides students with an understanding of key issues but is intended to pique their curiosity, motivating them to thoughtfully explore the topic of childhood language disorders, both now, as students, and in the future, as practicing professionals.

The author assumes that the audience is in the early stages of building the framework that is essential to future career growth and success. The book is appropriate for undergraduates who are enrolled in courses in either language disorders in children or methods for clinical practice, and it is assumed that students have completed introductory courses in communication disorders (i.e., "Introduction to Speech-Language Pathology," "Anatomy and Physiology of the Speech and Hearing Mechanism," "Voice and Phonetics," "Audiology I," and "Language Development") and core curriculum requirements (e.g., psychology, sociology, mathematics, and other science requirements). In order to accommodate learning needs of students at the intended level, the text includes clinical examples and illustrations as well as a comprehensive study guide series so that readers may have opportunity to assimilate each new concept as it is presented.

The study guide series is designed to assist readers as they acquire and internalize new information, further guiding those who benefit from instruction in how to highlight, organize, and retrieve information. In addition to answering each study guide question completely at the end of each chapter, it is suggested that students scan each chapter's study guide just prior to reading. By so doing, it is expected that they will be mentally prepared for each topic before it is presented. Further, professional terms are defined in the glossary and they are shown in boldface the first time they appear in the text.

Overall, the volume illuminates language development and disorders from birth through adolescence, focusing primarily on the needs of children from birth through the primary grades. Further, the disordered populations described here are comprised of those individuals who are traditionally included as well as several populations that are typically absent in editions on this topic.

The text is organized so that the most basic information is presented first, with subsequent chapters adding to and building on that groundwork. Part 1 is a discussion of language acquisition and the domain of language disorders (Chapters 1 and 2). Certain preliminary fundamentals are reviewed in the first chapter although modest prior knowledge is presumed. Language and its dimensions are defined and described, prerequisites to language acquisition (including anatomical and physiological, phonological, perceptual, cognitive, and social factors) are reviewed, and major developmental milestones and the process of language acquisition are highlighted. Chapter 1 is intended to briefly recapitulate information that is necessary for understanding the content of Chapters 2 though 6. It is assumed that students have access to more detailed information as a result of having successfully completed the prerequisite courses.

The second chapter defines language disorders and then expounds on a number of etiological factors that can lead to disordered language development. Language characteristics of a variety of special populations are summarized. These include individuals with mental retardation, learning disabilities, childhood aphasia, attention deficit disorder, reduced hearing sensitivity, central auditory processing disorder, developmental apraxia of speech, developmental dysarthrias, elective mutism, and autism, as well as multiple births. In describing each group, etiological, behavioral, and speech-language factors are all taken into consideration.

Part 2 (Chapters 3 and 4) outlines the basic clinical operations that apply to assessment and intervention procedures for children with language disorders, beginning with guidelines for clinical practice from an ethical perspective. Both screening and assessment procedures are described in Chapter 3. The general processes of a traditional language assessment are outlined in detail, from the time of initial contact to the writing of the assessment report. Modifications to the conventional language assessment protocol are suggested in order to facilitate assessment of taciturn and unintelligible children.

Chapter 4 explains procedures for planning and implementing traditional language intervention. Intervention options are introduced for preverbal children, as well as for those with disrupted form, content, and use; disrupted content-form interactions; separation of language dimensions; disrupted interaction between the dimensions; attention deficit disorder; and reduced hearing sensitivity. Intervention plans, lesson plans, and progress reports are also summarized.

Part 3 (Chapters 5 and 6) expands on the clinical ramifications discussed in Part 2 by describing implications for language-disordered children whose circumstances require modifications to the traditional model. In this part, the fundamentals from Chapters 1 through 4 are interfaced with prime issues such as family-centered intervention and multicultural concerns.

Chapter 5 introduces students to the notion of linking family resources with professional expertise, a notion that is central to family-centered assessment and intervention. This concept is at the very core of all practice with the birth-to-age-3 population and is applicable to clients and families of all ages.

Chapter 6 is a coauthored chapter (with Teri Mata-Pistokache), which provides introductory information about serving language-disordered children from a variety of cultural backgrounds. As a profession we have become more culturally sensitive in recent years. New information on multicultural concerns has become available, and in this chapter it is shared with students at a preliminary level.

In conclusion, the author wishes to acknowledge Bill Perison, for his endless patience and for his editorial comments; Alyssa Ann, for cooperating; Helen and Ray Johnson, for their encouragement throughout the years; and Charlena Seymour, for her mentorship and continuous support; the communication disorders faculties at UT-Pan Am for their cooperation throughout the project; and the many teachers, colleagues, students, clients and families who, together, enhanced my professional experience making it possible for me to complete this work.

PART I

Child Language and Language Disorders

CHAPTER 1

Language
A Review of Fundamentals

LEARNING OBJECTIVES

At the conclusion of this chapter, you should be able to:

- Define language and consider how it is used for communication, consider how ideas are communicated through language, and consider language as a code that is systematic and conventional;
- Describe and differentiate between each of the three dimensions of language (content, form, and use) and appreciate the three dimensions as an integrated whole;
- Identify and describe anatomical, physiological, audiological, neurological, perceptual, cognitive, and social conditions necessary for language acquisition;
- Discuss each prerequisite to language acquisition in relation to the three dimensions of language;
- Identify the approximate sequence and ages for developmental milestones associated with spoken language acquisition from birth through adolescence;
- Identify aspects of spoken language that continue to become more sophisticated through adolescence and adulthood;
- Discuss the process by which spoken language is usually acquired;
- Discuss some achievements associated with learning written language, and appreciate the relationship between spoken-language competence and academic success in reading and writing.

INTRODUCTION

Welcome to the study of language disorders in children. In preparation for discussions pertaining to disorders, it is expedient to review some basic concepts about **language** in general. This includes a definition of language, prerequisites to language, and the major milestones and basic **processes** of language acquisition. The first, and most fundamental, of these concepts is a definition of language.

DEFINITION OF LANGUAGE

Language can take a variety of forms, including spoken language, sign language, written language, and body language, as well as a variety of different languages and **dialects**. The scope of our discussion is limited to spoken language, its acquisition, its disorders, and basic implications for **assessment** and **intervention**.

The definition of language that we find most useful describes language as a *code*, whereby ideas about the world are expressed through a conventional system of arbitrary signals for communication (Bloom, 1988). An in-depth explanation follows.

Language Is Used for Communication

The purpose of language is communication with one's self and with others (Bloom, 1988). Communication that takes place with one's self is called **intrapersonal communication**. In this process, language is used for thinking, dreaming, imagining, and problem solving, to name a few examples.

In contrast, **interpersonal communication** is communication between people. People use language to make requests, ask questions, give commands, offer statements, make exclamations, engage in conversation, and perform a variety of other communicative acts. All of these interpersonal communication activities require the presence of at least two communicative partners—the listener and the speaker.

Language Is Used to Communicate Ideas

What we communicate through language is our ideas (e.g., thoughts) (Bloom, 1988). In order to understand or use language, one must have ideas. For example, to understand the word *cookie*, one must grasp the concept (or idea) that is represented by the word. Without this knowledge, the word *cookie* is only a sequence of sounds without meaning.

Concepts and ideas that are fundamental to language are gained through personal experience. That is, in order to realize the concept that is represented by the word *cookie*, a person first must have experiences with cookies. Experiences that result in ideas can be concrete (i.e., perceived through one of the five senses) or abstract.

In the act of intrapersonal communication (i.e., communication with one's self), it is our ideas that we mull over and resolve. Intrapersonally, the idea is not shared. By contrast, in the act of interpersonal communication, ideas cause us to ask questions, make statements, give commands, and make exclamations. Interpersonally, the idea is shared.

Language Is a Code

In a general sense, when a code is employed, one thing is used to represent another (Bloom, 1988). For example, the symbols on the controls of a VCR are a code representing the various functions of each button on the control board. One knows that in order to cause the tape to play in a forward direction, the arrow pointing to the right must be pressed. However, if one prefers to progress through part of the tape quickly, pressing the same arrow twice or pressing a button with two right arrows does the job, depending on the particular VCR. In each case, the symbols represent an action. This idiosyncratic symbol system, or code, is quickly learned by VCR users.

Similarly, and more specifically, language is a code. Words and combinations of words are used to represent objects (i.e., people, things, places), events (i.e., occurrences), relations between objects (e.g., possession, location), and relations between events (e.g., timing, location) (Bloom, 1988). Therefore, the word (or acronym) *VCR* is not an object but rather only *represents* the piece of equipment known as a VCR.

The Code of Language Is Systematic

The code can be learned because it is systematic; that is, it is ordered by a set of rules (Bloom, 1988). In any system, rules are followed. For example, to say we have a filing system means that there is a specific way to arrange the files, and that if they are placed in a different arrangement, the system will be broken, impeding file storage and retrieval.

Likewise, the code of language is systematic, or rule-governed. Words and combinations of words represent certain objects, events, and relations, categorizing language as a systematic code. For example, the word *VCR* always represents the same type of equipment, while the word *in* always represents the same locative relationship between objects.

Although some words and combinations of words may have a variety of meanings based on the context, there are rules that apply here as well. For example, the word *baby* may represent a newborn, a childish person, a sweetheart, or a doll belonging to a young child. However, regardless of the number of possible meanings, if the rules about **language content** are followed, the exact meaning intended by the speaker will be understood by anyone who is familiar with the language.

The Systematic Code of Language Is Conventional

Language can be understood by those who use it because the systematic code is a convention (Bloom, 1988). That is, knowledge of the code and its rules is shared by the users of the code. For example, the users of English agree that the word *baby* can represent any of a variety of people or objects, as mentioned, depending on the context. Further, users of the language also agree that certain changes in word order alter meaning (e.g., "The boy ate the cookie" is different from "The cookie ate the boy") and that certain **phoneme** combinations are allowable, while others are not (e.g., final [nts] is allowed [as in *mints*], but initial [nts] is not).

Therefore, language is a code whereby ideas about the world are expressed through a conventional system of arbitrary signals for communication.

DIMENSIONS OF LANGUAGE

The following discussion is intended as a brief overview of the three dimensions of language: form, content, and use (Bloom, 1988). It is expected that students who read this material have prior knowledge of these concepts and access to more detailed information as a result of having completed the prerequisite coursework in the area of language acquisition.

Language Content: Objects, Events, Relations

The first dimension of language to be discussed is language content (Bloom, 1988). Language content is the meaning, or **semantics**, of language. It is the objects, events, and relations about which we talk. The vast majority of children in all cultures have knowledge about objects, events, relations between objects, and relations between events, and they converse about these things.

Topic.   Content is constant across all cultures. For example, nearly all children have knowledge of the class of events that we call *play*. However, the specific objects, events, and relations that children experience may vary from culture to culture, and therefore, topics and vocabulary vary accordingly. Using the example of the class of events called *play*, the names assigned to the various play activities, the objects associated with play, the complexity or simplicity of the objects and activities, how objects are used, the way activities are carried out, and a variety of other variables may differ across age-groups and cultures, even within the same geographic region. Therefore, in a conversation about play, the overall concept of play comprises the content. However, the topic reflects the specific objects, events, and relations that occur in the speakers' social sphere or culture.

Semantic Categories.   Basically, semantics refers to the meaning conveyed by words, phrases, utterances, gestures, and body language. Specific **semantic categories** that may be used to sort words according to some aspects of language content are defined in Figure 1–1. They include existence, recurrence, nonexistence-disappearance, rejection, denial, attribution, possession, locative action, action, locative state, state, quantity, notice, dative designations, additive relations, temporal relations, causality, adversative contrasts, epistemic states, specification, and communication (Lahey, 1988). The terms in the figure that describe semantic categories are presented in approximate chronological order for learning. That is, those at the top of the list are generally acquired before those that appear further down. In addition, although each term is defined as a unique entity, there are areas of overlap between some terms, and some words within an utterance may share some of the features of more than one category (e.g., in some instances, attribution and possession may be difficult to clearly differentiate from state).

Language Form

Language form, or the shape of the language, includes all aspects that contribute to the surface features of the language, or the way that it is perceived auditorily and visually (Bloom, 1988). In spoken language, it is the device used for connecting sound with meaning and it comprises at least four parts: **phonology**, **prosody**, **morphology**, and **syntax**.

Surface Features.   When spoken, the **phonology** (i.e., sound system) and **prosody** (i.e., rhythm) of the language are perceived as the language's surface features. It is these surface features (i.e., phonology superimposed on prosody) that distinguish how a particular language sounds. Surface features are learned very early in the language acquisition process. That is, by about 10 months of age, the meaningless babble of most children sounds remarkably similar to the language of their parents. Surface features are not only learned very early, they are also transferred to a foreign language when it is learned adventitiously, such that a recognizable foreign accent is the result.

Phonology.   Phonology is described as the system of sounds and sound patterns that characterize the language (Bloom, 1988; Hodson and Paden, 1991). This division of language form consists of the rules that identify the phonemes and combinations of phonemes that the language allows. For example, the tapped *r* and trilled *rr* of the Spanish language are part of its phonology but not part of the phonology of Standard American English. Further, initial *tl* is allowed in Spanish, but not in English, while the many (i.e., 18) variations of

Existence. Utterances that serve to point out or identify the existence of objects. Early examples include looking at, touching, or pointing to an object while naming it (e.g., "bunny," "dog"). Eventually speakers identify existence more clearly (e.g., "That is a bunny," "That's my dog").

Recurrence. Utterances that make reference to the reappearance of an object or make reference to another instance of an object or event after the original instance is no longer apparent. Early examples are represented by the word *more* (e.g., "more," "more juice," "more zoo," "more jump"). Later examples of recurrence are more complex (e.g., "I want more candy," "I ride again").

Nonexistence-Disappearance. Utterances that make reference to the disappearance of an object or action, or the nonexistence of an object or action, in any context in which the object or event might be expected. A form of negation is necessary to express this content category. Some early examples include: "no," "all gone," "no more," "away." Later forms may also include complex sentences using *not* or a contraction of *not* (e.g., "I don't have any more juice," "The bunny is not here").

Rejection. Utterances that express that the child is opposing an action or refusing an object. A form of negation is necessary to code this content category. Early forms include the word *no* as in "no eat" and "no wash." Later forms also include more complex sentences containing the word *don't.*

Denial. Utterances that negate the identity, state, or event expressed in a prior utterance. The prior utterance may be the child's own utterance or the utterance of a communicative partner. Early denial utterances are coded by the response "no" (e.g., mother says, "Spinach is good for you;" and child responds, "No"). Later forms include contractions of *not* in more complex sentences.

Attribution. Utterances that make reference to properties of objects with respect to (1) *inherent state* of the object (e.g., "clean," "broken") or (2) *specification* of an object distinguishing it from others in its class (e.g., "blue," "small").

Possession. Utterances indicating that a particular object is associated with a given person. Associations may be permanent (e.g., "my foot") or temporary (e.g., "his crayon"), and the possessor may be coded with a noun (e.g., "Benji's toe") or a pronoun (e.g., "your shoe"). The *-s* possessive morpheme is not necessary to place an utterance in this category if possession is indicated by context (e.g., "Mommy hat"). In later forms it can also be coded by using a possessive pronoun and the copula form of the verb *to be* (e.g., "That boat is yours").

Locative Action. Utterances that refer to movement where the goal is to change the location of a person or object (e.g., "into the box").

Action. Utterances that refer to movement relationships among people and ob-

Figure 1-1. Semantic categories defined.

(continues)

jects where the goal is not to change the location. The movement may or may not affect another person or object (e.g., "I eat the cookie," "It spins").

Locative State. Utterances that refer to static spatial relationships. This category is used to establish location; no movement occurs. A preposition is not necessary in early examples (e.g., "Mommy work"). Later examples are coded by a preposition (e.g., "Baby in tub," "Mommy is at work," "Daddy is lying down").

State. Utterances that make reference to states of affairs. Four subcategories: (1) *internal state*, which codes feelings, attitudes, and emotions of animate beings toward objects and events, and may include verbs such as *like, want, should,* or *can;* (2) *external state,* which codes external conditions such as "hot" or "dark"; (3) *attributive state,* which refers to conditions or properties of an object (e.g., "dirty," "red," "broken"); and (4) *possessive state,* which codes a temporary state of ownership (e.g., "have," "mine," "got").

Quantity. Utterances that designate more than one object or person by using a number (e.g., "two"), plural -s, or adjective (e.g., *many, all, some*).

Notice. Utterances that code attention to a person, object, or event and include a verb of notice (e.g., "see," "hear," "look," "watch," "show").

Dative. Utterances that designate the recipient of an object or action, either with or without a preposition (e.g., "This toy is for you," "Give that to me").

Additive. Utterances that code a joining of two objects, events, or states without a dependence relation between them (e.g., "I have an apple and a banana," "I'll draw and you watch me"). A conjunction is not necessary (e.g., "That's big. That's little").

Temporal. Utterances that code the temporal contour of an event (timing), tense (temporal relations between the event and the utterance about the event), and temporal dependency between and among events (e.g., sequential and simultaneous events). Temporal utterances are coded by tense markers (e.g., -ed, -ing) and words denoting temporal information (e.g., *after, before, yesterday, now, when, as, first*).

Causal. Utterances that involve an implicit or explicit cause-and-effect relationship between states and/or events. Words that may indicate causality include *because* and *so.* Causality may also be coded using less obvious forms (e.g., "Put a bandage on it *and* it will feel better," "Don't do that. You might get hurt").

Adversative. Utterances that contrast the relations between two events and/or states. Usually, one clause negates, qualifies, or somehow limits the other (e.g., "This one is dirty, but the other one is clean," "The dog barks but he doesn't bite").

Epistemic. Utterances that describe mental states of affairs (e.g., including

Figure 1-1 (continued). Semantic categories defined.

(continues)

know, think, remember, or *wonder).* Utterances in this category are usually, but not always, complex sentences.

Specification. Utterances that indicate a particular person, object, or event. This may include contrastive forms of the demonstrative pronoun (*this* vs. *that*) and use of articles (*the* vs. *a*). Eventually, specification involves the joining of two clauses.

Communication. Utterances that direct the listener to communicate the utterance to another person (e.g., "Tell the doggie to stop barking").

Figure 1-1 (continued). Semantic categories defined.

vowel phonemes that are a part of English phonology are not included in the Spanish language, which has only 5 vowel phonemes.

Prosody. Prosody (also called the **suprasegmental** aspect) comprises vocal inflection, stress, intonation, pausing, and all other variables that contribute to the rhythmic contour of a language's phoneme combinations.

Morphology. Morphology includes the words and the **morphemes** (i.e., grammatical inflections) of the language. A morpheme is the smallest unit of language that carries meaning. For example, the phoneme [s] can be a morpheme in that, if added to a regular noun, it adds the meaning of plurality (e.g., book*s*); if added to a regular present-tense verb, it adds the meaning of third person singular (e.g., walk*s*), and if added to a person's name, it adds the meaning of possession (e.g., Susan'*s*). Other morphemes include, but are not limited to, *-ed* (verb ending), *-ing* (verb ending), *-tion* (suffix), and *re-* (prefix). Any phoneme, or combination of phonemes, which, when added to a word or sentence, can be shown to change the meaning or grammatical inflection of that word or sentence, is a morpheme.

Whole, single words are included in the division of language form called morphology. Words are divided into two broad classes, **content words** and **function words**. Content words (also called contentives or substantives) are the major building blocks of language (Brown, 1973). They include the nouns (i.e., people, places, things), verbs (i.e., actions and states), and adjectives and adverbs (i.e., modifiers). Content words carry the meaning of the sentence and, in fact, are able to carry meaning even when isolated.

Conversely, function words (also called functors) do not carry complete meaning when standing alone. Instead, function words are the "glue for holding the building blocks of a sentence together" (Bloom, 1988, page 13). They are the prepositions (e.g., showing location, direction, or relationship), articles, conjunctions, and pronouns that are used to connect the content words, and their exact meanings depend significantly on the content words that they connect. For example, the meaning of the word *my* depends entirely on who is the speaker and whether the possession is permanent (e.g., "my nose") or temporary (e.g., "my fork").

Syntax.   Syntax defines the way in which users of a language arrange the morphemes so that they are meaningful to other users of the same language. It is the system of rules for combining the linguistic units. For example, in order to change the sentence "We walk home" to a past-tense sentence, the *-ed* tense morpheme is added (i.e., "We walk*ed* home"). Individuals familiar with Standard American English know that the location of the *-ed* marker in the sentence is critical, and that apart from poetic license, the order of the words in the sentence is also consequential.

In order for any sentence to have conventional meaning, the arrangement of the words and morphemes follows certain rules. Simply speaking, these rules are the syntax of the language.

Language Content-Form Interaction

Note that in the discussion about language form, meaning is continually referenced. Further, recall that meaning is the significant feature of language content. Apparently, language form is the vehicle by which meaning (i.e., content) is customarily conveyed.

Therefore, in the context of real language, content and form are rarely separated. That is, meaning obligates distinctive linguistic forms. For example, if one desires to relate an event that already occurred, then in order to accurately represent the content (i.e., meaning), standard past-tense morphological markers are a necessary part of the form used to express the ideas. Because of this dependent relationship between form and content, the two dimensions of language are said to interact whenever content obligates the use of a particular form.

Language Use

Language use, also called **pragmatics**, is the language dimension that considers the function (i.e., goal, intent, or purpose) of the utterance and its context (i.e., speaker-listener relationship, situation, milieu) (Bloom, 1988). The exact form that an utterance takes and the ideas (i.e., content) that are expressed depend on the intended function and context.

Function.   The function of an utterance is described as the goal, intent, or purpose. What the utterance is intended to accomplish depends on the goal of the speaker and the message that the speaker intends to convey to the communication partner or listener. Categories of language function indicate that language may be used to comment, protest, reject, emote, regulate con-

Comment. Utterances that identify or describe objects, persons, states, or events with no other apparent function. Comments may or may not be directed to another person.

Regulate. Utterances that serve to regulate others and require a response. Six types of regulatory utterances are described: (1) *focus attention*: the child draws attention to self, an object, or an event; (2) *direct actions*: the child expresses a desire for some action to be carried out by another; (3) *obtain an object*: the child expresses a desire for an object that may or may not be in the immediate context; (4) *obtain response*: the child's utterance obliges a linguistic response from another; (5) *obtain information*: this is similar to obtaining a response, but here the child must obtain new information; (6) *obtain participation, or invite*: the child's utterance serves to request that the listener participate in some activity with the child.

Protest or Rejection. Utterances that express an objection or refusal of objects or actions of another person.

Emote. Utterances whose only function is to express emotion.

Routine. Utterances that are used for certain rituals (e.g., greetings, transferring objects, telephone manners, songs).

Report or Inform. Utterances describing objects or events not present.

Pretend. Utterances that set an imaginary scene.

Discourse. Utterances that serve to maintain and regulate conversational exchanges. Six subcategories are described: (1) *respond*: utterances that serve to provide a response that has been obligated by another person; (2) *affirm or acknowledge*: in a response to the utterance of another person, the child indicates "yes"; (3) *negate*: in response to the utterance of another person, the child indicates disagreement; (4) *feedback*: utterance that lets the speaker know that the listener is attending (e.g., "uh huh"); (5) *repair*: child responds to request for clarification or misunderstanding of the listener; (6) *initiate a topic or turn*: Child attempts to get the floor or change the topic.

Figure 1-2. Categories of language function defined.

versation, carry out a routine, report information, pretend, and accomplish discourse (Lahey, 1988). These terms are defined in Figure 1–2.

Context.   Context is the other dimension of language use. The context is determined by where the utterance takes place, what is present at the time, and, most important, to whom the utterance is directed. For example, in beginning a conversation, a pragmatic speaker considers information that the listener needs in order to respond. Since shared information may not need to be restated, objects, events, and relations are referenced differently depending on whether they are evident to both speaker and listener.

The speaker also considers the social needs of the listener and the speaker's relationship to the listener. For example, a different form may be selected to convey the same information to a student peer as opposed to a university professor or employer.

LANGUAGE COMPETENCE: INTEGRATING FORM, CONTENT, AND USE

In order for **language competence** to be achieved, a person must successfully integrate the three dimensions of language: form, content, and use (Bloom, 1988). Language form is highly dependent on content (i.e., what one talks about). This connection was described in the section on **content-form interaction**. Moreover, the purpose and context of the utterance (i.e., language use) strongly influence the form and content of the message.

Therefore, although the three dimensions are presented separately so that you may understand the contribution that each makes to the total picture, in reality language form, content, and use are not separate pieces but integral parts of the whole. Each dimension affects, and is affected by, the other two. By successfully integrating the three, a language user is competent to communicate with fellow communicators effectively, speaking and interpreting ideas accurately according to his or her intention.

PREREQUISITES TO LANGUAGE ACQUISITION

Having defined language with its three dimensions, let us begin considering how language is acquired, starting with a discussion of several conditions prerequisite to language acquisition. These include aspects of anatomical, physiological, audiological, **neurological**, perceptual, cognitive, and social conditions that are considered to be important to the conventional acquisition of spoken language. Since it is expected that the academic curriculum includes comprehensive courses in **anatomy** and **physiology**, audiology, psychology, and sociology, the information that follows is intended to be a basic overview, highlighting information that is available in more specific form through other sources.

Anatomy and Physiology of the Speech Mechanism: Prerequisites to Language

Anatomy refers to physical structure. The focus of this section is the anatomy of the speech mechanism (not to be confused with anatomy of the hearing mechanism and neuroanatomy, which are addressed in a later section).

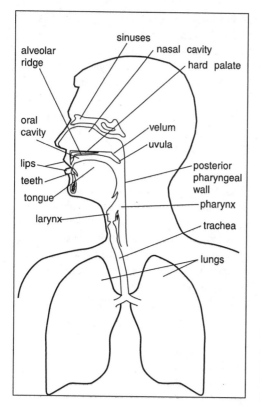

Figure 1-3. Anatomical structure that must be present and intact for conventional production of phonemes and segments.

In order to produce the phonemes and **segments** of the language (language form), certain physical structures (Figure 1–3) must be present, intact, and working properly. They are the lungs (air supply), trachea, larynx (sound source), resonating cavities (pharynx, nasal cavity, oral cavity, and sinuses), velopharyngeal valve (velum and posterior pharyngeal wall), and articulators (tongue, velum, hard palate, teeth, and lips).

Physiology is clearly related to anatomy in that it refers to the function of the anatomical structures, or what the structures actually do. Each structure has a particular primary biological function which, however important it is to life, does not contribute directly to language production. In addition to the biological purpose, each part has a communication function that, although secondary to the biological function, makes that structure indispensable to the production of the conventional language form. Thus, although communication function is secondary to biological function, the primary purpose of this discussion is to shed light on the secondary function of the structures, that is, spoken communication.

Air Supply.   The primary function of the lungs is to oxygenate the blood in order to maintain life. The secondary function of the lungs is to provide a moving air stream that can be set into vibration, producing the voice, which can be shaped into the phonemes and segments that are the building blocks for language form. Exactly how this occurs is described as follows.

Voice Production.   As the air is dispelled from the lungs, it passes through the trachea and then the larynx (pronounced [lar-ɪŋks]). If this airstream is used for speaking, voice is necessary for all vowels and more than half the consonants that characterize Standard American English.

Voice production is possible because the vocal folds in the larynx are set into vibration by air flowing out of the lungs. That is, when the vocal folds are in the abducted position, they serve to obstruct the moving air. Therefore, upon exiting the lungs, air molecules traveling upward through the trachea force the abducted folds apart. Those molecules traveling along the sides of the trachea are then forced to travel a greater distance than the air molecules traveling up the center, as they must travel around the obstruction of the vocal folds. Since air molecules traveling along the sides travel farther, they also travel faster, creating a situation in which the air pressure around the folds is less than the air pressure above and below them. Because of this pressure differential and because the vocal folds are pliable, the folds move toward the midline and close. The closing of the vocal folds in this manner is called the Bernoulli effect (Figure 1–4) (Boone and McFarlane, 1988; Colton and Caspar, 1990). Once closed, the subglottal air pressure (i.e., pressure below the larynx), which is caused by the moving air being dispelled from the lungs, blows the folds apart again and completes the cycle—which, in normal speak-

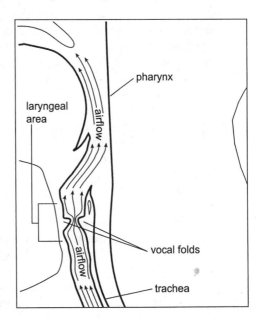

Figure 1-4. Bernoulli effect.

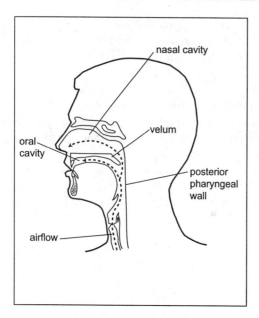

Figure 1-5. When the velopharyngeal valve is open, air may move through the nasal pathway, allowing production of the nasal consonants [m], [n], and [ŋ] and/or nasal resonance of other phonemes.

ing situations, may be repeated 100 to 500 times per second. This rapid opening and closing of the vocal folds results in the vibratory sound known as voice.

Resonating Cavities.   Having become an audible sound, the moving air continues upward, being further shaped and refined by the resonating cavities: first by the pharyngeal cavity and then by the oral and/or nasal cavities (Figure 1–3), depending on which path the sound takes. If the velopharyngeal valve is open (Figure 1–5), the velum does not approximate the posterior pharyngeal wall and the air makes its way through the nasal pathway. Nasal consonants ([m], [n] [ŋ]) or nasal **resonance** of any other (nonnasal) phoneme is produced when the velum and pharynx take on the open configuration. If, however, the velopharyngeal valve is closed (Figure 1–6), preventing air passage to the nasal cavity, the velum approximates the posterior pharyngeal wall in a sphincterlike action (i.e., like the closing of a muscular ring). The oral consonants (i.e., all consonants except [m], [n], and [ŋ]) and all vowels may be produced when the closed velopharyngeal configuration is assumed.

Speech-Sound Production.   The articulators offer the final influence on the air stream, producing the phonemes and segments of speech (part of language form). Tongue position, for example, determines the difference between a high front vowel (e.g., [i]) and a low back vowel (e.g., [ɔ]). The audible characteristics of the consonant sounds are determined by a combination of factors. These include the place where articulators constrict (e.g., bilabial, lingua-alveolar), the manner in which they constrict (e.g., stop, fricative, or glide), whether the velo-

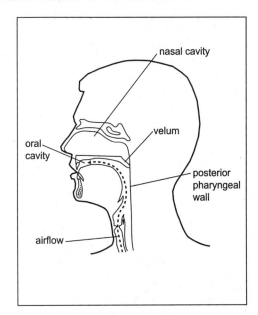

Figure 1-6. When the velopharyngeal valve is closed, it prevents air passage to the nasal cavity, which is necessary for the production of oral consonants (any consonant except [m], [n], and [ŋ]), vowels, and oral resonance.

pharyngeal valve is open or closed (i.e., nasal vs. oral resonance), and whether the vocal folds have been set into vibration (i.e., voicing).

Impact on Language Competence.   Although the structural integrity of the speech anatomy and its ability to carry out the characteristic physiology are both necessary for language to be produced in its conventional form, the impact of anatomy and physiology goes beyond the production of language form. It influences language content and use as well. For example, one who is able to produce the conventional form of the language has opportunities to practice using it, thus gaining exposure to concepts (content) and ways for representing concepts through language (use).

Further, **language competence**, or the integration of the three language dimensions, requires that all three dimensions develop adequately. When this occurs, the anatomical or physiological conditions enable one to produce the conventional language form so that it can be properly integrated with language content and use. Therefore, the health of the anatomical structures is important to the development of conventional language form, which in turn is critical to the ability to formulate and deliver messages effectively.

Anatomy and Physiology of the Hearing Mechanism: Prerequisites to Language

In order for one to interpret spoken language, the spoken language must be heard. The organ of hearing is the ear, and hearing is its primary function.

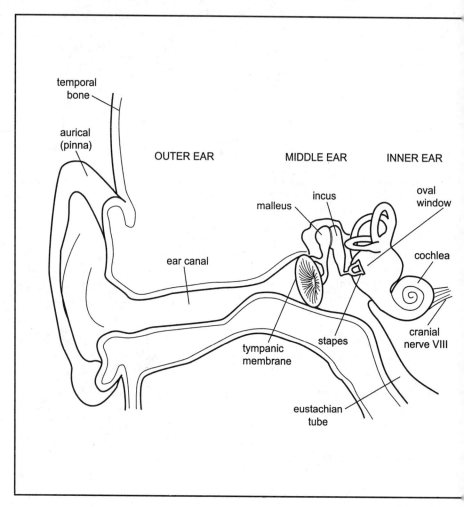

Figure 1-7. The parts of the ear.

Anatomically, the ear is comprised of three main parts which must all be present and intact to enable unaided hearing that is adequate for spoken-language learning. These parts are the outer ear (auricle and ear canal), middle ear (tympanic membrane and ossicles, including the malleus, incus, and stapes), and inner ear (oval window and cochlea) (Figure 1–7).

Outer Ear. The outer ear is comprised of the auricle, the ear canal, and the lateral surface of the tympanic membrane (Figure 1–7). In order for hearing to occur, a sound (i.e., disturbance in the surrounding air waves) must be present in the environment. Once the sound reaches the auricle, it is funneled into the ear canal. It then travels to the tympanic membrane where the airwave disturbance pushes against the lateral surface of the tympanic wall (Figure 1–7).

Middle Ear.

Ossicular Chain.   By viewing Figure 1–7, one can see that a chain of three tiny bones is attached to the medial surface of the tympanic membrane. As a group, the bones are called the **ossicles**; individually, they are called the malleus (hammer), incus (anvil), and stapes (stirrup). Their purpose is to magnify the mechanical energy produced by the sound waves that disturb the tympanic membrane.

They do this in much the same way as a lever and fulcrum amplify a physical force according to the laws of physical science. In a general sense, this phenomenon is demonstrated in Figure 1–8. A 150-pound rock cannot be moved by applying 75 pounds of force (Figure 1–8 A). However, by using a lever and fulcrum, the 75 pounds can be multiplied proportionately to the distance of the fulcrum (i.e., the small rock) from the force (75-pound child pushing). If the distance between the fulcrum (i.e., the small rock) and the force (i.e., the child pushing) is twice the distance between the fulcrum and the heavy object (i.e., the large rock), then the force will be multiplied by two, enabling one to budge the large rock with 150 pounds of force (Figure 1–8 B). The lever and fulcrum can be adjusted to magnify the affect of the force by moving the fulcrum closer to the heavy object and further from the force (Figure 1–8 C).

This physical phenomenon can be demonstrated further by a seesaw (Figure 1–9). If a heavy child and a light child are to play together on the seesaw, the board must be moved so that the fulcrum is closer to the heavy child. By so doing, the weight of the lighter child is magnified so that both children achieve balance, enabling them to enjoy the seesaw.

Similarly, in the middle ear, the joint between the incus and stapes serves as a lever and fulcrum. Therefore at the joint between these two ossicles, the displacement is increased so that by the time the sound reaches the end of the ossicular chain, it has tripled in magnitude.

Eustachian Tube.   Another important part of the middle ear is the eustachian tube (Figure 1–7). This anatomical part connects the middle ear with the oral cavity via the nasopharynx. Its influence on the sound pressure that travels through the middle ear is that of maintaining appropriate air pressure, minimizing fluid buildup, and preventing infection. These functions facilitate the conditions necessary for magnifying the sound pressure (i.e., free movement of the tympanic membrane, ossicular chain, and oval window).

Tympanic Membrane to Oval Window.   Not only does the ossicular chain (the lever and fulcrum) increase the force of the auditory signal by a factor of three, the force is further magnified by approximately 30 times as it is received by the oval window of the cochlea (Figure 1–7). This is because the force trans-

A

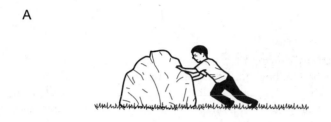

B

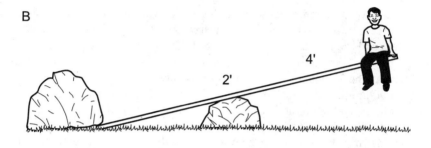

C

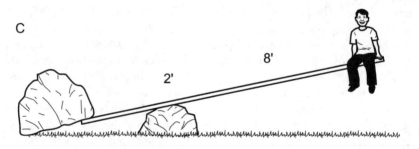

Figure 1-8. According to the laws of physical science, a lever is used to amplify physical force.

mitted from a greater area to a lesser area is always increased proportionately to the change in size (according to the laws of physical science).

A physical example of this is the pressure exerted on kitchen linoleum by a shoe having a flat heel 2 inches in diameter as opposed to the pressure exerted by a shoe having a conical heel with a ¼ inch diameter (Figure 1–10). Rarely do we see marks left on the linoleum as a result of a flat, wide heel. Instead, the marks are usually the shape and size of narrower, spikelike heels. This is because the pressure exerted on the linoleum through a flat, 2-inch heel is the same pressure as is applied by the foot to the shoe. Thus, 125 pounds across the 2 inches is reasonably well absorbed by the physical properties of the floor

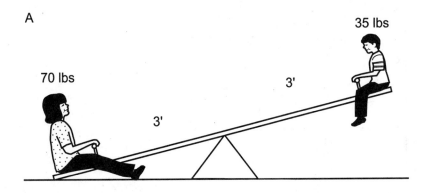

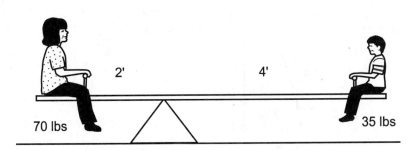

Figure 1-9.   The physical phenomenon of the lever and fulcrum effect can be demonstrated by a seesaw.

(Figure 1–10 A). However, the same 125 pounds applied to a conical heel is multiplied by the difference between the wide upper surface of the heel and the narrow lower surface. Thus, if the upper surface is 2 inches in diameter and the lower surface is ¼ inch in diameter, the same pressure is applied to an area only one-eighth the size, and therefore, it is magnified eightfold. The 125 pounds across 2 inches becomes equivalent to 1,000 pounds across ¼ inch, and this force is what leaves a mark on the floor (Figure 1–10 B).

The same principle applies to sound pressure as it travels from the tympanic membrane across the ossicles to the oval window of the inner ear. Since the surface area of the tympanic membrane is approximately 30 times greater

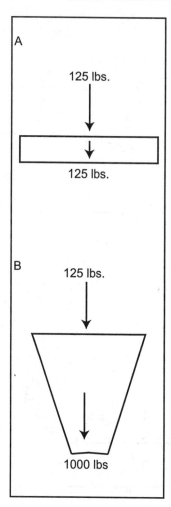

Figure 1-10. The force transmitted from a greater area to a lesser area is always increased proportionately.

than the surface area of the oval window, the resulting sound pressure is multiplied by a factor of 30 (Figure 1–11). Further, the movement of the ossicles results in a pistonlike action, applying this amplified pressure to the oval window in pressure surges.

Inner Ear. The amplified mechanical pressure that is transmitted from the tympanic membrane to the oval window is immediately transformed into hydraulic pressure when it reaches the fluid-filled cochlea. The tiny cochlea is approximately the size of the tip of the little finger and it requires only a fraction of a drop of perilymph (fluid) to fill it. This small amount of perilymph is set into motion by the vibration that reaches it through the oval window of the cochlea. It is in the cochlea that the hydraulic disturbance (i.e., sound) is differentiated for physical characteristics such as frequency and intensity. Sim-

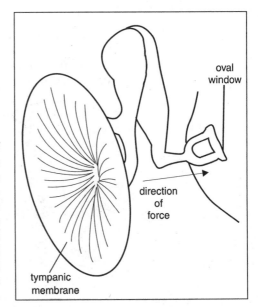

Figure 1-11. The area of the tympanic membrane is approximately 30 times greater than the area of the oval window. Therefore, the sound pressure force that is applied to the tympanic membrane is magnified 30 times as it is transferred to the cochlea through the oval window.

ply speaking, the acoustic information is received by the eighth cranial nerve (Figure 1–7), which transmits it to Heschl's gyrus in the temporal lobe of the brain (see Figure 1–12) for further interpretation.

Impact on Language Competence.   The hearing of spoken language impacts all three language dimensions. The form of spoken language is, by definition, how the language sounds. The content of the spoken language chiefly comprises the symbols representing objects, events, and relations, and the use of spoken language requires the selection of form and content in order to effectively accomplish some communicative goal in a way that is appropriate for the communicative context.

Therefore, since the form, content, and use of spoken language are all conveyed by acoustic events, the development of all three is highly dependent on access to adequate hearing. Further, since spoken-language competence depends on one's ability to integrate the three dimensions and one's ability to advance and integrate the three dimensions depends on hearing spoken language, competence in spoken language depends on the healthy structure and function of the auditory mechanism, and/or one's ability to compensate through amplification (e.g., hearing aids).

Neurological Prerequisites to Language

The cortex of the brain comprises two hemispheres—termed left and right. Although both contribute to language, the left hemisphere dominates for most

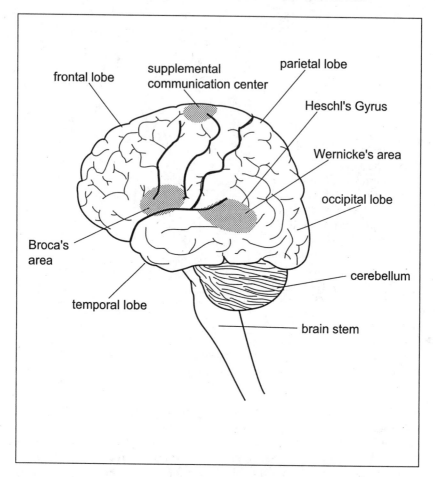

Figure 1-12.   Neuroanatomy.

people. For that reason, all diagrams here depict the left hemisphere, and the remainder of the discussion of neurology describes left hemisphere function predominantly.

Each hemisphere comprises four cortical lobes: the frontal, parietal, occipital, and temporal (Figure 1–12). The lobes that concern our discussion are the frontal and temporal. Relevant noncortical areas of the brain include the cerebellum, arcuate fasciculus, and basal ganglia.

Language Production.   All the anatomical structures necessary for speech, language, and hearing are in communication with the brain through nerve supply. Therefore, the health of certain cortical structures and their associated cranial nerves is critical to the production of spoken language. Language formulation, speech-sound production, and production of language are all discussed in the following pages in relation to contributions from neuroanatomy and neurophysiology.

Speech-Sound Production. Broca's area is located in the frontal lobe at the third frontal convolution (Figure 1–12). It is primarily responsible for formulating and programming the oral movements required for speech and language, with the help of the supplemental communication area, cerebellum, and basal ganglia. The supplemental communication area, which is also located in the frontal lobe (Figure 1–12), at the upper end of the motor strip, assists in carrying out the movements that are planned in Broca's area. The cerebellum is located below the occipital lobe and behind the brainstem (Figure 1–12). It coordinates the movements that are planned in Broca's area. The basal ganglia (not pictured) are located beneath the cerebral cortex and they inhibit meaningless, unintentional movements.

Formulating Language. In the formulation of language, topics and words are selected (language content and use) and sentences are organized (content-form). In order for these activities to take place, Broca's area of the frontal lobe and Wernicke's area of the temporal lobe (see Figure 1–12) work cooperatively. They are each involved in planning and producing language, and the two structures communicate with each other through a bundle of subcortical fibers called the arcuate fasciculus (not pictured).

Producing Language. The areas of the brain described in the preceding section transmit neural messages to the speech mechanism through cranial nerves. To simplify an explanation of the event, the neurological commands are given at the level of the cortex (i.e., Broca's area and Wernicke's area) and then carried by cranial nerves to the appropriate anatomical structures. The structures carry out the command and the outcome is communicated back to the cortex, again via cranial nerves.

Language Comprehension. In addition to speaking, language includes the hearing and understanding of incoming linguistic messages. Some of the same areas of the cortex that are involved in speaking are also involved in the hearing and understanding of language. It is primarily Wernicke's area of the temporal lobe (Figure 1–12) that receives and interprets spoken language, with Broca's area of the frontal lobe (Figure 1–12) playing a less significant role.

Again, cranial nerves are involved. Cranial nerve VIII (the acoustic nerve) (Figure 1–7) receives information from the ear (i.e., spoken language) and transmits that information to Wernicke's area (Figure 1–12) for interpretation and response. To a lesser degree the cranial nerves that innervate the articulators also participate in the comprehension of spoken language.

Phonological Prerequisites

Phonological maturation requires two areas of skill development: (1) The phonemes that are included in the language are acquired and produced accurately. (2) Then, the phonemes are skillfully produced in combination, according to the phonological rules of the language. Individuals who learn to produce spoken language must acquire skill in both these areas. That is, prior to the **comprehensible** production of a first word and subsequent words, a child must become able to produce several vowels and at least a few consonants with such accuracy that they are recognizable by adults who use the language and, further, the child must be able to combine at least two phonemes in sequence (consonant-vowel [CV] or vowel-consonant [VC]) at will and consistently (Oller, 1976, 1980).

Perceptual Prerequisites

In order for one to learn a spoken language, one must hear the language and perceive it. Exactly how spoken language is perceived is not fully understood. However, we do know that language is perceived mostly in the dominant (usually the left) hemisphere of the brain, most actively utilizing Wernicke's area, Broca's area, the arcuate fasciculus, and the supplemental communication center (Figure 1–12).

Identification.   In order to understand **perception**, one must first understand **identification** and **discrimination**, two intimately related concepts. (Indeed, some scholars do not differentiate between the two.) In the identification of anything, one is aware of that thing's characteristic properties. For example, if one is to identify a ball, one must know the properties that characterize objects in the word class, "ball."

Likewise, in the identification of speech sounds, one must be aware of auditory, visual, and tactile-kinesthetic properties that characterize speech-sound patterns (Secord, 1989). In other words, one must have knowledge of what speech sounds like, looks like, and feels like when produced. By knowing the auditory, visual, and tactile-kinesthetic properties of the sounds, one establishes a set of internal models for the sound system that characterizes the language (Winitz, 1989). These internal models include an internal auditory model (i.e., knowing what speech sounds like), an internal visual model (i.e., knowing what speech looks like), and an internal tactile-kinesthetic model (i.e., knowing what speech feels like when produced).

Discrimination.   Conversely, discrimination involves comparing one thing to another (Secord, 1989). In speech discrimination, one compares the target sound to other sounds using the same auditory, visual, and tactile-kinesthetic criteria that are used for identification. Further, one compares sounds to internal auditory models, focusing on their most relevant acoustic characteristics (Winitz, 1989). This applies to sounds produced by oneself (intrapersonal discrimination) as well as sounds produced by others (interpersonal discrimination).

Prosody.   Language perception may possibly be explained by attention given to certain prosodic elements from which an overall interpretation is gleaned. We know that for the developing infant, the prosodic features (or musical aspects) of the language are of greater import than the actual spoken words (Bloom & Lahey, 1978; Hodson & Paden, 1991; Wells, 1986). Even for adult listeners, research has shown that poorly articulated speech with good prosody is easier to understand than accurately articulated speech with inappropriate prosody (Oller et al., 1987). It is possible, then, that this melodic aspect of spoken language is critical to language perception.

Production and Perception.   Although it is most likely that one must first perceive the sounds and patterns of a language accurately in order to produce them, perception and production continue to influence one another throughout language and phonological development. A sound or pattern may be perceived and imitated, but it is production practice that refines a person's internal model of that sound or sound pattern, enabling him or her to produce and perceive sound patterns according to the conventions of the language system (Hodson & Paden, 1991; Winitz, 1989).

Perceptual Bias.   Perceptual bias probably contributes to language perception. That is, what we perceive is often influenced by expectations. For example, for some people the phoneme sequence perceived depends on which language was anticipated (Flege & Eefting, 1987). In order for language to be perceived as others perceive it, it is important, then, for individuals to share and expect the same internal models (Winitz, 1989).

Impact on Language Competence.   The perception of language goes beyond the perception of the surface features of the language discussed thus far (i.e., phonology and prosody). That is only the first level of language perception. Even if surface features are perceived accurately, the message (language content) is still subject to further interpretation depending on the context in which the utterance is heard (language use), the expectations that one has concerning the utterance (language use), one's familiarity with the information being communicated (language use), and one's relationship to the speaker (language use) (Weiss, Gordon, & Lillywhite, 1987).

The cerebral event of language perception impacts all three dimensions of language in much the same way as the auditory event of hearing spoken language. All three dimensions and their potential integration are highly dependent on one's exposure to the language. This includes how the language sounds (form), the characteristic symbols representing concepts (content-form), and the context and function of the utterances (use). If one is to be exposed to a spoken language, one must not only hear but also perceive each element as others hear and perceive it.

Cognitive Prerequistes to Language

Cognition means knowledge and the ability to use it. It includes linguistic knowledge and nonlinguistic knowledge—two domains that overlap and are not identical in shape. Both domains develop as one acquires experiences, with the size of the domain and degree of interface changing as one experiences the world. A complete match between the two domains is never achieved, even for adults. For example, most individuals always have knowledge that is difficult to express in words, such as knowing how to ride a bike (nonlinguistic knowledge), and most individuals always have knowledge that is not applicable outside the domain of language, such as knowing how to order words in a sentence (linguistic knowledge).

However, even for small children, a large area of overlap exists between the domains of linguistic and nonlinguistic knowledge. That is, nonlinguistic knowledge can be expressed linguistically as one uses words and sentences to express ideas. Further, linguistic knowledge changes as one applies it to nonlinguistic experiences. Both types of knowledge are necessary for language to be acquired (Rice & Kemper, 1984).

Returning to our definition of language (Bloom, 1988), language is used to communicate ideas or knowledge. One gains knowledge through experiences. This is true of both linguistic and nonlinguistic knowledge, and both types of experiences are prerequisites to language learning. We must have experiences with the world to have something to talk about (language content). We must have experiences with the language so that we have a means for expressing this knowledge (language form and content) and so that we know the acceptable and appropriate way to go about expressing our knowledge (language use).

Therefore cognition, or knowledge, is essential to the development of all three dimensions of language. Nonlinguistic knowledge is essential to the development of language content and use; linguistic knowledge is fundamental to language form, content, and use. Moreover, both types of knowledge are required if the three dimensions are to be integrated such that the person becomes a competent user of the language.

Cognitive Concepts Prerequisite to Language Learning.   Certain cognitive concepts are essential to language learning. Two important concepts are the concept of recognizing that one thing can be used to represent another and the concept of object permanence.

Using One Thing to Represent Another.   Language is a system of symbols (i.e., a code), and in order for one to begin learning any linguistic referents (i.e., words and gestures), one must recognize that one thing can be used to represent another. Infants begin to recognize this as shown by their use of symbolic gestures beginning in the second half of their first year of life (e.g., "waving bye-bye"). By the end of the first year, most children have begun to express certain wants and needs by using approximations of conventional words—nonconventional linguistic symbols that represent objects, events, and relations (e.g., "baba" may represent "bottle").

Object Permanence.   Another example of a cognitive concept that is important to language learning is object permanence. In order to learn the linguistic referents for the many objects, events, and relations that one experiences, one must know that the objects, events, and relations either exist or can occur even when they are not in the immediate context. By recognizing that experiences exist or can occur outside one's immediate realm, one is led to recognize that labels (linguistic referents) are important in order to request experiences that are not present in the immediate context. Therefore, the development of the cognitive concept of object permanence is important to the accelerated vocabulary growth that takes place in the second year. Moreover, the emergence of this concept is important to at least two semantic categories of language content: recurrence and nonexistence-disappearance (Figure 1-1). In turn, these two categories are important to the development of two-word sentences. Therefore, it is not likely that coincidence can account for the remarkable vocabulary growth and the emergence of two-word sentences that coincide with the mastery of the cognitive concept of object permanence.

Social Prerequisites to Language

The preceding discussion presents information regarding anatomical, physiological, perceptual, and cognitive factors that contribute to the acquisition and maintenance of language. Each is necessary and prerequisite to language. However, the final factor to discuss, socialization, is perhaps the most critical. Further, it is the only variable over which we are able to exert some measure of control (noninvasive) in our efforts to facilitate language acquisition and the integration of the dimensions of language.

Interpersonal language is a social phenomenon. It is an essential element of relationships between people. If one is to acquire conventional language, integrate all three language dimensions, and experience enjoyment and satisfaction as a direct result of social interchange, one must experience language in the context of social situations and view interpersonal communication as a meaningful, purposeful, and desirable event.

Examples of early social behaviors that are fundamental to language acquisition include engaging in eye contact with a social partner, attending to the same object or event of interest (e.g., mother and child both engage in feeding or both attend to the auditory and visual characteristics of a rattle), and taking turns in a social activity (e.g., cooing, blowing, clapping).

As a result of social interchange, the infant learns the conventional labels for various objects, events, and relations because significant adults repeatedly label the same objects, events, and relations for them as these occur in the child's presence. Social interchanges in which objects, events, and relations are labeled in an atmosphere of acceptance and encouragement are fundamental to language learning. Through these interchanges, the child learns language form (i.e., the surface features and syntax of words and sentences), language content (i.e., how to describe objects, events, and relations), and language use (i.e., the context and function of such communicative events).

MAJOR LANGUAGE ACQUISITION MILESTONES

As a future professional in the field of speech-language pathology, it is important for you to have a working knowledge of the process and approximate sequence of language acquisition so that you may optimally serve the individuals who seek to benefit from your professional expertise. For example, in conducting screenings or diagnostic evaluations, your handy knowledge and understanding of linguistic expectations for people at all levels of language development is required for determining whether further services are needed. Moreover, in providing services, you are effective only if you plan for your clients to acquire behaviors for which they are developmentally prepared and if you provide opportunities for your clients to engage in language-learning activities that naturally facilitate progress in language acquisition.

For that reason, you may use the following narration as a guide while you continue to become familiar, in a practical way, with the stages of language performance and the process of language learning. It is by taking opportunities to observe and interact with normally developing individuals, at all levels, that developmental milestones will become meaningful to you. Furthermore, it is by directly and consciously observing the interactions of people in the process of acquiring a first language that you will come to understand the natural process of language acquisition and how the principles of that process may be applied to strategies for language facilitation and intervention.

Therefore, in reading about each stage or age-group, it is your personal responsibility to make the effort to (1) think about real people relative to each stage, (2) arrange to observe and interact with children, adolescents, and adults, and (3) observe young children interacting with their primary caretakers. By doing these three things, you will experientially verify the milestones and processes of language acquisition.

The major milestones that are typically achieved in the process of language acquisition are briefly summarized in Table 1–1. Refer to it as you read. The table is intended to provide a sense of perspective regarding both the approximate sequential order of major achievements and simultaneous achievements across content-form and use dimensions.

Table 1-1. Stages of Language Development Summarized

Ages	Content-Form Characteristics	Use Characteristics
0–6 weeks	Reflexive vocalizations. Sounds include prevowels (resonants) and preconsonants, mostly nasals.	Perlocutions (0–4 months). Actions intentionally communicate a need and thereby result in a change in caretaker behavior such that the need is met.
6–16 weeks ($1\frac{1}{2}$ to 4 months)	Cooing and laughing. Resonants and constrictions may be produced alternately, but syllable units are not recognizable.	
16–30 weeks (4 to $7\frac{1}{2}$ months)	Vocal play. Marginal babbling begins at about 6 months. Vocalizations seem to be reinforced by tactile-kinesthetic sensation and social pleasure.	Illocutions (4–10 months). Socially recognized nonverbal signals are used intentionally to convey requests and guide adult attention.
31–50 weeks ($7\frac{1}{2}$ to $11\frac{1}{2}$ months)	Reduplicated babbling. Resonants and constrictions more closely resemble true vowels and consonants. Prosody begins to resemble adult language pattern. By about 8 months, babbling appears to be under auditory control.	
10–14 months	Variegated babbling. Strings of syllables closely resemble adult prosodic pattern. Early single-word utterances begin at 10–12 months. Single-word utterances are used to represent objects, events, and relations. Words are utterances that resemble adult words or phrases and are used consistently by the child in reference to a particular situation or object. Most words are simplifications of the adult pattern. Vocables may be substituted for words.	Locutions. Child begins to use meaningful words purposefully. By the time first words are spoken, child uses language for purposes of regulating other people, interacting socially, calling attention, initiating new topics, taking turns with a conversational partner, and maintaining topic for a maximum of one or two conversational turns.
14–20 months	Successive single-word utterances, rapid increase in vocabulary, and increased frequency of talking. Many words are simplifications of the adult pattern.	

(Continues)

Table 1-1 (continued). Stages of Language Development

Ages	Content-Form Characteristics	Use Characteristics
16–31 months (1⅓ to 2½ years)	Onset of true two-word utterances. Two-word utterances begin to dominate late in the stage, with noun phrases and main verbs being used with regularity. Use of phonological processes (simplification patterns) is rapidly decreasing.	By age 2 years, a child can maintain a topic for a few conversational turns, initiate a new topic, change topic, express imaginative concepts, and express personal feelings. Child does not yet consider the needs of the conversational partner.
21–35 months (1¾ to 3 years)	Two-word utterances are used proficiently. Three- and four-word sentences are used. Expressive vocabulary is several hundred words. Few simplification patterns remain. Uses regular plural -s, present progressive -ing, copula form of verb to be, no and not for negation, some prepositions (in, on), routine forms of what and where questions.	
24–41 months (2 to 3½ years)	Uses demonstratives, articles, quantifying modifiers, possessive modifiers, adjectives, present-tense auxiliary verbs, additional negative forms (no, not, can't, don't), and more complex wh- question forms (who, why, how).	By age 3, the child engages in longer dialogues and demonstrates awareness of social aspects of discourse by verbally acknowledging comments of conversational partner and by code switching. Conversational cohesion is not yet accomplished.
28–48 months (2⅓ to 4 years)	Sentences include a subject comprising a noun phrase with one or more elements. Child uses regular -ed past tense both appropriately and inappropriately; also present progressive (is —ing), auxiliary verbs in yes/no questions, inverted syntax and/or rising intonation to mark questions, and when questions. Most phonological processes (simplification patterns) have been suppressed.	
35–52 months (3 to 4⅓ years)	Child uses irregular past-tense verbs, regular third-person singular verbs, articles, and contractible copula (be). The child	

(Continues)

Table 1-1 (continued). Stages of Language Development

Ages	Content-Form Characteristics	Use Characteristics
	may negate a sentence by forming a contraction with a negative and auxiliary verb, past tense of verb *to be*, or some of the past-tense modals (would have, could have, should have).	
41 months (3¼ years) kindergarten	Child uses contractible auxiliary *be* and irregular third-person singular, and may begin to use past perfect tense and past-tense modals.	By the end of preschool years, child depends much less on conversational partner to carry the dialogue, audible monologues are replaced by inaudible monologues, and skill with narration has developed substantially. By kindergarten, language is used for all of the following purposes: (1) regulating others, (2) interacting socially, (3) calling attention, (4) initiating new topics, (5) maintaining several turns of conversations, (6) providing adequate information so that the conversational partner is able to respond without seeking clarification, (7) expressing feelings and emotions, (8) responding to comments of the communication partner with utterances that relate to the topic of conversation, (9) code switching when the situation requires, (10) phrasing indirect requests, (11) using some deictic terms, and (12) talking to one's self both audibly and inaudibly.
6 years	Child uses and understands adverbial conjunctions. Child comprehends, but does not use, passive sentences. Change in word-association skill is under way (syntagmatic-paradigmatic shift).	Child responds to indirect hints, tries to repair misunderstood utterances upon request, is beginning to view circumstances or perspective of conversational partner, and is beginning to develop fundamentals for dealing with languages at the metalinguistic level.

(Continues)

Table 1-1 (continued). Stages of Language Development

Ages	Content-Form Characteristics	Use Characteristics
7 years	Child comprehends causality inconsistently, understands and uses many spatial opposites, understands and uses most deictic terms, can manipulate sounds to create rhymes, and can recognize unacceptable sound sequences and replace them with acceptable ones.	Child is skilled at making desires known through indirect request. Child tells narrative stories that have a plot that is characterized by main character with a problem to solve, a plan for overcoming the problem, and a resolution to the problem.
8 years	Child understands and uses passive sentences, and understands comparative relationships. Morphological marker -*er* is used to denote that a person performs an action. All Standard English phonemes are produced at all levels of conversation for native speakers. All rules for patterning phonemes and syllables are accurately applied. Any persisting articulation errors are not likely to resolve spontaneously. Simple morphophonemic rules are applied accurately.	Child is capable of sustaining concrete topics, is beginning to consider perspective of other people. Proverbs are interpreted literally. Most children benefit from metalinguistic instruction.
9 years	Word-association skills resemble adult skill.	Metaphoric language is partially understood. Child uses deictic terms for conversational cohesion and a variety of cohesive markers. Child repairs conversational breakdowns effectively. Child is metalinguistically sophisticated.
10 years	Child uses *in* and *on* to express temporal concepts.	
11 years	Child comprehends and uses the word *because* consistently and accurately. Instrumental -*er* and adjectival -*y* are understood and used.	Figurative language is interpreted more accurately. Abstract concepts are sustained in conversation.
12 years	Child uses adverbial conjunctions and disjunctions.	

(Continues)

Table 1-1 (continued). Stages of Language Development

Ages	Content-Form Characteristics	Use Characteristics
13–15 years	Adolescent uses and understands *unless* and *at* for expressing temporal concepts.	Figurative language is interpreted accurately. Abstract language is used and comprehended.
16–18 years	Morphophonemic shifts are made skillfully.	Sarcasm, jokes, and double meanings are used effectively. Metaphoric language is used deliberately. Humorous comments are created skillfully. Command of abstract language approaches adult skill. Adolescent is aware that each person's perspective is different.

The First Year of Life

For most children, the first intelligible words are spoken just prior to the first birthday. The experiences that are accumulated in the 10 to 12 months antecedent to that milestone are essential and preparatory, as the process of acquiring language begins not with the onset of speech but with the birth of the child (Gleason, 1989; Sachs, 1989).

Prespeech Development of Form and Content.   Six stages occurring in the first year of life (Stark's stages) are used to describe a sequence of developmental milestones that precede spoken language (Stark, 1980). Most agree about the general nature and order of these stages, while also recognizing their considerable overlap, which occurs because one stage does not definitively end before the next begins.

Reflexive Vocalizations.   Stark's stage one takes place from birth to approximately six weeks of age and is characterized by **reflexive vocalizations**, or vocalizations that are automatic in nature (Table 1–1). They occur in response to stimuli (e.g., sensations such as pain, hunger, and discomfort), and they seem to require no mental processing. Some examples include reflexive crying, fussing sounds associated with discomfort, and a variety of primitive or vegetative sounds that typically disappear soon after birth (Stark, 1980).

Sounds at this stage are predominantly nasal. **Resonants** (i.e., **pre-vowels** or vowel approximations) outnumber **constrictions** (i.e., **pre-consonants** or consonant approximations) by about five to one. Control of voice and nasal-oral resonance is gross. However, control of all structures advances quickly at this very young age (Oller, 1976, 1980).

Cooing and Laughing.   Stark's stage two begins at approximately 6 weeks and ends at about 16 weeks of age (1½ to 4 months) and is characterized by cooing and laughing (Table 1–1). Although some reflexive sounds may continue, the child also begins to make sounds of contentment and pleasure. Usually, the cooing and laughing sounds are elicited initially by attention from an adult or older child, and later they may occur in situations that lack any social stimulation, such as when the child engages in **self-play** (Stark, 1980).

Resonant (i.e., vowel-like) sounds continue to dominate, with a few constrictions (i.e., consonantlike sounds) being introduced. Although these pre-vowels and pre-consonant sounds may be produced alternately, they are vague, and **syllable** units are not recognizable (Oller, 1976, 1980).

Vocal Play.   Stark's stage three takes place from approximately 16 to 30 weeks of age (4 to 7½ months) and is characterized by **vocal play** (Table 1–1). During these months, the infant experiments with pitch and volume extremes. The limited vocal repertoire of reflexive and responsive utterances is expanded to include such spirited sounds as squealing, growling, yelling, raspberries (a precursor to fricatives), and nasal murmurs.

Although the child's playful expressions may not have any clear communicative intent, they appear to be deliberate and are frequently made in conjunction with social interplay or as a part of nonsocial self-play (Stark, 1980). However, the vocalizations are probably reinforced and controlled by tactile-kinesthetic sensations combined with social pleasure. It is only later that the auditory sensations associated with producing sounds become a source of pleasure and reinforcement (Oller, 1976, 1980).

As the vocal play stage (Stark's stage three) begins to come to a close (after about six months of age), the phenomenon called **marginal babbling** begins (Oller & Smith, 1977). Marginal babbling is characterized by long series of syllabic segments that resemble adult syllables only in that they are composed of both consonants and vowels. A notable difference between adult syllables and the syllables of marginal babbling is that the phonemes and combinations of phonemes either may or may not be the same ones heard in the adult language model. (Pre-vowels, or resonants, and pre-consonants, or constrictions, may be used instead.) Further, the prosody of marginal babbling does not characteristically resemble adult language. That is, the sounds and sound patterns, the duration of the syllables, the frequency and duration of the pauses between syllables, and the pitch, inflection, and stress patterns of marginal babbling are clearly different from those heard in adult language.

Reduplicated Babbling.   Stark's stage four can be observed between approximately 31 and 50 weeks of age (7½ to 11½ months) and is predominantly characterized by **reduplicated babbling** (Table 1–1). Reduplicated babbling, also called **canonical babbling**, is recognized easily as a series of repeated consonant-vowel (C-V) syllables (e.g., "ba ba ba . . ." "dee dee dee . . ."). In reduplicated babbling, the syllables begin to take on the features of adult speech production. That is, resonants and constrictions begin to more closely resemble true vowels and true consonants, respectively. Further, the syllable duration, the duration and frequency of pauses, and the pitch, inflection, and stress patterns of the syllables begin to resemble adult language patterns. By approximating the prosodic patterns of adult language while speaking reduplicated syllables that are not intelligible words, the child's vocalizations may seem to mimic adult language, especially when this behavior is superimposed on the child's developing ability to take appropriate turns with an interested conversational partner (Oller, 1976, 1980; Stark, 1980).

By about 8 months, babbling appears to be under auditory, rather than tactile-kinesthetic, control. It is at this time that children with reduced hearing sensitivity often fall behind their peers in language development (Oller, 1976, 1980).

Variegated Babbling. Stark's stage five takes place from approximately 10 to 14 months of age (Table 1–1). In this stage, the child moves on to nonreduplicated babbling, which also may be called **expressive jargon** or **variegated babbling**. Variegated babbling is different from the reduplicated babbling of the previous stage in that the child begins to use a variety of consonants and vowels within each syllable series and the repertoire is not limited to C-V patterns. Vowel (V), vowel-consonant (V-C), and consonant-vowel-consonant (C-V-C) syllables are heard as well. Further, greater variety is taken on in the stress and intonation of nonreduplicated utterances such that the strings of syllables very closely resemble the stress and intonation patterns of adult speech and nearly all phonemes used are standard to the adult language model. With an increased variety of articulatory patterns and closer approximations to adult phonemes and prosody, the child may speak in an unintelligible tongue that convincingly resembles the adult model in all respects except comprehensibility (Stark, 1980).

Early Single-Word Utterances. Stark's stage six begins between 10 and 12 months of age. It is characterized by the onset of **single-word utterance**s, and ends when the child begins to use utterances that exceed one word (at about 18 months of age) (Table 1–1). "Words," at this stage, are expressions that are similar in form to adult words or phrases and are consistently used in reference to a particular situation or object (Owens, 1992). For example, the word *baby* may refer to the child speaking or to a child younger than the one speaking, while the word *goggie* may refer to the family pet or any other four-legged creature. The word *monsit* (combined with an appropriate gesture) may be used in a situation where the child is making the request, "Come on, sit."

In order to produce the first real words, the child must have sufficient control over the articulatory mechanism so that at least two adjacent phonemes (a consonant and a vowel) can be produced in a consistent manner. Further, in order for adults to recognize the first real words, the C-V combinations must be repeatedly produced in a similar manner and context (Oller, 1976, 1980).

For many children, some utterances may not resemble the form of any adult word but may be used repeatedly and consistently by the child to represent the same object, event, or relation. An example may be the child who always says [bɛp] when requesting a cracker or [son] when asking to be picked up. These wordlike utterances are called **vocables** or **phonetically consistent forms (PCFs)**, and their appearance is consistent with the onset of early single-word utterances.

Further, the emergence of single-word utterances does not necessarily mark the end of variegated babbling, and in fact, the expressive jargon that predominates the child's vocal repertoire generally continues for some time.

Prespeech Development of Language Use.   Three stages describing the preverbal development of language use have been identified (Bates, 1976; McCormick & Schiefelbusch, 1984). They are the perlocutionary stage, the illocutionary stage, and the locutionary stage. Each is described as follows.

Perlocutionary Stage.   The perlocutionary stage partially corresponds to Stark's stages one and two (Table 1–1). The perlocutionary stage is characterized by **perlocutions**, which are actions that unintentionally communicate a need and thereby result in a change in caretaker behavior such that the need is met.

For example, the infant experiences hunger and therefore cries. As a result, the adult caretaker provides nourishment. Although the crying initiated by the child is not intended to result in satisfying the hunger sensation, the response of the adult caretaker serves to reinforce the child's unintentional communicative behavior. Eventually, when the child recognizes the hunger sensation, crying is repeated *intentionally* in order to achieve the desired effect of satisfying the biological need for food.

Similarly, the child whose needs have been met may feel content and happy and therefore coo, with no communicative intent whatsoever. The cooing, however, may result in adult attention and social interchange, and eventually the child makes sociable noises for the purpose of initiating social interaction.

Illocutionary Stage.   The realization of the perlocutionary stage leads to the illocutionary stage, which generally corresponds to Stark's stages three through five and is characterized by **illocutions** (Table 1–1). Illocutions are conventional, socially recognized **nonverbal** signals that are intended to convey requests and guide adult attention. Continuing with the examples used previously, intentional crying for the purpose of satisfying the biological need for food and intentional cooing for the purpose of initiating social interchange are both illocutionary acts. At the illocutionary stage (approximately 4–10 months), an infant begins to use nonverbal communication purposefully, as directed by his or her own interests and needs.

Locutionary Stage.   The accomplishment of completing the illocutionary stage prepares the child for the locutionary stage, which begins at about the same time as Stark's stage six and corresponds to the onset of the child's first words (Table 1–1). **Locutions** are meaningful words that are used purposefully. By the time the child begins to use meaningful, conventional words purposefully, the child has already learned to use nonverbal language for regulating the behavior of other people, for interacting socially, and for calling attention to one's self, an object, or an action (Bruner, 1978; Wetherby, 1991). Further, children who are beginning to utter their first meaningful words are already skilled at initiating new topics either verbally or nonverbally, although they are limited to topics represented by objects that are present. In addition, they are adept at taking turns with a conversational partner and capable of maintaining a topic for a maximum of one or two conversational turns (Owens, 1992).

In other words, at about the time that the first words are spoken, the foundation for becoming an effective user of the language has been laid and the process of becoming a skilled communicator has begun. It is now through consistent practice with the language that the child learns how to use conventional forms for effective social and purposeful communication.

Prespeech Development of Comprehension.   Whether comprehension of language precedes production or whether production precedes comprehension has been a topic of debate for a number of years and does not appear likely to be settled in the immediate future. If comprehension precedes production, then children understand words and concepts that they do not yet express verbally. Conversely, if production precedes comprehension, children verbally express words and concepts that they do not yet fully understand.

Both propositions appear to have a measure of validity for children who are learning their first language. That is, although it may be true that children who have not yet spoken their first words appear to comprehend several words and even some sentences, it is perhaps the act of processing and comprehending words and sentences that facilitates the eventual production of comprehensible utterances. Further, it may also be true that the first words are not completely understood by the child, and that the process of speaking the words in context is necessary in order for the child to begin to more fully understand the meaning of what is said. For example, it is not uncommon for a child beginning the second year of life to demonstrate incomplete understanding of the word *dada* by using it to reference a number of adult males, much to the frustration of Daddy himself. By continuing to hear the word spoken in context *and* by continuing to say the word in appropriate and partially appropriate contexts, the child eventually gains a more complete understanding of the word.

The Preschool Years

For the purpose of this discussion, we consider the preschool years to begin with the second year and to be completed when the child enters school. Therefore, language acquisition and the behavior of children ages 1 through 5 years are described in this section.

Early Development of Content and Form.   We generally accept that first words are spoken at approximately the first anniversary of the child's birth. From the onset of the first word, seven stages of language acquisition are labeled according to Brown's Stages: Pre–Stage I, and Stages I, II, III, IV, V, and V+ (Brown, 1973; Miller, 1981). As with all stages of linguistic development, overlap is extensive in that the end of one stage is by no means prerequisite to the beginning of the next.

Brown's Pre–Stage I.   The beginning of Brown's Pre–Stage I apparently corresponds to the beginning of Stark's stage six and the beginning of the locutionary stage (Table 1–1), both of which are described in the previous section. Brown's Pre–Stage I describes the typical language performance of the majority of children between the ages of 10 and 20 months.

Pre–Stage I has two phases, the first of which is described as the *Early One-Word phase*. Children who linguistically function within the Early One-Word phase of Pre–Stage I have just begun to linguistically represent objects, events, and relations by using single-word utterances. "Words" at this stage (as defined in a previous section) resemble adult words or phrases and are consistently used in reference to a particular situation or object. At this level of language acquisition, single-word utterances may occur in combination with, or in juxtaposition to, the expressive jargon that is also typical of children who have just added approximations of adult words to their linguistic repertoires (Brown, 1973; Miller, 1981).

The second phase of Brown's Pre–Stage I is described as the *Middle One-Word phase* (Table 1–1). The onset of the Middle One-Word phase is marked by the emergence of successive (or chained) single-word utterances, a rapid increase in vocabulary (from a handful of words to a few hundred by the close of the stage), and increased frequency of talking (Brown, 1973; Miller, 1981).

Since your exposure to some of the concepts related to language acquisition may be limited at this time, you may not understand what is meant by "successive single-word utterances" without an explanation. Therefore, consider the following two successive single-word utterances: "Goggie. Gone." In this example, the child says the word *goggie* to report that a four-legged creature was seen. Immediately after saying, "Goggie," the child says "Gone," to register that the animal is no longer within view. In this case, the two words are considered to be two successive, single-word utterances rather than a single two-word utterance because the child marks the end of each utterance by a downward inflection and the end of the first utterance by a brief, but noticeable, pause. The completion of Brown's Pre–Stage I is distinguished not only by the child's attempts to use single words for the purpose of representing objects, events, and relations, but also by the milestone of beginning to recognize that two spoken words may be loosely juxtaposed to express a combination of ideas (Brown, 1973; Miller, 1981).

Brown's Stage I.   In its turn, the beginning of Brown's Stage I is recognized by the onset of true two-word utterances. The average utterance length for children in this stage is 1.01–1.99 morphemes, and the typical chronological age is 16–31 months (i.e., 1⅓ to 2½ years) (Miller, 1981). (See Table 1–1.)

The exact nature of two-word utterances is clarified by expanding on the previous example of successive single-word utterances. Having learned to successively chain single-word utterances such as "goggie" and "gone," the child eventually begins to create short sentences, of two words in length, that represent both concepts previously represented by the two shorter (one-word) sentences. For example, the single two-word utterance, "Goggie gone," performs both functions of representing that a four-legged creature was seen or heard *and* that the four-legged creature has disappeared. Prosodically, a two-word utterance is different from a set of successive single-word utterances because the downward inflection marking the end of the sentence is applied *only* to the second word (*gone*) and no noticeable pause is detected between the two words.

Although the child in early Stage I has begun to combine words in order to produce very simple sentences, the single-word utterances and successive sets thereof continue to take the lead for some time. Toward the end of Brown's Stage I, two-word utterances begin to dominate, with noun phrases and main verbs used with some regularity. Examples of two-word utterances having noun phrases include "My cookie" and "Big doggie." Examples of two-word utterances having a main verb include "Baby look" and "Bobby eat." Children who have completed Brown's Stage I use two-word utterances with proficiency, have begun to generate some three- and four-word sentences, and possess an expressive vocabulary of several hundred words (Brown, 1973; Miller, 1981).

Brown's Stage II.   At Brown's Stage II, children demonstrate an average utterance length of 2.00–2.49 morphemes and are typically between the ages of 21 and 35 months (i.e., 1¾ to almost 3 years) (Table 1–1). The increase in utterance length can be accounted for by the emergence of the regular plural form -*s* (e.g., "cats"), the present progressive -*ing* verb form (e.g., "boy running," which lacks the auxiliary verb *is*), the **copula** form of the verb *to be* (e.g., "cat *is* big."), use of the words *no* and *not* for the purpose of negating an entire sentence (e.g., "Michael *no* eat spinach"), other forms of negation (the occasional use of *can't* and *don't*), some prepositions (e.g., *in* and *on*), and, routine and eventually, novel forms of *what* and *where* questions (Brown, 1973; Miller, 1981).

Brown's Stage III.   Brown's stage III is characterized by utterances that are 2.50–2.99 morphemes in length on the average, and it is within normal limits when it occurs between the ages of 24 and 41 months (i.e., 2 to 3½ years) (Table 1–1). The increase in utterance length can be accounted for by the emergence of demonstratives (e.g., *this, these, those, that*), articles (e.g., *a, the*), quantifying modifiers (e.g., *some, a lot, two*), possessive modifiers (e.g., *his, mine, hers*), adjectives (e.g., *big, red, hot*), present-tense auxiliary verbs (e.g., *can, will, be*), frequent use of additional negative elements (e.g., *no, not, can't, don't*), and more complex *wh-* forms (e.g., *who, why,* and *how* forms) (Brown, 1973; Miller, 1981).

Brown's Stage IV.   Brown's stage IV is typically characterized by utterances that are 3.00–3.74 morphemes in length, on the average; this stage is within normal limits for children when it occurs between the ages of 28 and 48 months (i.e., 2⅓ to 4 years) (Table 1–1). At this level, it is **obligatory** for sentences to include a subject or noun phrase (e.g., "*Cookie* all gone," and "*That* is my boat"). Although sentences must contain a subject or noun phrase, the noun phrase most frequently consists of only one element. Articles, adjectives, possessives, and demonstratives may be included occasionally but are not obligatory (Brown, 1973; Miller, 1981).

Further, in Brown's Stage IV, the regular *-ed* past-tense marker may be used both appropriately and inappropriately. For example, the child will have learned to add the past-tense *-ed* marker in order to express the past tense of regular verbs (e.g., walk*ed*, patt*ed*, cook*ed*), and the child is likely to express the past tense of irregular verbs using the same marker (e.g., go*ed*, buy*ed*, eat*ed*). Also in regard to verbs at the Stage IV level, the child will have learned to use the present progressive verb form (e.g., "The dog *is* runn*ing*") and have begun to use at least one past-tense modal (e.g., *could, would, should, must, might*) (Brown, 1973; Miller, 1981).

Auxiliary verbs (e.g., *be, can, will, do*) are used in the phrasing of yes/no and *wh-* questions. Although Stage IV children begin to use inverted syntax to mark such questions ("*Are* you *going?*" as opposed to "You *are going?*"), they continue to use rising intonation as an alternative method for marking questions. In addition to the other *wh-* question forms that appear in the earlier stages (*what, where, why, who,* and *how*), *when* questions emerge at Stage IV (Brown, 1973; Miller, 1981).

Brown's Stage V.   At Brown's Stage V, the average utterance length is 3.75–4.50 morphemes, and Stage V is within normal limits for children between the ages of 35 and 52 months (i.e., 3 to 4⅓ years) (Table 1–1). It is at this level that we expect correct use of irregular past-tense verbs (e.g., *came, bought, went*), regular third-person singular verbs (e.g., "The dog *walks*"; "The boy *eats*"), articles (e.g., *a, the*), and the contractible copula *be* (e.g., "Mary *is* thin"; "The cat *is* fluffy") (Brown, 1973; Miller, 1981).

Further, at Brown's Stage V, the child may negate a sentence by forming ¡ contraction with the auxiliary verb and the negative ("We *aren't* running"; "They *can't* go"). Negative contractions may also be applied to the past tense of *be* (e.g., *wasn't*, *weren't*) and to some past-tense modals (e.g., *wouldn't*, *couldn't*, and *shouldn't*) (Brown, 1973; Miller, 1981).

Brown's Stage V+.   Brown's Stage V+ applies to children with an average utterance length of at least 4.51 morphemes, generally preschool children ages 41 months and older (i.e., 3¼ years) (Table 1–1). It is at this level that children use the contractible auxiliary form of *be* (e.g., "We*'re* running"), the uncontractible auxiliary form of *be* (e.g., "Are you going? I *am*"), the uncontractible copula form of *be* (e.g., "Is the cat fluffy? He *is*"), and the irregular third-person singular (e.g., "John *has* some," "The cow *says* moo," "Mary *does* that"). Moreover, some children who have command of longer utterances begin to use the past perfect tense (e.g., *have eaten*, *have written*) and past-tense modals (e.g., *would, could, should, must*, or *might*) (Brown, 1973; Miller, 1981).

Early Phonological Development.   Throughout the preschool years, children increase their ability to produce the phonological structure of the language (Table 1–1). The phonological structure has two components: (1) the sounds used by adult native speakers of the language and (2) the rule system that defines how the sounds can be arranged to form syllables and words (Hodson & Paden, 1991).

Regarding the development of the sounds or phonemes that are used by adult native speakers (Hodson & Paden, 1991), children hear and begin to process these phonemes (i.e., consonants and vowels) from birth, and even perhaps prenatally. Children produce approximations of adult phonemes (i.e., pre-consonants, or constrictions, and pre-vowels, or resonants) from birth, and sound production evolves such that most children actually begin producing identifiable true phonemes at about 6 months of age (i.e., near the end of Stark's stage three). Marginal babbling (at Stark's stage three) and reduplicated babbling (at Stark's stage four) include both the standard phonemes that are common to the language and the phoneme approximations that developmentally precede the production of standard consonants and vowels.

Throughout phonological development, the proportion of nonstandard phonemes decreases such that by the time children begin to use variegated babbling (at Stark's stage five), standard phonemes predominate. The mastery of standard phonemes continues throughout the preschool years and into the primary grades. Under typical language-learning circumstances, we can expect that by the age of 3, most children will have mastered all standard vowels and a few of the consonants (i.e., [p], [b], [m], [h], and [w]), such that they use them consistently and with accuracy. Although other phonemes may be articulated accurately at this age, it is completely within normal limits for them to be inconsistent or somewhat distorted. The typical progression of phoneme mastery can be observed in Table 1–2. It is generally accepted that

Table 1-2. Mastery of Phonemes.

Age Level	Phonemes Mastered
30 to 36 months (2½ to 3 years)	all vowels except [ɚ] and [ɝ] rising diphthongs: [aɪ], [aʊ], [oʊ], [eɪ]; consonants: [p], [b], [m], [w]; 75% intelligible in connected speech.
36 to 54 months (3 to 4½ years)	centering diphthongs: [ɔɚ], [aɚ], [eɚ], [ɪɚ], [ʊɚ]; consonants: [n], [ŋ], [j], [t], [d], [k], [g]; some stops substituted for fricatives (e.g., [p/f], [t/s], [d/z]).
54 to 66 months (4½ to 5½ years)	consonants: [f], [v], [j], [θ], [ð], [l].
66 to 78 months (5½ to 6½ years)	[ɚ], [ɝ] (vowels); all centering diphthongs; consonants: [r], [s], [z], [ʃ], [ʒ], [tʃ], [dʒ].
84 months (7 years)	all consonant clusters

Source: Weis, C.E., Gordon, M.E., & Lillywhite, H.S. (1987). Williams & Wilkins: Baltimore, Md.

all standard consonants and vowels are mastered by most children by the age of 7 years.

The second component of the phonological structure is the rule system that defines how the phonemes are arranged to form syllables and words (Hodson & Paden, 1991). Returning to prespeech linguistic development, it appears that children are capable of combining pre-consonants and pre-vowels alternately as early as 6 to 16 weeks of age (at Stark's stage two). Then, at about 6 months of age (during Stark's stage three), they begin to combine consonants and vowels to create recognizable syllables, although the rules that define how these phonemes are combined are not necessarily the same rules that govern adult language. By 7½ months (at Stark's stage four), reduplicated babbling demonstrates that the child has learned to combine consonants and vowels in order to form C-V syllables. At about 10 months (Stark's stage five), the consonants and vowels are combined with greater variation, such that the unintelligible variegated babbling impressively mimics the mother tongue.

Further, at 10 to 12 months (Stark's stage six and Brown's Pre–Stage I), an emerging system of phonological rules can be identified. For example, most jargon-syllables and first words resemble adult words in that standard phonemes are used and the vowels and consonants are conventionally juxtaposed. However, other rules for arranging the phonemes are often simplified by very young children. For example, some words may not contain the standard number of syllables (e.g., [ba]/"bottle") and others may lack initial or final consonant phonemes (e.g., [ak]/"sock"; [no]/"nose"), while still others may simplify or reduce combinations of phonemes (e.g., [bu]/"blue"). These patterns, which appear to simplify the adult patterns for ordering phonemes, are called **phonological processes**. They occur naturally in most early words of very young children (at about 12 to 18 months) and gradually come to occur less frequently, disappearing as the more complicated, standard phonological rules are acquired. Most simplification patterns (i.e., phonological processes) are completely suppressed by age 4 years in most children (Hodson & Paden, 1991).

Early Development of Use.   As mentioned in the previous section, preverbal children achieve certain milestones with regard to language use, or pragmatics. By the time the first words are spoken, children have learned to use language for the purposes of regulating other people, interacting socially, calling attention, initiating new topics, taking turns with a conversational partner, and maintaining a topic for a maximum of one or two conversational turns (Table 1–1).

Development of Social Discourse.   Preschool children build on these skills such that by 2 years of age they are able to maintain a topic for a few conversational turns, initiate a new topic, change the topic of conversation, and express imaginative concepts and personal feelings. Two-year-olds, however, do not generally consider the needs of a conversational partner in that they rarely provide enough background information for a listener to enter the conversation without seeking clarification (Owens, 1992).

At age 3, children engage in longer dialogues and demonstrate awareness of the social aspects of discourse by verbally acknowledging comments made by a conversational partner and by code switching (Owens, 1992). Verbal acknowledgments of comments made by others in many cases may be minimal (e.g., "uh-huh," "oh").

Code switching proficiency in 3-year-olds varies from individual to individual. However, children at this level may demonstrate that they recognize the appropriateness of changing the communication mode according to the perceived needs of a communication partner. This may be accomplished by changing to **Motherese** when speaking to an infant or by changing dialects when conversing with an individual who is perceived to be a member of a particular culture.

However, for 3-year-olds, maintaining a cohesive conversation continues to present problems. As a group, 3-year-olds do not spontaneously produce a large number of utterances that are **contingent** to (i.e., related to) the utterance most recently spoken by a communication partner. Instead, most statements relate to the child's most recent utterance or a new topic.

Throughout the preschool years, children depend on adults to take the lead when engaging in discourse, such that conversations are usually somewhat imbalanced or asymmetrical (Kay & Charney, 1981). This dependence on the contributions of others decreases as the child progresses toward becoming a full conversational participant.

Development of Self-Talk.   Another characteristic of preschool language use that decreases with age and maturity is the pattern of engaging in long, audible, private, self-directed **monologues** which are characterized by behaviors such as verbal play, songs, rhymes, accounts of imaginative stories and events, and expressions of emotions. These monologues are termed **self-talk**. Such audible, private monologues decrease substantially throughout the preschool years, and they appear to be replaced by inaudible monologues, or talking to one's self (Kohlberg, Yaeger, & Hjertholm, 1968). Apparently, people learn at a very young age that when conversing with one's self, it is best to mutter quietly so as to conceal the content of one's private ruminations.

Development of Narration.   A third form of language use that is understood and used by preschoolers is **narration** (Oller, 1980). A narration is an uninterrupted monologue that is generated for the purpose of entertaining or informing a listener. Narrations include four types (Owens, 1992).

The *recount* is one type of narration. In a recount the child tells about a past experience, usually at the request of an adult who shares knowledge of the experience (Owens, 1992). For example, the child's recount may begin with the adult request, "Tell me about our trip to the zoo."

An *eventcast* is an explanation of an ongoing or expected event. This form of narration may be used by children for the purpose of directing imaginative play (Owens, 1992). For example, the eventcast may begin with the child's suggestion, "Let's pretend that you're Cinderella and I'm the fairy godmother."

An *account* is a spontaneous exposition (unrequested by the listener) about an experience that was not shared by the listener (Owens, 1992). For example, the account may begin with the child's exclamation, "Guess what!"

A *story*, the fourth type of common narrative, is a monologue describing some fictional event. Although stories may begin with the traditional introductory statement, "Once upon a time," there are a variety of methods for introducing story narrations. Generally, stories have a plot that is composed of a main character who has a problem, a plan for surmounting the problem, and a series of events leading to successful resolution of the problem. However, stories told by preschoolers often lack many of these characteristics, as story narration is one aspect of language that becomes much more fully developed during the school years (Owens, 1992).

In general, narration requires that the speaker provide all of the information to the listener in an organized whole (Roth & Spekman, 1985), and thus places more demands on the speaker than does dialogue or private monologue. For that reason, although most 3-year-olds use, and are capable of understanding, all four types of narration, even 4- and 5-year-olds create narrations that lack a cohesive plot. Skill with narration continues to develop for a number of years and is used more effectively by school-age children and adults.

Although children in most cultures are exposed to, and use, all four types of narration, the proportion of each type varies from culture to culture (Heath,

1986). For example, in some white, working-class families in the South, preschool experiences with narrative language are predominantly limited to recounts that are firmly regulated by an examining adult. In the same group, preschool experiences with narrative accounts and stories are quite limited. By contrast, also in the South, in some African-American working-class families, children typically have preschool experiences with accounts and eventcasts but not necessarily with recounts. These differences among cultures may place some minority children at a perceived disadvantage when they enter school if teachers expect them to have had experiences with each of the four standard narrative types.

Language Use Accomplishments at the Preschool Level.   At the age of 5, most children are ready to begin kindergarten. In general, kindergartners are able to use language for all of the following purposes: (1) regulating other people, (2) interacting socially, (3) calling attention, (4) initiating new topics, (5) maintaining several turns of conversation, (6) providing adequate information so that the conversational partner is able to respond without seeking clarification, (7) expressing feelings and emotions, (8) responding to the comments of the communication partner with utterances that relate to the topic of conversation (contingency), (9) code switching when the situation requires a variation on the language, (10) phrasing indirect requests, (11) using some **deictic terms** such as *this* and *that* or *here* and *there*, and (12) talking to one's self, both audibly and inaudibly (Table 1–1).

Early Development of Comprehension.   This discussion of the preschooler's development of language comprehension is strongly influenced by the interactive relationship between language comprehension and production. It appears that at all levels of language achievement, individuals may be able to comprehend more language than they are able to speak. Apparently, language learners are also capable of verbalizing certain aspects of language that are beyond their immediate spontaneous comprehension.

At all levels of language acquisition it may be the process of producing partially understood language that facilitates more complete understanding, while the process of comprehending complex language may be what facilitates advances in one's ability to express one's self. Therefore, it is likely that the achievement of the expressive milestones described in this chapter is facilitated by, and facilitates, the achievement of the corresponding receptive milestones.

The School-age Years and Adolescence

This discussion of school-age children begins with 6-year-olds, as most children at that age are enrolled in kindergarten or first grade. By the time children enter school, they are capable of producing and understanding complex language, have a receptive and expressive vocabulary of several thousand words, and use language proficiently and for a variety of purposes. However, their language acquisition is not yet complete. In fact, the process continues through the school-age years and into adulthood.

In general, school-age children increase in their abilities to produce longer utterances, use and comprehend indirect questions and requests, communicate with appropriate levels of politeness, switch codes appropriately according to a variety of situations, maintain a topic, talk about language (i.e., use language *metalinguistically*), and access an increasingly large vocabulary. Further, throughout these years children deepen their understanding of words and grammatical forms and they improve in their ability to comprehend and use **figurative** language (Table 1–1).

6-Year-Olds. At 6, children who are acquiring Standard American English as a first language under uninterrupted circumstances have achieved all milestones mentioned in the preceding section. Further, they speak in utterances that are estimated to be approximately 7.5 to 9.5 morphemes in length and have taken on a number of additions to their linguistic repertoires. That is, grammatically, most 6-year-olds are capable of using and understanding adverbial conjunctions such as *now*, *then*, *so*, and *though* (Scott, 1988), and they are beginning to comprehend, but not use, passive sentences (e.g., "The boy was kissed by the girl") (Bridges, 1980).

Pragmatically, children at this age respond to indirect hints. Further, when asked to repair miscommunications (make a **conversational repair**), it is at about the age of 6 that children *begin* to truly repair their misunderstood utterances (Owens, 1992). Prior to 6, when informed that an utterance is not understood, children generally repeat the misunderstood utterance verbatim. However, 6-year-olds will make limited changes in an attempt to address the difficulties encountered by the listener or conversational partner.

Also from a pragmatic perspective, 6-year-olds are just beginning to learn to view circumstances from the perspective of other people, making it easier for them to provide adequate information to communicative partners. Therefore, fewer requests for additional information and clarification are necessary in order for people to enter into discourse with children at this level (Konefal & Fokes, 1984).

Up until the age of 6, most children are *incapable* of dealing with language at a metalinguistic level. That is, they do not participate well in conversations about language and do not benefit remarkably from most instructions about grammatical form. However, at about the age of 6, many children begin to develop some fundamental abilities for dealing with language at the metalinguistic or instructional level such that they can discuss differences between regular and irregular forms. Metalinguistic instruction combined with experiential learning can be successful with some 6-year-olds when teaching certain basic linguistic concepts.

7-Year-Olds. Even more can be expected of children who have passed the 7th birthday. For one thing, by 7, mean utterance length has increased such that for many children, utterances of 9 to 11 morphemes are estimated as average.

Further, at 7, children comprehend the concept of causality only inconsistently. In like manner, the word *because* is understood in part, but not fully (Kuhn & Phelps, 1976) Additionally, spatial opposites, such as *left/right* and *front/back*, are understood and used by children at this level.

Children at 7 years use and understand most deictic terms. Deictic terms are words whose meanings depend on speaker's perspective as a point of reference (Owens, 1992). For example, the exact meaning of the words *here* and *there* depends entirely on the speaker's point of reference. *Bring* and *take* are other examples of deictic terms in that the speaker's word choice depends on the direction that the object moves in relation to the speaker. The word *bring* is chosen when something is to move in the direction of the speaker, with the speaker being the point of reference (e.g., "*Bring* the book to me"). By contrast, the word *take* is chosen when something is to move away from the speaker (e.g., "*Take* these toys to your room"). *Me* and *you* and *mine* and *yours* are also examples of deictic pairs, as the word of choice depends on the speaker's perspective.

Grammatically, 7-year-olds typically order their words in sentences using the adult pattern. However, for children at this level, maintaining sentence rhythm is more important than including all the necessary words and phonemes, so that many comprehensible sentences are produced that lack some morphemes and function words (Holden & MacGinitie, 1972).

Phonologically, at 7, most children are capable of manipulating sounds for creating rhymes (Owens, 1992). For example, 7-year-old children are typically able to generate a number of words rhyming with a simple word such as *cat* (e.g., *hat, bat, mat, rat*). Further, 7-year-olds typically recognize unacceptable sound sequences and replace them with acceptable sequences when given the opportunity (Owens, 1992). For example, if an adult were to label an object with a nonsense word containing an unacceptable sound sequence for the English language (e.g., "tsno") the 7-year-old is likely to recognize that the sound sequence is not standard, and is further likely to exchange it for one that is (e.g., "snow" or "to snow").

Pragmatically, by this age, most children are skilled at making their desires known through indirect requests (Garvey, 1975). For example, most 7-year-olds are completely capable of letting the adult in charge know that it would be nice to go outside to play simply by stating that it is a beautiful day outside. Certainly, the skill with indirect forms begins before the age of 7, given that younger children are capable of requesting a drink by declaring that they are thirsty. However, it is not until approximately 7 that most children demonstrate consistent skill with indirect forms (Garvey, 1975). Even beyond 7, the skill and flexibility with which a person uses the indirect forms continues to improve.

With regard to narrative skill (discussed in the section on preschoolers), by the age of 7 children begin to tell narrative stories with a plot that is characterized by a main character with a problem to be solved, a plan for overcoming the problem, and some sort of resolution to the problem (Oller, 1980).

8-Year-Olds.   At 8 years, children may speak in utterances that are between 10.5 and 12.5 morphemes in length, on average. (Obviously, some longer and shorter utterances are produced, but it is within normal limits for utterance length to fall within this estimated range.)

By the age of 8, children not only understand most passive sentences (e.g., "The boy was kissed by the girl"), they use them properly as well (Baldie, 1976). Further, they understand comparative relationships such as *funnier than* and *as fuzzy as* (Owens, 1992). The morphological marker *-er* denoting that a person or thing is used to perform an action, is also partially understood by 8-year-olds (Derwing & Baker, 1977). At 8, most children are consistently able to understand and use the *-er* marker to denote a *person* who performs an action (e.g., teacher, painter) but not to consistently denote a *thing* used to perform an action (e.g., eraser, printer).

Phonologically, at this age, all Standard American English phonemes are typically produced by native speakers at all levels of conversation and all rules for patterning phonemes in syllables are accurately applied. It may be assumed that any articulation errors persisting to this point are not likely to resolve spontaneously.

Morphophonemic development, which is an advanced aspect of phonological development, is under way as well by 8 years of age. **Morphophonemic rules** are the rules that govern changes in pronunciation as morphemes are added. At 8, most children abide by the language's basic morphophonemic rules. For example, they recognize that when the past-tense morpheme *-ed* is added to a word that ends in a voiceless consonant other than [t], *-ed* is pronounced as [t] (e.g., "laughed" is pronounced "[læft]), that when *-ed* is added to a word that ends in a voiced consonant other than [d], that *-ed* is pronounced as [d] (e.g., "sneezed" is pronounced "[snizd]"), and that when *-ed* is added to a word that ends in [t] or [d], *-ed* is pronounced as a separate syllable [əd] (e.g., "started" is pronounced "[staɚtəd]").

Pragmatically, 8-year-olds are capable of sustaining concrete topics and are beginning to consider the intentions of other people (Owens, 1992). These developments improve their ability to participate effectively as conversational partners.

Proverbs are interpreted literally by 8-year-olds (Owens, 1992) so a statement such as, "A bird in the hand is worth two in the bush," is interpreted as a comment about the value of birds in hands as compared to the value of birds in bushes, and not as an analogy meant to discourage impulsively risking what one has on the chance of gaining what one does not have.

At 8, most children who learn language under natural circumstances have the benefit of reasonably sophisticated metalinguistic awareness (Saywitz &

Cherry-Wilkinson, 1982). This enables them to increase their knowledge of language through discussions about it. Although direct experiential practice is still necessary in teaching language concepts, at 8, children of at least average intelligence are able to gain linguistic insight through instruction.

9-Year-Olds.   At 9, children's utterances are estimated to be between 12 and 14 morphemes in length. Regarding language content, 9-year-olds are able to associate words in a way that more closely resembles adult word-association skills. It seems that for very young children, words are associated syntactically, such that if asked to think of a word prompted by a stimulus word, the young child usually produces a word that is likely to occur next in a phrase or sentence. For example, the stimulus word "run" may result in the associative response, "away."

On the other hand, for older children (i.e., approximately age 9 and older) and adults, words are not usually associated according to anticipatory syntactic relationships, but rather according to semantic relationships. Therefore, older children and adults, if asked to associate the word "run," may offer a word in the same grammatical class with a similar meaning, such as "hurry" or "race."

Actually, between the ages of 5 and 9, children make rapid changes in their word-association skills. Evidently, it is at about 5 that children begin to make the shift from syntactic word associations to semantic word associations. By the age of 9, word-association skills are apparently more semantic in nature than syntactic. Word-association skills continue to develop through adulthood, such that for adults, spontaneous word associations are nearly all semantic. This shift from syntactic to semantic word associations is called a "syntagmatic-paradigmatic shift" (Ervin, 1961).

Some **metaphoric** language is partially understood by 9-year-olds (Owens, 1992). For example, certain psychological states are described metaphorically, such as "purple with rage," "feeling blue," and "a warm greeting." Prior to 8 or 9, children interpret these metaphors quite literally, with negligible appreciation for the figurative meaning, such that if asked to interpret a saying such as "feeling blue," younger children are inclined to say that the person likes blue or is wearing blue clothing. On the other hand, by the time children are 8 or 9, they show some signs of beginning to appreciate that the saying is not to be interpreted literally. However, because of limitations in their ability to fully appreciate the relationship between the psychological state and the metaphor, at 9 a fully accurate interpretation of such metaphoric language is still unlikely. Thus, although "feeling blue" is no longer interpreted literally, the exact figurative meaning may not be clearly understood.

Deixis is described in the section about 7-year-olds, as at age 7 the majority of children are able to use and understand *most* deictic terms. However, as with many aspects of language, deixis continues to develop over a number of years, and at 9 children are usually becoming able to use deictic terms for the purpose of **conversational cohesion** (tying parts of the conversation together).

Several types of **cohesive markers** are used by children at this level. Simply speaking, cohesive markers are words that serve to link the parts of the conversation together. One type of cohesive marker is the use of pronouns for the purpose of anaphoric reference (i.e., for the purpose of referring to a previously specified object, event, or relationship). For example, the pronoun *he* may be used to refer to a male person who was previously identified by the speaker, or the demonstrative pronoun *that* may be used to reference an event that was already described (e.g., "When that happened").

Pragmatically, when **communication breakdown** occurs in discourse and a speaker is asked to repair a misunderstanding, up until about the age of 9, the type of repair that can be expected is minimal and may be as ineffective as a verbatim repetition with increased loudness. Most 9-year-olds, however, are able to identify the source of the breakdown and provide the needed information in order to accurately clear up the confusion (Brinton, Fujiki, Loeb, & Winkler, 1986). Metalinguistically, 9-year-olds are sophisticated enough to discuss the process of noticing the misunderstanding, identify the source of the communication breakdown and the information needed by the listener, and execute the repair (Brinton et al., 1986). In addition, most nine-year olds are adept conversationalists, often sustaining topics through at least a dozen turns.

10-Year-Olds.   The average length of utterance for most 10-year-olds may be between 13.5 and 15.5 morphemes. Of course, variation between individuals is expected.

The prepositions *in*, *on*, and *at* may be used to express temporal concepts. For example, generally, *in* and *on* are used to express certain specific periods of time (e.g., "in December"; "in the afternoon"; "on Thursday") and *at* is used to express an exact time (e.g., "at noon"; "at 3:00"). Most 10-year-olds are capable of comprehending and using the preposition *in* for its temporal function in addition to the **locative** function that was initially learned many years prior (Owens, 1992).

11-Year-Olds.   The estimated mean length of utterance for 11-year-olds may be between 15 and 17 morphemes, although individual performances vary. At 11 years, children consistently and accurately comprehend and use the word *because*, which is quite a sophisticated accomplishment. In order to fully comprehend the causal relationship expressed by the word *because*, the child must not only realize the relationship between two events but also grasp the temporal ordering of the two events. Children who do not fully understand these causal and temporal concepts often substitute the conjunction *and* or *then* for *because* (e.g., "I need a bandage *and* I cut my knee") or use the word *because* with a reversed causal relationship ("I cut my knee because I need a bandage"). This pattern of misexpressing causality usually dissipates by the age of 11 (Corrigan, 1975).

Some morphological markers are acquired by the age of 11. For example, in English the -*y* marker is often added to nouns and verbs in order to form adjectives (e.g., runn*y*, past*y*, shin*y*). This pattern is generally understood and used by the age of 11 (Owens, 1992). Another marker that is usually acquired by age 11 is the instrumental -*er* marker. That is the use of the word ending -*er* for the purpose of denoting a thing that is used to accomplish a task (e.g., eras*er*, print*er*). Although the -*er* marker denoting a human to perform an action has been understood for some time, it is not until about 11 that we can expect most children to use it accurately for the instrumental purpose, to denote a thing that is used to perform an action (Clark & Hecht, 1982).

Figurative language is more fully understood by 11-year-olds than by younger children. For example, we examined the difficulties experienced by 9-year-olds who are faced with comprehending certain metaphors, such as physical terms used to describe psychological states. At 11, children no longer misinterpret such metaphors (Owens, 1992), so a statement like "feeling blue" is now interpreted accurately to mean a state of melancholia or sadness rather than as a color descriptor.

Most 11-year-olds are able to sustain abstract topics (Owens, 1992). Abstract topics may include events that have already taken place or have not yet taken place, as well as discussions about thoughts and ideas.

12-Year-Olds. For most 12-year-olds, utterance length, on the average, is estimated to be between 16 and 19 morphemes. Individual differences are expected. Typically, 12-year-olds are capable of using the following adverbial conjunctions: *otherwise, anyway, therefore,* and *however.* They also use two disjunctions: *really* and *probably.* However, the development of adverbial conjunctions and disjunctions is nowhere near completion, as we can expect to hear only 4 disjunctions per 100 utterances at the age of 12, in contrast to the 12 disjunctions that we can expect to hear per 100 utterances at the adult level (Scott, 1988).

Younger Adolescents. As language continues to develop through the junior high school years, individuals from age 13 to 15 years speak in utterances that are estimated at between 18 and 23 morphemes on the average. Morphologically, in English, the -*ly* marker is used to denote many adverbs (e.g., *quickly, barely*). This grammatical marker is now consistently and accurately used and fully understood (Owens, 1992).

Further, young adolescents are able to comprehend and use language on a much more abstract level than previously. Words such as *unless* and the temporal form of the word *at* are now understood and used accurately. Also during these early adolescent years, individuals begin to fully comprehend the figurative meanings of proverbs. Therefore, the "bird in the hand" that was misunderstood by the 8-year-old is interpreted accurately by most 13- to 15-year-olds (Owens, 1992).

Older Adolescents.   Adolescents between the ages of 16 and 18 years may use utterances that are quite lengthy, perhaps more than 25 morphemes in length. Further, individuals at this level are continuing to learn to use and understand language, becoming increasingly adultlike in their performance.

Although adolescent language learners have been using the standard system of phonology with proficiency for a number of years, it is during the later adolescent years that people become skilled at making morphophonemic shifts, enabling them to correctly pronounce grammatical variations on most words (Hodson & Paden, 1991). For example, the word *photograph* is pronounced with the primary stress on the first syllable, and the vowel in the second syllable is pronounced [ə]. A morphological variation, *photography*, results in a few prosodic and phonemic differences, such that the word *photography* has the primary stress on the second rather than the first syllable, and the vowel in the second syllable is not pronounced [ə], but [ɔ] or [a]. Understanding the morphophonemic rules that govern these changes in pronunciation enables older adolescents to correctly pronounce unfamiliar variations of words. Many words have morphophonemic variations (e.g., "tele-graph/tele*graph*ic," "cosmetic/cosme*tol*ogy," and the verb and noun forms of the word refuse, "re*fuse*/refuse), and it is in the later adolescent years that people become sophisticated in their ability to make phonemic adaptations for such morphophonemic changes in words.

Pragmatically, older adolescents are likely to use sarcasm, jokes, and double meanings effectively (Shultz, 1974). Along the same lines, they make deliberate use of metaphors (Gardner, Kircher, Winner, & Perkins, 1975). The ability to skillfully and creatively generate humorous comments and stories is one that does not suddenly emerge at this late date but rather gradually evolves over a period of many years. For example, even preschoolers are able to appreciate simple humor generated by others or even make occasional humorous comments. Further, many very young school-age children tell jokes and generate humorous remarks. By the time most people reach the later years of adolescence, the ability to understand and apply abstract concepts of humor is both skilled and spontaneous. Moreover, older adolescent language learners are capable of explaining complex behavior and natural phenomena (Elkind, 1970), demonstrating a command of abstract language that approaches adult-level skill.

In addition, many older adolescents are aware that each person's perspective is different (Owens, 1992), enabling them to fully participate in discourse. Individuals at this level provide enough information to satisfy their conversational partners' needs, take turns appropriately, sustain topics with skill, and change **communication style** as situations demand.

Adulthood

Language development continues throughout adulthood for most, with the exception of individuals who lose some level of command due to a disease process or brain injury. Adult language becomes more elaborate with experience, and the way in which an individual adult uses the language becomes more diverse. The language experiences and communication needs of the individual are the primary factors that determine the extent to which language continues to develop and the amount of diversity that is achieved (Owens, 1992). For example, as an adult who has selected to further your formal education by pursuing a career in speech-language pathology, you have communication needs and experiences that are remarkably different from the experiences and needs of adults who have chosen to pursue a different set of goals.

As a result of communication needs and experience, adults tend to develop a rather complicated network of communication styles (Owens, 1992). This phenomenon is one that develops over a period of years, beginning at the preschool level. The system is adequately developed by the time one enters adulthood, and continues to undergo refinements throughout one's life. For example, adult communication style may vary according to a number of variables. Different styles may be called on depending on whether one is on the job, with an intimate partner, among strangers, friends, or business associates, at a social function such as a wedding, funeral, party, or sports event, or with individuals who are members of a specific ethnic heritage or social group. Adults have access to a variety of **communication registers** that are applied according to the situation.

To complicate matters, one's overall choice of words or choice of communication style may depend on one's political, social, or religious orientation. For example, in describing particular groups of people, the choice of words often reflects a person's beliefs, values, or political orientation. These word choices do not necessarily change from situation to situation as do communication registers, and they communicate to a listener something about an individual's identity in relation to the groups. These variations in communication style are called **communication codes.** Some examples of word choices that may characterize a person's overall thinking pattern are: "pro-choice/pro-abortion," "birth parents/real parents," and "single parent/unwed mother."

THE PROCESS OF LANGUAGE ACQUISITION

Having read the preceding sections, you now have a sense of the milestones that characterize language acquisition in children who acquire Standard American English as a first language. Although it is important for you as a student of speech-language pathology to have a knowledge of the milestones along with their approximate sequences and ages of emergence, it is equally important to have a clear understanding of the processes or natural phenomena that result in the achievement of the milestones. It is by your understanding of the approximate sequences and ages associated with the milestones that you can accurately evaluate, diagnose, and plan intervention for individuals who come to you for assistance. Similarly, it is that knowledge, combined with your understanding of the natural process of language acquisition, that enables you to effectively provide intervention for the same individuals.

Several natural phenomena that typically result in first language acquisition are discussed in the sections that follow. These are contextual phenomena, behavioral phenomena of primary caretakers, behavioral phenomena of language learners, and experiential phenomena contrasted to metalinguistic phenomena.

Contextual Phenomena

Basically, we are concerned with three contextual phenomena. They are the social context, the context of personal need, and the context of individual mental activity.

Social Interaction and Opportunity.   A first language is learned in a social context that incorporates the activities of everyday life. Infants are exposed to a first language during daily routines of eating, bathing, preparing for sleep, dressing, being comforted, playing, and the like. Since infants are not capable of taking care of any routines independently, all daily activities are performed in the presence of another human being and thus provide the opportunity for socialization between the infant and primary caretaker. Thus, the context of early exposure to language is described as social. Beyond infancy, language continues to develop in a social context. That is, when the first words are spoken, adult caretakers and older children respond, demonstrating to the child how language is useful for social interaction. Throughout life, language is experienced and acquired in the presence of social interchange.

Personal Need and Interest.   Beyond the social purpose, language is a vehicle by which needs and desires are communicated and thereby met. Therefore, a critical secondary context that influences the development of language is the context of need and personal interest. The needs and desires that young children experience certainly impact the words and combinations of morphemes that they acquire. The intensity with which one experiences a need or desire, combined with the realization that language is the medium by which these needs and desires can be communicated and thus satisfied, influences the rate of language acquisition.

Mental Activity.   A third context of language acquisition is the context of mental activity. Language is the medium by which our thoughts and ideas are expressed to individuals who matter to us. Therefore, a person who has thoughts and ideas has something to communicate, creating a need or desire to interact. Although the communication of thoughts and ideas is abstract and cannot be done expertly until the adolescent years, even preschool children begin to develop skill in this abstract area by such linguistic activities as making requests for things that are not readily available (e.g., "Mommy, can we take out the paints and color?" or "I want to watch Beauty and the Beast").

The very concept of using language for the purpose of expressing ideas and thoughts brings us back to the idea that language is learned in a social context, because it is by sharing thoughts and ideas that the very young child enhances the social relationship with the primary caretaker and the older child initiates and strengthens new social relationships.

Language Facilitation: Primary Caretaker's Role

During the social events that are also called daily routines, a child's needs and desires are met by primary caretakers. Exactly what the primary caretakers do and say during these activities naturally facilitates the acquisition of the first language. One very important thing that primary caretakers do is talk directly to the child, making the assumption that the child is a participating communication partner. Linguistic adaptations are made by the caretaker in order to accommodate the child socially, linguistically, and contextually.

The linguistic adaptations made by primary caretakers have certain identifiable characteristics, such that the language of caretakers has been given a name, *Motherese*. The language of Motherese differs from standard adult language along all three language dimensions (described below).

Adaptations to Language Form.   In talking to the child, caretakers tend to adapt the form of the language, using simplified linguistic structures, a slightly elevated pitch, and imitations of the child's utterances. Each of these adaptations of form has a purpose. For example, by using simplified structures, the adult clearly demonstrates to the child exactly how to combine words to make short sentences. By imitating the utterances of the child, the adult relates socially on the child's own level. Finally, by elevating pitch, the adult draws the child's attention to the social interchange.

Adaptations to Language Content.   Primary caretakers also adapt the content of their language, selecting topics that have the attention of the child and therefore are assumed to be of interest. Caretakers talk most about what the child is looking at, listening to, or doing. By selecting topics that have the immediate interest and attention of the child, caretakers provide the child the opportunity to form clear associations between what is being said and the subject of the child's attention.

Adaptations to Language Use.   Finally, caretakers tailor the use of language so that it addresses the pragmatic needs of the language learner. Attempts at participation in sociable exchanges are met with acceptance and encouragement, regardless of whether the child's utterances approximate the adult language model. Not only does the adult caretaker not require the infant to conform to the adult standard, the adult conforms to the language of the child. One needs to observe a new mother for only a short time to see a clear demonstration of behavior that communicates total acceptance of immature attempts at social discourse.

Further, what primary caretakers do naturally to reinforce comprehensible language is important and worthy of being imitated by those who facilitate language learning professionally. That is, the rewards caretakers usually offer for successful communication are of the highest and most powerful level of reinforcement. (See the section on reinforcement in Chapter 4.) They are not edibles, tangibles, praises, nor activities. Instead, when communicating with a primary caretaker, successful attempts at communication are typically met with (1) a verbal or physical response that communicates that the message is understood and appreciated, (2) a verbal response that is contingent to the child's utterance, and (3) the encouragement to continue in the social exchange.

For example, an 11-month-old child is engaged in a social exchange with the mother. The child picks up a toy telephone and says, "Gauk" (an approximation of *talk*). The mother pretends to use her hand as a telephone, places her thumb and small finger near her ear and mouth, and says: "You want to talk? Hello." Note that the mother does not correct the child's articulation; she does not say, "Good speech!" or "I like the way you talk!"; she does not give the child a sticker or a piece of candy for having said a word; and she does not give the child the opportunity to add a block to a tower as reward for communication. What the mother does instead is far more powerful. She communicates that what the child says is understood, she models how to continue a conversation with another person, and she communicates that continued social communication is a desirable activity.

Language Learning: The Child's Role

With language acquisition being a social phenomenon, it is not only necessary for the primary caretaker to perform certain acts, it is important for the child to participate. Primarily, the child's role is to *enjoy* the socialization that surrounds the activities of daily living. It is by this socializing and by the enjoyment of it that the child encounters language and learns what language can do for one personally.

Through language, needs and desires are communicated and thereby satisfied, ideas are expressed and thereby shared, and socializing is accomplished, which provides a source of great pleasure. If a child is to participate in the process of acquiring a first language, he or she must at least subconsciously recognize that language is an effective and preferred means for accomplishing these ends.

In addition, most children naturally imitate their significant others. Daily routines, rituals, expressions, and mannerisms are examples of adult behaviors that children duplicate with astounding accuracy. This natural tendency to copy the individuals who care for them may serve to facilitate the acquisition of the conventional form of the language.

Metalinguistic and Experiential Phenomena

Metalinguistics is language about language. Accordingly, the metalinguistic phenomena that contribute to language acquisition and development are the natural conversations about language that deepen one's understanding of it. Further, under natural language-learning circumstances, among children who are acquiring language without interference, some may benefit in a limited way from metalinguistic conversations as early as age 6, and most children are capable of participating in, and benefiting from, direct language instruction by the age of 8.

For that reason, one may assume that metalinguistic phenomena do not play a significant role in natural language acquisition prior to the age of 6. Although some normally developing 6-year-olds benefit from direct instruction on certain simple linguistic contrasts, usually any metalinguistic instruction at this level is naturally combined with experiential learning as described in the section on the caretaker's role in language facilitation.

Further, it is not until the age of 8 that most children are able to benefit fully from early metalinguistic instruction. However, even under natural language-learning circumstances, metalinguistic instruction is also strongly associated with experiential learning and examples.

For example, the child who continues to say *bringed* instead of *brought* may be metalinguistically instructed by a significant other that the word has been used incorrectly and an example may be given to correct the verb form. The following conversation might be heard under such circumstances, and it exemplifies metalinguistic instruction in the absence of experiential demonstration.

Child: "Mommy, I bringed you a flower."

Adult: "Michael. You *brought* me a flower."

Child: "What?"

Adult: "It's not 'I *bringed* you a flower.' It's 'I *brought* you a flower.'"

Child: "Oh. I brought you a flower."

Adult: "Thank you."

Although as a result of the above conversation, the typical young child may recognize that *brought* is the correct past-tense inflection of the verb *to bring*, one might also consider the other **consequence**s of such extemporaneous metalinguistic instruction. In addition to the correct past-tense inflection of the verb, the child learns very little from the interchange. Nothing is learned about maintaining the topic or making contingent responses to the comments of others. Michael is given no reason to believe that what he says is important enough to deserve a related response. Moreover, he learns nothing about making appropriately polite responses upon receiving gifts.

Thus, although metalinguistic instruction can be used to improve a child's command of language structure, it does not predominate in natural language-learning opportunities, even of older children, and it does not usually promote the pragmatic use of language. Experiential opportunities are preferred. Perhaps the experiential phenomena occur in natural language learning because language use is nearly always compromised when metalinguistic instruction predominates the language-learner's exposure to linguistic elements. Therefore, the following conversation may prove more effective.

Child: "Mommy, I bringed you a flower."

Adult: "Oh, how nice, you *brought* me a flower. Thank you, Michael. Can you bring me another flower?"

(Michael goes to pick another flower and returns.)

Child: "Here." (presents flower.)

Adult: "Thank you. You *brought* me another flower. You *brought* me two flowers."

Adult: (Walks to Michael and gives a flower.) "And I *brought* you a flower."

In this second exchange, Michael does not receive direct instruction in the inflection of the verb *to bring*. However, he hears the irregular past-tense form used correctly four times, the natural and appropriate pattern of discourse is not interrupted, and he is not criticized but rather is shown respect by his conversational partner.

READING AND WRITING

The comprehension and production of spoken language does not necessarily develop through direct instruction but rather through experience and enjoyment in a social context, and it begins to develop long before actual performance can be measured. In much the same way, the reading and writing of printed language begins long before the formal instruction that takes place in school, through the social and interactive context of storytimes, bedtime stories, and pretending to read while turning the pages of a picture book. It is in these highly interactive, sociable, and enjoyable contexts that a child begins to recognize that the orderly marks on the page correspond to the pictures and message of the story. It is also in these contexts that the child begins to take hold of the personal benefits that can be derived from accessing information through books. However, learning to read and write is quite different from learning to understand and produce spoken language, as most people learn reading and writing though formal, systematic, metalinguistic instruction and planned experiential practice.

Reading

Learning to read requires that one master a progression of complex skills. These include the visual recognition of letter shapes, auditory recognition of letter sounds, and formation of a clear mental connection between the visual shapes and auditory sounds associated with each letter. To complicate this achievement, in English a number of letter shapes are associated with multiple sounds. The letter *c* is an example. It is pronounced [k] when followed by the vowels *a*, *o*, and *u*, and also when it is followed by the consonants *k*, *l*, and *r*; but it is pronounced [s] when followed by the vowels *e*, *i*, and *y*. Many other consonants and all vowels have more than one sound that is associated with the visual letter symbol.

Another set of visual symbols that must be learned and associated with auditory sounds are called digraphs. Digraphs are the combinations of two letters that, when they appear together in written form, are associated with a single sound. For example, when the letters *ch* appear together they sound like [tʃ] or [k], when the letters *sh* appear together they sound like [ʃ], when the letters *th* appear together they sound like [θ] or [ð], and when the letters *ph* appear together they sound like [f].

Silent letters, short and long vowels, and rules for letter combinations are among the other factors that must be addressed when one is learning to read. In addition to the multiple and complex network of auditory-visual associations that are made, one must also develop skill in sound blending and complex pattern recognition. Beyond that, a person who learns to read must comprehend the meaning of the written words and sentences that are read, even though the words and their meaning are disconnected from any meaningful context.

Writing

All the previously mentioned auditory-visual associations are also necessary for learning to write. Further, rules for spelling in English are complicated and have many exceptions. Thus, in addition to knowing the rules that exist for spelling, a person must also have sufficient experience with viewing the written language so that one can recall the spelling of words that do not fit neatly into the highly irregular rule system. Therefore, the fact that a particular sound may be represented by any number of letter combinations must be appreciated. For example, the auditory sound "uh" ([ə] or [ʌ]) may be **orthographically** transcribed as *u* in the word *tub*, *o* in the word *love*, *oo* in the word *flood*, and *a* in the word *alone*.

In addition to the auditory-visual associations, sound sequencing, and rules for spelling, writing requires that one develop sufficient fine motor coordination to accurately reproduce the letter shapes with a writing instrument. Further, in order to write, one must have something to write, an idea.

CONCLUDING REMARKS

This chapter focused on spoken and written language as it applies to Standard American English when acquired under uninterrupted circumstances. However, for a small group of children, language acquisition is interrupted by conditions such as cognitive limitations, sensory-input reduction, motor skill deficit, deficiency in socialization, and lack of learning opportunity. It is under these circumstances that the stages and processes of language acquisition proceed at a different rate and/or take a different course. The next chapter describes these circumstances and how they may impact language acquisition across all three dimensions: form, content, and use.

REFERENCES

Baldie, B. (1976). The acquisition of the passive voice. *Journal of Child Language*, *3*, 331–348.

Bates, E. (1976). *Language and context: The acquisition of pragmatics*. New York: Academic Press.

Bloom, L. (1988). What is language? In M. Lahey (Ed.), *Language disorders and language development*. New York: MacMillan.

Bloom, L., & Lahey, L. (1978). *Language development & language disorders*. New York: John Wiley & Sons.

Boone, D. R., & McFarlane, S. C. (1988). *The voice and voice therapy*. Englewood Cliffs, NJ: Prentice-Hall.

Bridges, A. (1980). SVD comprehension strategies reconsidered: The evidence of individual patterns of response. *Journal of Child Language*, *7*, 89–104.

Brinton, B., Fujiki, M., Loeb, D., & Winkler, E. (1986). Development of conversational repair strategies in response to requests for clarification. *Journal of Speech and Hearing Research*, *29*, 75–81.

Brown, R. (1973). *A first language, the early stages*. Cambridge, MA: Harvard University Press.

Bruner, J. (1978). From communication to language: A psychological perspective. In I. Markova (Ed.), *The social context of language*. Chichester, UK: John Wiley & Sons.

Bryant, P., Bradley, L., MacLean, M., & Crossland, J. (1989). Nursery rhymes, phonological skills and reading. *Journal of Child Language*, *16*, 407–428.

Clark, E., & Hecht, B. (1982). Learning to coin agent and instrument nouns. *Cognition*, *12*, 1–24.

Colton, R. H., & Casper, J. K. (1990). *Understanding voice problems: A physiological perspective for diagnosis and treatment*. Baltimore, MD: Williams & Wilkins.

Corrigan, R. (1975). Ascalogram analysis of the development of the use and comprehension of "because" in children. *Child Development, 46,* 195–201.

Cox, M. (1989). Children's over-regularization of nouns and verbs. *Journal of Child Language, 16,* 203–06.

Derwing, B., & Baker, W. (1977). The psychological basis for morphological rules. In J. MacNamara (Ed.), *Language learning and thought*. New York: Academic Press.

Elkind, D. (1970). *Children and adolescents*. New York: Oxford University Press.

Ervin, S. (1961). Changes with age in the verbal determinants of word-association. *American Journal of Psychology, 74,* 361–72.

Fey, M. E. (1986). *Language intervention with young children*. Austin, TX: Pro-Ed.

Flege, J. E., & Eefting, W. (1987). Cross-language switching in stop consonant perception and production by Dutch speakers of English. *Speech Communication, 6,* 185–202.

Gardner, H., Kircher, M., Winner, E., & Perkins, D. (1975). Children's metaphoric productions and preferences. *Journal of Child Language, 2,* 125–141.

Garvey, C. (1975). Requests and responses in children's speech. *Journal of Child Language, 2,* 41–63.

Gleason, J. B. (1989). *The development of language*. Columbus, OH: Merrill.

Heath, S. (1986). Taking a cross-cultural look at narratives. *Topics in Language Disorders, 7*(1), 84–94.

Hodson, B. W., & Paden, E. P. (1991). *Targeting intelligible speech*. Austin, TX: Pro-Ed.

Holden, M., & MacGinitie, W. (1972). Children's conceptions of word boundaries in speech and print. *Journal of Educational Psychology, 63,* 551–57.

Kay, K., & Charney, R. (1981). Conversational asymmetry between mothers and children. *Journal of Child Language, 8,* 35–49.

Kohlberg, L., Yaeger, J., & Hjertholm, E. (1968). Private speech: Four studies and a review of theories. *Child Development, 39,* 691–736.

Konefal, J., & Fokes, J. (1984). Linguistic analysis of children's conversational repairs. *Journal of Psycholinguistic Research, 13,* 1–11.

Kuhn, D., & Phelps, H. (1976). The development of children's comprehension of causal direction. *Child Development, 47,* 248–51.

Lahey, M. (Ed.), (1988). *Language disorders and language development*. New York: Macmillan.

McCormick, L., & Schiefelbusch, R. L. (1984). *Early language intervention*. Columbus, OH: Merrill.

Miller, J. F. (1981). *Assessing language production in children*. Austin, TX: Pro-Ed.

Norris, J., & Bruning, R. (1988). Cohesion in the narratives of good and poor readers. *Journal of Speech and Hearing Disorders, 53*, 416–23.

Oller, D. K. (1976). Analysis of infant vocalizations: A linguistic and speech scientific perspective. Miniseminar presented at the annual convention of the American Speech-Language-Hearing Association, Houston, TX.

Oller, D. K. (1980). The emergence of speech sounds in infancy. In G. Yeni-Komshian, J. A. Kavanagh, & C. A. Ferguson (Eds.), *Child phonology: Vol. 1. Production.* New York: Academic Press.

Oller, D. K., Moeller, M. P., Leutke-Stahlman, B., Osberger, M. J., Robbins, A., Eilers, R., Brackett, D., Johnson, C., & Carney, A. (1987). Communication development in hearing-impaired children. A miniseminar presented at the annual convention of the American Speech-Language-Hearing Association, New Orleans.

Oller, D. K., & Smith, B. L. (1977). Effect of final syllable position on vowel duration in infant babbling. *Journal of the Acoustical Society of America, 62*, 994–997.

Owens, R. E. (1992). *Language development: An introduction.* Columbus, OH: Merrill.

Rice, M. L., & Kemper, S. (1984). *Child language and cognition.* Austin, TX: Pro-Ed.

Roth, F., & Spekman, N. (1985). Story grammar analysis of narratives produced by learning disabled and normally achieving students. Paper presented at the Symposium on Research in Child Language Disorders, Madison, WI.

Sachs, J. (1989). Communication development in infancy. In J. B. Gleason (Ed.), *The development of language.* Columbus, OH: Merrill.

Saywitz, K., & Cherry-Wilkinson, L. (1982). Age-related differences in metalinguistic awareness. In S. Kuczaj (Ed.), *Language development: Vol. 2. Language, thought and culture.* Hillsdale, NJ: Erlbaum.

Scott, C. (1988). Producing complex sentences. *Topics in Language Disorders, 8*(2), 44–62.

Secord, W. A. (1989). The traditional approach to treatment. In N. A. Creaghead, P. W. Newman, & W. A. Secord (Eds.), *Assessment and remediation of articulatory and phonological disorders.* Columbus, OH: Merrill.

Shultz, T. (1974). Development of the appreciation of riddles. *Child Development, 45*, 100–105.

Stark, R. E. (1980). Stages of speech development in the first year of life. In G. H. Yeni-Komshian, J. F. Kavanagh, & C.A. Ferguson (Eds.), *Child phonology: Vol. 1. Production.* New York: Academic Press.

Weiss, C. E., Gordon, M. E. & Lillywhite, H. S. (1987). *Clinical management of articulatory and phonologic disorders.* Baltimore, MD: Williams & Wilkins.

Wells, G. (1986). The conversational requirements for language training. A special session delivered at the annual convention of the American Speech-Language-Hearing Association, Detroit.

Wetherby, A. M. (1991). Profiling pragmatic abilities in the emerging language of young children. In T. Gallagher (Ed.), *Pragmatics of language: Clinical practice issues*. San Diego, CA: Singular Publishing Group.

Winitz, H. (1989). Auditory considerations in treatment. In N. A. Creaghead, P. W. Newman, & W. A. Secord (Eds.), *Assessment and remediation of articulatory and phonological disorders*. Columbus, OH: Merrill.

STUDY GUIDE 1

A. Define each of the following terms and provide an appropriate example of each.

1. language	14. relations between events
2. interpersonal communication	15. syllables
3. semantics	16. segments of language
4. intrapersonal communication	17. prosody
5. objects	18. suprasegmental aspects
6. communicative acts	19. morphology
7. events	20. morphemes
8. communication partner	21. content words
9. language form	22. function words
10. language content	23. syntax
11. phonology	24. language use
12. relations between objects	25. pragmatics
13. phonemes	26. function of an utterance
	27. context of an utterance
	28. language competence

B. Describe what is meant by each statement.
   1. Language is used for communication.
   2. What we communicate through language is our ideas.
   3. Language is a code.
   4. The code of language is systematic.
   5. The systematic code of language is a convention.
   6. Content is constant across all cultures, while topic and vocabulary vary from culture to culture.

C. Name and describe each:
   1. categories of language content
   2. categories of language function

D. Address each of the following.
   1. Differentiate between anatomy and physiology.
   2. Discuss the difference between biological function and communication function.
   3. Which dimension of language is directly affected by the structure and function of the speech mechanism? How is it affected? And how are the other two dimensions affected indirectly?

4. Describe how anatomical and physiological limitations might impact language competence.
5. How is hearing necessary for the conventional development of form, content, and use?
6. Which cerebral hemisphere is usually dominant for language?
7. Discuss language perception in relation to identification and discrimination.
8. Discuss the role of prosody in language perception.
9. How may perceptual bias impact language perception?
10. Contrast linguistic knowledge and nonlinguistic knowledge.
11. Describe what is meant when one says that certain cognitive concepts are essential to language learning.
12. Why is social interaction necessary for language learning?

E. Be able to locate each of the following structures on a diagram.

1. lungs	17. auricle
2. trachea	18. ear canal
3. larynx	19. tympanic membrane
4. pharynx	20. malleus
5. nasal cavity	21. incus
6. oral cavity	22. stapes
7. sinuses	23. oval window
8. velopharyngeal valve	24. cochlea
9. tongue	25. eustachian tube
10. velum	26. Heschl's gyrus
11. hard palate	27. Wernicke's area
12. teeth	28. Broca's area
13. lips	29. supplemental communication area
14. outer ear	
15. middle ear	30. cerebellum
16. inner ear	

F. Describe each of the following anatomical structures with regard to its contribution to production of language form.

1. lungs	4. resonating cavities
2. trachea	5. velopharyngeal valve
3. larynx	6. articulators

G. Describe each of the following anatomical structures in regard to its contribution to hearing.

1. tympanic membrane	5. eustachian tube
2. ossicles	6. Heschl's gyrus
3. oval window	7. cranial nerve VIII
4. cochlea	

H. Describe each of the following neuroanatomical structures in regard to its contribution to speech production.

1. Broca's area
2. supplemental communications area

    3. cerebellum

    4. basal ganglia

I. Describe each of the following neuroanatomical structures in regard to its contribution to language formulation.

    1. Broca's area

    2. Wernicke's area

    3. arcuate fasciculus

J. Define the following terms.

    1. identification   4. perceptual bias

    2. discrimination   5. cognition

    3. phonology

K. Questions about language acquisition.

    1. How will your knowledge of developmental milestones and the process of language acquisition enhance your ability to serve those who seek to benefit from your professional expertise?

    2. Describe in detail each of Stark's six stages of prespeech linguistic development.

    3. What are "resonants" and "constrictions"?

    4. Differentiate between marginal babbling, reduplicated babbling, and variegated babbling.

    5. Differentiate between single-word utterances, successive single-word utterances, and two-word utterances.

    6. Stark's stage six corresponds to which of Brown's stages?

    7. Describe in detail the three stages of preverbal development of language use.

    8. By the time the child begins to purposefully use meaningful, conventional words, he or she has already achieved a number of pragmatic skills. What are they?

    9. Describe the relationship between language comprehension development and language production development.

    10. Describe in detail each of Brown's seven stages of language acquisition.

    11. For the purpose of early language acquisition, define the term *word*.

    12. What are the two components of phonological structure?

    13. Describe the development of skill in producing phonological structure, as it takes place in the preschool years.

    14. What are phonological processes?

    15. At what stage of development are phonological processes normal and why do they disappear?

    16. Describe the preschooler's development of language content and use.

    17. Describe the four types of narration.

    18. When children enter kindergarten, they are able to use language for a number of purposes. What are they?

19. Describe language acquisition milestones that are achieved by the ages of 6, 7, 8, 9, 10, 11, and 12, and by early adolescents, later adolescents, and adults.
20. What are deictic terms?
21. What are metalinguistic abilities and at what age should we expect children to be able to benefit from metalinguistic instruction?
22. Why is causality difficult for children to understand?
23. What are morphophonemic shifts? At what age should we expect people to be able to make these adaptations in pronunciation?
24. Describe the adult use of communication registers.
25. Describe the phenomena that typically facilitate language acquisition.
26. Differentiate between metalinguistic and experiential phenomena that characterize language learning.
27. Why should speech-language pathologists be concerned about the learning of reading and writing?
28. What can be done by speech-language pathologists in order to potentially minimize the risk of future difficulties with reading when providing early language intervention for some preschool-aged children?

CHAPTER 2

Childhood Language Disorders

The Domain

LEARNING OBJECTIVES

At the conclusion of this chapter, you should be prepared to:

- Define language disorders;
- Describe the potential effects of language disorders on each of the three dimensions of language and on the way in which the dimensions interface;
- Describe circumstances that result in disordered language and how these conditions impact language development across all dimensions.

INTRODUCTION

In order to assist in preparing you to address the specific atypical language behaviors that you will encounter as a **speech-language pathologist**, this chapter
begins by defining the term **language disorder**. The three dimensions of language (described in Chapter 1) are then discussed, each dimension in terms of
language behaviors that may be observed when disruptive patterns occur in a particular dimension or in the way in which the dimensions interact. This is followed
by a discussion of several circumstances that regularly result in language disorder
and how each condition may impact language development across dimensions.

LANGUAGE DISORDER: A DEFINITION

The term *language disorder* is used to describe a heterogeneous group of children whose language behaviors are different from, and not superior to, the
language behaviors of their same-age counterparts (Lahey, 1988). Thus, children whom we describe as having a language disorder exhibit language that
is qualitatively and/or quantitatively different from that which is used by same-
age children who have no **language impairment**, or they exhibit language
that is similar to, but developing more slowly than, the language of their non–
language-disordered peers.

    Language disorder is one of many terms used to describe such children.
Other terms associated with the same concept include **language delay**, **language disability**, language impairment, **deviant language**, **specific language disability**, and **specific language impairment** (**SLI**). Some terms
may seem to imply late development while others seem to imply a qualitative
or quantitative difference in performance. However, no one term is able to
specify the exact nature of a particular child's performance and all are found
to be used interchangeably (Lahey, 1988).

    Therefore, regardless of which term is chosen to label a child's condition, one
may assume *only* that his or her language behaviors are different from, and not
greater than, those expected at a particular chronological age. Beyond that, no
additional assumptions are reasonable, regardless of the term chosen to label
the condition. Without fail, the specific language behaviors are explicitly outlined
in order to provide accurate and complete information about the individual child's
language performance across the three dimensions. Some examples that more
completely describe disordered language are summarized in the following sections. For academic purposes, each is presented as a separate entity. However,
in reality dimensional disturbances rarely occur singly, or in isolation.

Late or Slow Development of All Three Dimensions

When language development is delayed across all three dimensions, language
acquisition occurs in the same sequence as for normally developing children.

However, it begins later and/or proceeds more slowly (Lahey, 1988). Under circumstances of delay, language performance is different from that of the child's peers only in that it lags behind, yet it is similar to the language expected from younger children in both quality and quantity.

An example of late or slow language development is a 7-year-old child whose language performance, both expressively and receptively, is that of a 4-year-old, a condition identified and documented by both formal and informal tests. In addition, a child with late or slow language development may or may not display symptoms of disturbances of specific language dimensions. There may also be differences between expression and reception with regard to the degree of involvement. However, in every case of late or slow development, all behaviors associated with each of the three language dimensions emerge late and/or develop slowly.

Disrupted Content

A **diagnosis** of disrupted language content may be assigned if the child produces well-articulated, grammatically correct, and socially appropriate utterances that do not make much sense (Lahey, 1988). Language form is well developed, such that articulation is clear, intonation and stress patterns are typical of the child's familiar language and culture, and syntax and morphology are accurate. Language use is also adequately developed, meaning that language is used for an apparent purpose with appropriate social interaction. However, language content is disrupted, such that the child's ideas, concepts, and knowledge are insufficient for meaningful communication.

The child's portion of the following conversation is an example of disrupted language content. Notice that the child's sentences are grammatically accurate and that he or she interacts appropriately with the adult. However, there are serious difficulties with the content of the child's utterances. Substantive ideas are absent or do not make sense, especially when considered in relation to the adjacent adult comments.

Adult: Tell me about your painting.

Child: (Pointing to a painted picture of a cat): Red paint and blue paint are over here. I like to paint.

Adult: (Pointing at the cat): Look here! Tell me about this part.

Child: (Pointing to the same place as the adult): Do you like it?

Disrupted Form

When language form is disrupted, the child's ideas about the world, as well as his or her ability to communicate these ideas to a conversational partner, are well beyond the child's knowledge of the linguistic system that is used for representing and communicating these ideas (Lahey, 1988). Language content is relatively intact. That is, the child has age-appropriate knowledge about objects, events, and relations and can use language to express ideas about the world. In addition, language use is adequate in that the child uses purposeful language with satisfactory social skill.

However, the child may use articulation, phonology, syntax, morphology, and/or prosody that are not age-appropriate for the conventional language system, or the child may be nonverbal. Yet it may be evident that the child has something to say because clear messages are frequently communicated through gestures and other unconventional or primitive means.

An example of a child with disrupted language form may be one with a desire to communicate the need for a drink but, who instead of using words (e.g., "May I have some juice?" or "I'm thirsty"), secures the mother's attention and then stands at the refrigerator door holding a cup. Although the message is precisely communicated in a socially appropriate context, the form of the message is unconventional and primitive. This type of communicative behavior is typical of a preverbal or nonverbal child.

Another example of disrupted language form is manifest in the following conversation about a spotted mouse and a brown mouse.

Um, um Spotted One is the spotted one's name. Spotted one the is girl one. The boy the brown.

Clearly the child has ideas to express including the name of the spotted animal and the gender of both. Further, the child communicates this information in an appropriate conversational format. The language form, however, is unconventional. That is, words are transposed in the second sentence (*is* and *the*), some necessary words are omitted in the third sentence (*is* and *one*), and some disfluencies are evident at the beginning of the utterance (*um, um*).

Disrupted Interaction between Content and Form

When a disruption occurs in the interaction that normally takes place between language content and form, the child attempts to express an idea that obligates a particular form but either omits the obligatory form or substitutes an inappropriate form in its place (Fey, 1986). Language use is intact, as the language is purposeful and the context is socially appropriate.

An example of a disruption in the content-form interaction is the child who wishes to express an ongoing activity of brushing one's own teeth, obligating the words, "I am brushing," yet omits the word *am* or the -*ing* morphological ending or substitutes an inaccurate verb form. This results in a form that does not accurately represent the intended idea (e.g., "I brushing"; "I am brush"; "I brush"; "I brushed").

Disrupted Use

When language use is disrupted, the child has a message or idea that is communicated clearly through a conventional linguistic system, but the style of delivering the message is somehow inappropriate. Language content may be intact, as evidenced by age-appropriate ideas and knowledge, and language form may be intact, as evidenced by phonology, morphology, syntax, and prosody that are typical of the language that is common to the child's culture. Nonetheless, the child has a problem with using language purposefully, with varying the content and form of the language to suit the circumstances, or with considering the needs of the communication partner.

Children whose language difficulty lies with the dimension of language use may exhibit a variety of communication difficulties. For example, some children experience problems with assuming the roles of both speaker and listener. As a result, these children may not initiate communication or may not respond readily to the communication attempts of other people (Prutting & Kirchner, 1987).

Children with language-use disorders may also experience difficulties with selecting, introducing, maintaining, and changing topics. For example, they may rarely select or initiate topics for discussion. They may be reluctant to participate in conversation or contribute to an ongoing topic so that it can be maintained. Furthermore, they may change topics without appropriately warning their conversational partner that a new topic is about to be introduced (Prutting & Kirchner, 1987).

A disorder of language use may also manifest itself in difficulties with conversational turn taking. The children may hesitate to initiate or respond to opportunities to take a conversational turn. They may neglect to request clarification when needed or they may neglect to repair a miscommunication. Pause time between turns may be too long or too short, and they may interrupt or attempt to speak over the conversational partner. Some children may provide ambiguous feedback or fail to provide feedback at all so that the conversational partner cannot tell whether clarification is needed. They may make contributions to the conversation that are not related to the immediate topic, or they may make comments that do not follow a logical sequence. In general, children with disrupted language use often lack skill in adapting their communication to the requirements of the specific listener or situation (Prutting & Kirchner, 1987).

Paralinguistically, intelligibility may be depressed, vocal intensity or vocal quality may be inappropriate, prosodic patterns may be unsuited for the language and culture, or the form of the message may be **disfluent**. Nonverbally, a child may assume a physical position that is either too close or too far in relation to the conversational partner, or a child may make an inappropriate number of physical contacts or may make physical contacts that are socially unsuitable. The body posture may be too far forward or slouching, or a child may make excessive foot, hand, and arm movements. Appropriate gestures may be lacking or inappropriate gestures may be used. The face may lack expression, the expression may be forced or artificial, or eye contact may be either excessive or absent (Prutting & Kirchner, 1987).

Occasionally, any or all of these characteristics may be observed in most children, which does not indicate disordered language use. However, when these patterns pervade a child's communication style, a disruption of the dimension of language use should be investigated.

Disrupted Interactions between Form, Content, and Use

When interactions between form, content, and use are disordered, it is possible that all three dimensions of language are individually disrupted to some extent as well (Lahey, 1988). Regarding language form, messages may be well formed, with appropriate phonology, morphology, syntax, and prosody, and the conventional linguistic system is generally the one that is used by the child. Regarding language content, the child may use language to express some complex ideas about the world, and some element of content may relate the message to the situation in which the message is generated. Regarding language use, messages may be expressed for a specific purpose and in appropriate situations, and language may be used for interpersonal interaction.

However, the disordered interactions between the dimensions is evident when a *contradiction* exists between the content of the message and the way in which the message is delivered, and another contradiction exists between the content of the message and the form that carries the message. An example of disordered interaction between the three dimensions is the child who says, "Don't spank the baby. Be nice to the baby," while at the same time hitting a rag doll. The sample utterance may be one that was heard previously by the child in a similar situation and, therefore, is remotely related to an idea that the child is expressing. Yet the idea expressed is inconsistent with the child's actions and the remark is not particularly appropriate for the context or situation.

Separation of Form, Content, and Use

For some children, the three dimensions of language do not appear to relate well to one another (Lahey, 1988). The content, or idea, is so far removed from the situation or context that any relationships among content, form, and use are concealed to the listener.

A child may repeatedly utter a comment that has been heard previously. For example, suppose a child habitually goes through the daily routine repeating the sentence, "Put the bear on Mary's bed, Suzy." This sentence is most likely one that the child has heard in some appropriate context in which Suzy was being directed to put a stuffed bear on Mary's bed. However, by repeating the sentence throughout the day, while the bear, Suzy, and Mary's bed are all absent from the context, the child expresses an idea that is not related to the situation. Further, the form is precisely memorized, and it is related neither to the idea nor the situation. Form, content, and use are therefore separated.

Echolalia is another speaking pattern that exemplifies a separation of form, content, and use. Echolalia is said to occur when the child repeats an utterance or part of an utterance that has just been said by another person, with no apparent intent to convey, emphasize, or elaborate on the information communicated by the previous speaker. The following is an example of echolalia.

Adult: Put the clown away now.

Child: Clown away now.

Note that the form of the echolalic utterance is exactly the same as the form of the utterance just said by the adult. Therefore, the form is accurate to the extent that the adult's utterance is accurate. Since the form does not represent an idea that the child is trying to express, content and form do not interact properly. Furthermore, the echolalic utterance is not an appropriate response to the remark made by the adult. Appropriate responses to the adult's remark might be, "OK," "No," "Not now," or "I don't want to." Therefore, the way in which the utterance is used is also disconnected from the meaning.

Perseverative speech also exemplifies how one's language may be characterized by separated form, content, and use. **Perseveration** is the meaningless repetition of a behavior that may at one time have been useful, meaningful, or contextually appropriate. In the case of perseverative speech, it is the meaningless repetition of a remark that the child has already said. The first time the child made the comment, it may have been appropriate. However, for some reason the child repeats the utterance in contextually inappropriate situations. The reason for the continued repetitions may be that the child was reinforced the first time the utterance was used, so that the comment (content-form) was strengthened regardless of the context (use). However, external reinforcement is not necessary for perseveration to occur. An example of perseverative speech follows.

Adult: (Playing with the toy farm animals and a toy barn): Oh look! A cow! What does the cow say?

Child: (Child takes the cow and looks at it): *Cow say "moo."*

Adult: (Visibly pleased): That's right!

Adult: (Picks up another cow, pretending that it is talking to the one that the child holds): Moo! Moo!

Adult: (Gives the second cow to the child and picks up the horse. Allows child to play with the cows for a few moments. Child puts down the cows): Here's the horse. What does the horse say? (Gives horse to child.)

Child: (Holding horse in hand, looking at the horse): *Cow say "moo."*

In the example, the second time the child says the utterance, the exact form of the first utterance is repeated. Although the form represents a meaningful and appropriate reply to the first adult remark, it does not represent a meaningful response to the last remark. Therefore, form and content are separated. Further, the form and meaning of the child's second utterance do not represent a contextually appropriate response to the contingent adult remark. Consequently, language use is separated from content and form.

Other common examples of children whose language suggests a fragmentation of content, form, and use are those whose language repertoires consist of recitations of radio and television ads, phrases commonly used by individuals in the child's environment, and phrases used by radio and television broadcasters. Like the other examples, these represent language form that is not particularly meaningful in terms of the context at hand.

Comprehension and Production Deficits

It has already been suggested that language comprehension and language production develop simultaneously, for the most part, with comprehension practice probably facilitating advances in language production and production practice probably facilitating language comprehension development (Chapter 1). However, in some children with language disorders, differences between comprehension and production have been identified such that one may lag behind the other.

Production Lags behind Comprehension.   Generally, when a disparity exists between language comprehension and production, it is usually production performance that is found to trail comprehension (Lahey, 1988). This pattern makes sense, since in order for a child to *produce* language, the child must access, encode, and generate a well-developed set of linguistic representations, including phonologic, morphologic, syntactic, prosodic, semantic, and pragmatic options for coding the concepts that he or she wishes to express linguistically.

On the other hand, *comprehending* language requires a less completely developed set of linguistic representations since it is not necessary to access representations and create sentences. By contrast, comprehension can be accomplished by merely recognizing, differentiating, and associating the linguistic units that are heard.

Comprehension Lags behind Production.   Some children are able to produce utterances that appear to be beyond their own comprehension abilities. This is generally the case when the interaction between the three language dimensions is disrupted and the three dimensions are separated as described just prior to this section. In disrupted dimensional interaction, the message (content) *contradicts* form and context (use), whereas in separated dimensions, there is *no clear relationship* between the message (content) and its form or between the message and its context (use). In either case, utterances do not seem to be comprehended or appreciated by their speaker.

LANGUAGE DISORDERS: ETIOLOGICAL FACTORS

In addressing the topic of language disorders, it is important to discuss why some children experience difficulty with language acquisition while the vast majority acquire language without complications. Generally, when language is not acquired normally, we may presume that something has interfered with language learning (Lahey, 1988). Exactly what it is that interferes is called the **etiology** (cause) of the language disorder. A variety of etiologies may potentially result in language disorder.

Five etiological categories are identified (Lahey, 1988). These include cognitive limitations, sensory input deficits, motor skill deficits, deficient social relations, and lack of linguistic opportunities in the environment. Some specific conditions from each category are discussed, with each condition selected for discussion being one associated with a high incidence of language disorder. For each, we describe some likely circumstances under which the condition develops, characteristics of the condition, and language behaviors that most typically result.

It can also be assumed that, unless otherwise indicated, individual language performance varies and should be specifically assessed and described on an individual basis. Further, always bear in mind that for many individuals, a number of disorders will be found to occur together.

Cognitive Limitations

Cognitive skill deficits are distinguished by low intelligence, difficulties with symbolic thinking, and/or difficulties with pattern recognition and identification (Lahey, 1988). This etiology category includes, but is not limited to, individuals with **mental retardation**, learning disabilities, childhood aphasia, and attention deficit disorder.

Mental Retardation.   Mental retardation is identified when an individual's cognitive, intellectual, and behavioral skills are below that of same-age peers. Language disorder is a basic characteristic of mental retardation (Hegde, 1991).

Mental retardation ranges in severity from mild to profound. However, most individuals with mental retardation are mildly affected (i.e., approximately 89 percent), with intelligence quotient (IQ) scores between 55 and 69. Preschoolers who have a mild form of mental retardation achieve developmental milestones somewhat later than their peers, and upon reaching school they lag significantly behind their peers in achieving academic goals and therefore are usually placed in special programs for at least part of their formal education. Adults with mild retardation are usually capable of holding down simple jobs and living independently (Lahey, 1988).

Moderately retarded individuals account for approximately 6 percent of all retarded people and have IQ scores between 40 and 54. Most moderately retarded people are identified at the preschool level because of obvious developmental lags. Although they may eventually learn to talk, moderately retarded people often experience difficulties with some or all three dimensions of language. As adults, many can learn to carry out routine and repetitive tasks with supervision (Lahey, 1988).

The remaining 5 percent of retarded people are divided between two categories, severe and profound. Individuals with severe retardation have IQ scores between 25 and 39 and make up about 3.5 percent of the retarded population. Those with profound retardation have IQ scores below 25 and comprise approximately the remaining 1.5 percent. Individuals with severe and profound retardation are very late in achieving developmental milestones, including speech and language accomplishments. Indeed, some milestones are not achieved at all by individuals in these two categories. Severely and profoundly retarded people experience difficulties across all three language dimensions and rarely achieve competence in conversation. Independent living is unlikely, as nearly all require close supervision throughout their lives (Lahey, 1988).

Around 2 percent of all children born at any one time are born with some degree of mental retardation or a condition that is likely to result in mental retardation (Hegde, 1991). Most likely, the children who are born under these circumstances are mentally retarded as a result of brain injury, chromosomal disorder, or genetic disorder.

Brain Injury.   Factors that may result in brain injury include excessively premature birth, low birth weight, difficult and prolonged labor and delivery, accidents, disease, and toxic chemicals. Premature birth and low birth weight are factors that leave a child vulnerable to a number of health problems. Therefore premature and low–birth weight children are frequently at risk for developing conditions that may interfere with normal cognitive development and maturation of neuroanatomical structures. Difficult and prolonged labor and delivery may result in brain injury as a result of oxygen deprivation and stress applied to the infant.

Although accidents sometimes occur at birth, accidents that result in brain injury can happen later as well. Car accidents are the most common accident to result in brain injury. Serious falls and other accidental events resulting in closed-head or open-head trauma also can result in injury to the brain. Prenatal diseases and diseases that strike infants and very young children also may result in mental retardation secondary to brain injury. Some examples are cytomegalovirus (CMV), meningitis, syphilis, rubella, mumps, and measles. Finally, children who are exposed to toxic chemicals, such as lead, or those with prenatal exposure to drugs and alcohol may be at risk for mental retardation.

Mental retardation that occurs secondary to brain injury ranges from mild to profound, depending on the extent and location of the injury. **Lesion** locations that result in reduced language performance are usually in Broca's area, Wernicke's area, the supplemental communication center, the cerebellum, and/or the brainstem (Figure 1–12). However, with mental retardation, although the injury may include these specific sites, the lesion is usually diffuse (i.e., not confined to one small area of the brain).

Further, although language characterized by late onset and slow development of language (i.e., delay) is a universal factor, any or all of the disruptions of specific linguistic dimensions may be observed as well. No specific disorder pattern is universally associated with the mental retardation that results from brain injury.

Cytomegalovirus (CMV) is the most common viral disease among the newborn. Further, it is the most common viral disease that results in brain injury and, thus, mental retardation. It is estimated that approximately 3,000 children each year are damaged by CMV. Mental retardation results because of brain injury, which is the outcome of direct tissue destruction secondary to infection (Sever, 1983). CMV is especially dangerous to infants if it is contracted prenatally, with less effect resulting from **perinatal** and postnatal infection (Gerber, 1991). Infants born with the CMV infection have a high mortality rate. Those who survive are severely and multiply handicapped, with mild to severe mental retardation, motor disabilities, seizures, blindness, and deafness (Myers & Stool, 1968).

The exact nature of the communication disorder resulting from CMV varies depending on the degree of mental retardation and nature of hearing loss. Behavioral descriptions based on individual language performance are essential to understanding the idiosyncratic language-learning needs of a person with language disorder secondary to CMV.

Fetal alcohol syndrome (FAS) is another example of brain damage that occurs prenatally and may result in a type of mental retardation (Young, 1987). FAS is likely to occur when a woman consumes alcohol when pregnant—and not necessarily in excessive amounts. No differences have been found in the frequency or severity of FAS in children born to alcoholic mothers as opposed to mothers who drink only socially.

FAS is among the most common birth defects and one of the leading causes of mental retardation (Gerber, 1991). The symptoms of FAS include three features. First, FAS babies are likely to be small in size and have a low birth weight, a condition that persists throughout postnatal development. Second, individuals born with FAS have permanent developmental delay and microcephaly (i.e., small brain circumference) below the third percentile. Other central nervous system disorders are also likely to occur. Finally, FAS results in characteristic facial features. These include microphthalmia (i.e., abnormally small size of one or both eyes), underdeveloped philtrum (i.e., a medial groove on external surface of the upper lip), thin upper lip, and maxillary hypoplasia (i.e., an underdeveloped maxilla, or upper jaw). If all three symptoms are observed, then FAS is the diagnosis. If only two of the three physical symptoms are observed, the diagnosis is fetal alcohol effect (FAE) (Gerber, 1991).

Regarding communication, a language disorder that correlates to the degree of mental retardation is expected (Gerber, 1991). The language disorder may be characterized by an across-the-board delay in language acquisition, or it may be characterized by any number of difficulties with any combination of the three language dimensions. In addition, there is a high incidence of craniofacial anomaly among children born with FAS (Gerber, 1991), and some evidence supports that FAS is characterized by articulation disorders and disfluency (Sparks, 1984).

Chromosomal Disorders.   Chromosomal disorders may also cause mental retardation. Chromosomal disorders bear some similarity to genetic disorders since the genes that code specific genetic information reside on the **chromosomes**. However, the chromosomal disorders are quite different from genetic disorders in that genetic disorders are always **inherited** as genes carrying a particular trait are passed down from one generation to the next, whereas chromosomal disorders are *not* inherited.

Instead, a chromosomal disorder is a disorder of the number or structure of the chromosomes as they are distinctively arranged for a particular individual (Gerber, 1991). Each living organism has its own characteristic chromosomal pattern and number, which distinguish it from all other living organisms. This unique genetic pattern that identifies the individual's chromosomal pattern has a particular genetic map indicating the exact location that each **gene** assumes on every chromosome (Gerber, 1991). The two types of chromosomal disorders are aberrations in chromosomal number and in structure.

Disorders of chromosomal number are discussed first. The appropriate number of chromosomes for human beings is 46 (i.e., 23 from each biological parent). Therefore, in humans, 46 chromosomes reside in all cells throughout the body with the exception of the red blood cells. (Red blood cells have no chromosomes because they have no cell nuclei.) The number 46 is the only number that is normal for human chromosomal arrangement. Any other number is abnormal and results in deformity.

Counting the exact number of chromosomes in a given cell is a relatively simple procedure for skilled professionals. Chromosomes are extracted from the body for the purpose of examination by taking a very small sample of blood or skin. In the case of a fetus, chromosomes are extracted by taking a small amount of amniotic fluid from the intrauterine space.

Disorders in the number of chromosomes occur at conception, which is the stage of development when the chromosomes disjoin (i.e., separate). When a pair of chromosomes fails to separate, the outcome is an abnormal number of chromosomes for 1 of the 23 chromosomal pairs. This mishap results in a chromosome number that is not 46 and not a multiple of 23. Usually, the resulting pattern is called **trisomy**, which means that 1 of the 23 chromosomal "pairs" has three members instead of the standard two.

Trisomy 21 (Down syndrome) is the most common trisomy. The term *Trisomy 21* means that at the location of the 21st chromosome, there are three members instead of the customary two. Trisomy 21 is most often caused by late maternal age. Individuals with Trisomy 21 generally have the following characteristics: generalized hypotonia (i.e., reduced muscle tone) that extends through the oral cavity, resulting in an open-mouth posture and protruding tongue, hyper-flexibility (i.e., increased flexibility) of joints, universal mental retardation, which is usually mild or moderate in degree; a characteristic face with brachycephaly (i.e., a disproportionally short head with a reduced front-to-back dimension), occasional eye discoloration; characteristically shaped outer ears; characteristic hypoplasia (i.e., underdevelopment) of the fifth finger (60 percent), simian crease (45 percent) (i.e., a crease on the palm of the hand similar to that found in some monkeys), heart malformation (40 percent), dry skin accompanied by fine, soft, sparse hair (75 percent), universal hypogonadism (i.e., small testicles), and occasional seizures, strabismus (i.e., sporadic eye movements), and cataracts (Gerber, 1991).

With regard to communication, individuals with Trisomy 21 present a number of difficulties (Gerber, 1991). Mental retardation is inevitable, so delayed and disordered acquisition pervades all language dimensions. The severity of the language disturbance varies, as does the severity of the cognitive limitations. Some individuals with mild intellectual involvement display language abilities that approximate normal limits, while others whose involvement is more serious are either nonverbal or quite primitive in their language performance. All combinations of language disturbance between the two extremes are possible as well. Therefore, in order to identify the exact nature of the language disorder, a complete diagnosis is necessary including detailed descriptions of behavior.

In addition to the wide range of possible language disturbances that may be manifest in Trisomy 21, a number of additional variables may serve to complicate the communication impairment. For example, upper respiratory anomalies, which include external ear malformations and probable middle ear malformations, make the individual particularly susceptible to recurrent **otitis media** (Gerber, 1991). (For details on this condition refer to the section on otitis media and hearing loss later in this chapter.)

A number of physical traits and physiological idiosyncrasies generally lead to problems with articulation. These include a characteristic head shape that results in a short distance between the front and back of the mouth, and a short vocal tract. Consequently the tongue may appear to be too large for the short oral cavity, and it may even protrude. When this occurs, articulation is usually affected (Gerber, 1991).

Trisomy 13 (Patau syndrome) and Trisomy 18 (Edwards syndrome) are examples of other disorders of chromosome number that may result in mental retardation. However, individuals with an abnormal number of these larger chromosomes generally do not survive postnatally. If they do survive, life expectancy is short and their handicaps are multiple and severe (Gerber, 1991).

Disorders of chromosome structure may also result in mental retardation. Diagnosis involves the analysis of a tissue sample, as is required for a diagnosis of abnormal chromosome number. However, determining the structure of chromosomes is far more complicated than simply counting the chromosomal members. Each chromosome is approximately X-shaped, with four "arms," two short and two long. Most disorders of structure occur when an arm of a chromosome is found to be missing or added (Gerber, 1991).

Cri du Chat syndrome (5 p-) is one example of a disorder of chromosome structure. *Cri du Chat* syndrome is diagnosed by determining that a short arm of the fifth chromosome is lacking. The cause of this particular chromosomal anomaly is yet unknown.

With regard to communication, a typically narrow oral cavity may result in articulation problems. Further, mental retardation can be expected, and the degree of language disorder generally correlates with, or is greater than, the degree of cognitive disability (Gerber, 1991). The exact nature of the language impairment with regard to the impact on all three dimensions of language is determined by diagnostic evaluation. A detailed description of individual language behavior is required in order to accurately describe the individual's idiosyncratic language characteristics.

Other structural deletion syndromes that result in mental retardation have been identified (e.g., 9 p-) (Gerber, 1991). However, they do not occur as often as *Cri du Chat*. Individual language behavior is generally related to the degree of mental retardation, and the exact nature of the language disorder is idiosyncratic to the individual person.

Genetic Disorders.   **Genetic** disorders are different from chromosomal disorders in that chromosomal disorders occur when a chromosome is damaged or fails to disjoin at about the time of conception. This condition *cannot* be inherited. By contrast, genetic disorders are the result of an abnormal gene being passed from one generation to the next. Genetic disorders are always inherited. However, they are not always congenital, as the symptoms of the genetic disorder may not manifest themselves until a number of years after birth.

Fragile X syndrome (fra X), also called Martin-Bell syndrome, is the most common hereditary (or genetic) form of mental retardation, and it is among the leading causes of mental retardation overall (Wolf-Schein et al., 1987). Fra X accounts for 2 to 6 percent of all mentally retarded males (Nielson, 1983). It occurs in 1 in every 1,000 live male births (Carmi, Meryash, Wood, & Gerald, 1984) and 1 in every 2,000 live female births (Wolf-Schein et al., 1987).

Fra X occurs when an abnormal gene resides on the long arm of an X sex chromosome (Scharfenaker, 1990). The inheritance pattern of fra X is similar to the inheritance pattern of most X-linked genetic traits. Briefly, female children inherit two X sex chromosomes, one from each biological parent. Male children, on the other hand, inherit one X sex chromosome from the biological mother and one Y sex chromosome from the biological father.

If the fra X genetic trait resides on one of the biological mother's two X sex chromosomes, there is a 50 percent chance that each of her children will inherit the syndrome, with male offspring being more seriously affected by the disorder than female offspring. This difference is due to the fact that the defective X sex chromosome is the only X sex chromosome inherited by the male children, whereas the female children with one abnormal X have a second normal X, which typically masks fra X symptoms to some degree (Scharfenaker, 1990).

If the fra X genetic trait resides on the biological father's only X sex chromosome, then there is no chance that he will pass the syndrome on to his son because a son will receive no X sex chromosomes from him. However, he will pass the fra X genetic trait on to all his daughters (Scharfenaker, 1990).

The physical characteristics of fra X are not apparent at birth. However, a number of features become increasingly evident as the child with fra X matures (Wolf-Schein et al., 1987). These features include large head circumference, prominent forehead, long and narrow face, narrow distance between the eyes, high palatal arch, some facial asymmetry, prominent and long ears, and postpubescent macro-orchidism (i.e., exceedingly large testicles).

The speech-language impairments of children with fra X may range from very mild to very severe. Speech-language delay is often the first symptom to be noticed, and with proper referral it may lead to the diagnosis. For that reason, all children who present with mental retardation of unknown etiology, autism, or four or more of the following characteristics should be referred for chromosomal analysis to determine whether the cause is fra X. The fra X checklist includes: mental retardation, perseverative speech, hyperactivity, short attention span, negative reaction to physical contact, hand flapping, hand biting, poor eye contact, hyperextensible (i.e., abnormally flexible) finger joints, large and prominent ears, large testicles, simian crease (i.e., a crease on the palm of the hand similar to that found in some monkeys), and family history of mental retardation (Hagerman, 1987).

Unlike many other forms of mental retardation, the symptoms of the language disorder are *not* accounted for by the degree of mental retardation alone. This is demonstrated when fra X males are compared to Trisomy 21 males with similar cognitive abilities, as the language of fra X males is significantly more seriously impaired. For example, regarding language content-form interactions, fra X males use more **jargon** (i.e., unintelligible strings of syllables). Regarding the way in which the three dimensions of language interact, fra X males perseverate more and use more echolalia. Further, concerning language use, fra X males make more inappropriate comments (i.e., off topic), they talk to themselves more, and they make fewer appropriate nonverbal gestures to support or enhance their attempts at verbal communication. In general, the identified fra X language characteristics are typical of autistic language, and in fact there is a high incidence of fra X among individuals with autism (Wolf-Schein et al., 1987).

In planning speech-language intervention for individuals with fra X, a team approach is suggested, which should include all professionals who assist in addressing the medical and educational needs of the child. In carrying out a speech-language program, it may be beneficial to consider that, typically, visual memory is strong while auditory memory is weak. For that reason, in devising and implementing an intervention program, a clinician is wise to represent materials visually whenever possible (Scharfenaker, 1990).

Learning Disabilities.   A learning disability is identified when a school-age child performs below grade expectations (i.e., usually lagging by at least two grade levels) in the understanding and use of spoken language, written language, mathematics, and/or reasoning abilities, and when these difficulties are not attributable to an identified handicapping condition (Hammill, Leigh, McNutt, & Larsen, 1981). Since the learning-disabled population is defined partially by the absence of an explanatory condition, accuracy in diagnosing a learning disability largely depends on success in identifying handicapping conditions that may explain performance lags. Weaknesses that exist in our ability to properly isolate children who truly have no accompanying explanatory condition (e.g., recurrent otitis media, mental retardation, hearing loss, access to poor instruction, or lack of motivation) may cause the disorder to appear to be more common than it really is. In many schools, the diagnosis appears to have reached epidemic proportions and is on the increase (Lahey, 1988).

According to the Education of All Handicapped Children Act (also called Public Law 94-142), the classification of learning disabilities may include conditions such as "perceptual handicaps, brain injury, minimal brain dysfunction, dyslexia, and developmental aphasia," indicating that there is substantial overlap between the condition of language-related learning disability and the condition of language disorder. One way to differentiate between the two is, first, to view *language-related learning disabilities* as the difficulties that one experiences with the academic language skills that are customarily learned through academic instruction and, second, to view *language disorders* as the difficulties that one experiences in the acquisition of nonacademic language skills that are usually achieved through exposure to caregiver interactions, and not the result of direct instruction (Lahey, 1988).

Even by separating the two definitions in this way, a number of school-age children diagnosed as language disordered in the preschool years often experience academic difficulties and become categorized as learning disabled during the school years (Boone & Plante, 1993). It may be that the same factors that contribute to the language-learning difficulties, if not remediated, will continue to interfere with the learning process at the academic level.

For that reason, perhaps in our treatment of preschool-aged children with language disorders, we should keep in mind that the children are in a high-risk category for experiencing academic difficulties as well. This may require that we give special attention to any language-related preacademic skills that are identified as troublesome for the language-disordered child and that we refer the preschool child to the schools for assistance if impending academic difficulties are apparent.

Knowledge of specific difficulties associated with learning disabilities can assist in making referrals and planning remediation for high-risk children. Therefore, speech-language pathologists should know that children with learning disabilities often experience motor coordination problems that may be exhibited in difficulty with rapid alternating finger movements, difficulty with imitating motor movements (in the absence of an explanatory perceptual disability) (Rudel, 1985), and inaccurate production of polysyllabic words (Kahmi & Catts, 1986). Further, learning-disabled children also are likely to experience difficulties with concentration and attention, a condition that is often accompanied by hyperactivity.

Although attention deficits and motor problems improve somewhat with maturation, learning-disabled children continue to lag behind their age-matched peers and the gap widens with increasing age (Rudel, 1985). If, therefore, in the process of treating a preschool child with a language disorder, we discover attentional and/or motor difficulties such as described here, we should take the proper steps toward addressing these concerns at the preschool level, whether by referral or by making adaptations to the intervention program.

Childhood Aphasia. When a child experiences normal language development for a period of time and then incurs damage to the left hemisphere of the brain, acquired childhood aphasia is a probable result (Aram, Ekelman, Rose, & Whitaker, 1985). The cause of the damage to the left cerebral hemisphere is usually a traumatic injury due to an accident that results in closed-head or open-head trauma. However, stroke, infectious disease, tumor, and seizures are other possible etiologies for acquired aphasia in children.

Linguistically, children with aphasia experience language comprehension difficulties that cannot be attributed to hearing loss or cognitive limitations. Comprehension problems include difficulties with understanding complex sentences, following directions, and reading. Academic difficulties can be expected as a result (Cranberg, Filley, Hart, & Alexander, 1987).

Research indicates that the expressive language of children who acquire aphasia is most often the **nonfluent** type. It seems to begin with a period of extreme nonfluency, which is so severe that the child may even be nonverbal at first. As spoken language emerges, it can be described as agrammatic and telegraphic due to the omission of morphemes, rearrangement of words, and omission of function words (Satz & Bullard-Bates, 1981; Swisher, 1985).

Less often, children experience fluent aphasia. When they do, expressive language comprises easily produced, but unintelligible, words, phrases, and sentences that are spoken with a normal prosodic pattern. Whether the disorder is fluent or nonfluent, expressive difficulties primarily affect content-form interactions, and they are always accompanied by disturbed comprehension. The severity of the disorder ranges from mild to profound, depending on the extent, type, and location of the lesion.

Further, for a period of time immediately following the cerebral insult, consistent recovery can be anticipated. It is during this acute stage of the illness that the young person with aphasia is particularly responsive to clinical intervention. However, the exact length of the amenable recovery period ranges from a few months to several years, depending on the type of lesion and severity of the disorder (Lees & Urwin, 1991).

Regarding intervention, it is important to evaluate the individual child and address the idiosyncratic needs that are evident for the specific case. Complete recovery is not to be expected, as most children with aphasia experience a number of residual difficulties (Lees & Urwin, 1991). A continual reassessment of performance and progress is needed in order to determine whether the client is likely to benefit from continued intervention.

Some prognostic indicators (defined in Chapters 3 and 4) have been identified. That is, children who gain two standard deviations on formal testing, as measured at the end of the first six months, are likely to regain more skill than those who gain less than two standard deviations in the same time period (Lees & Urwin, 1991). Younger age of onset and traumatic injury (as opposed to a **vascular lesion**) are positive prognostic signs. Persistent paraphasia, persistent perseveration (Lees & Urwin, 1991), later age of onset, vascular etiology, and the experience of a coma for more than seven days (van Dongen & Loonen, 1977) are all negative prognostic indicators. These measures are helpful in ascertaining expectations for progress. However, in making a decision regarding whether treatment is to continue, actual benefits that the child experiences from the intervention program are always given priority.

Attention Deficit Disorder.   Children with attention deficit disorder (ADD) are highly distractible and inattentive, find it difficult to focus and sustain their attention on a topic or activity, and often act impulsively. Academically, children with ADD are at risk because their behavioral characteristics interfere with ability to listen to instructions, follow directions, and complete assignments (Boone & Plante, 1993).

Linguistically, children with ADD have disrupted language use, which is secondary to the other symptoms. For example, children with ADD are apt to interrupt while others are talking, attempt to talk over others, make comments that are inappropriate or unrelated to the discussion, and shift topics without warning. ADD may occur concomitant to other conditions that also result in language disorder, and when that is the case, language content and form may be impaired as well (Boone & Plante, 1993).

In children, the symptoms of ADD can often be controlled by medication. Although symptoms subside with maturation for many individuals, ADD may persist into adulthood. For that reason, medicating a child with ADD is not enough. In order to prepare for the challenges of adult life, the child with ADD must be helped to learn strategies that minimize the effects of distractions and maximize one's ability to focus and to follow tasks through to completion (Boone & Plante, 1993). (Some suggestions are included in Chapter 4.)

Sensory Input Deficits

Hearing loss and central auditory processing disorder are the two sensory channel deficits that are likely to result in serious communication disorders. Blindness is a third significant sensory channel deficit, but its effect on communication development is slight when compared to the extreme effects that can result from the other two.

Hearing Loss.   In general, hearing loss is defined as reduced hearing sensitivity (Northern & Downs, 1991). The term *loss* is applied loosely in that it by no means implies that hearing was once present and has actually been lost, as the condition can be either congenital or acquired. The only sense that the term *loss* carries here is that hearing sensitivity is lower than that of most people.

The terms *hearing loss* and *reduced hearing* are used interchangeably for the sake of this discussion, even though a number of other terms are often used to describe the condition. The terms *hearing impairment* and *hearing defect* may be seen in the literature and in a number of clinical reports. However, I do not advise using them because many individuals with reduced hearing capacity object to being described as "impaired" or "defective."

Although *deafness* is the term preferred by those in a cultural community that comprises mostly individuals with severe or profound reduction in hearing, the term *deaf* is more meaningful when used to describe cultural phenomena than as a descriptor of hearing level and capacity for spoken communication. (Cultural phenomena associated with deafness are described in Chapter 6.)

Speech-language pathology issues associated with reduced hearing sensitivity (i.e., hearing loss) are the topic of this section, and we feel that they are best described by the terms that we have chosen. Distinctions among groups of individuals within the population are defined by specifying the degree of reduced sensitivity (i.e., mild, moderate, severe, or profound).

The impact of reduced hearing sensitivity on spoken language development depends on a number of factors. These include the degree, age of onset, type, configuration (as shown on an audiogram), and stability of the hearing loss. For children, additional contributing factors include the amount of training available, age at which training begins, age at which hearing amplification is provided, and consistency with which amplification is used. Family attitudes and availability of visual communication systems may also impact the effect of reduced hearing on the outcome of a child's spoken communication development and training.

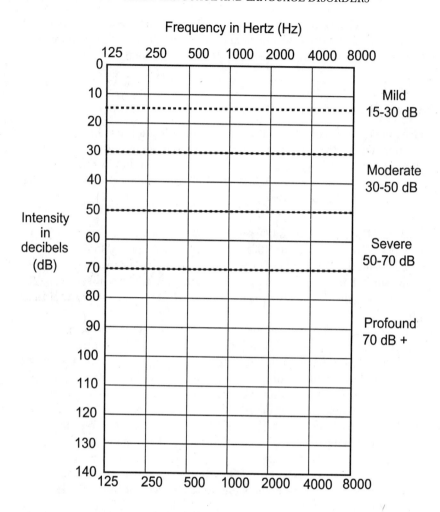

Figure 2-1.   Levels of reduced hearing as shown on an audiogram. A hearing loss is considered mild if unaided thresholds are between 15 and 30 dB, moderate between 30 and 50 dB, severe between 50 and 70 dB, and profound exceeding 70dB.

The Degree of Hearing Loss.   Four levels of severity are described. They are mild, moderate, severe, and profound hearing losses.

A mild hearing loss is indicated when a person has a 15 to 30 **decibel (dB)** reduction in hearing sensitivity (see the audiogram in Figure 2–1). This condition has a mild impact on spoken language learning since the vowel sounds and many consonants are often heard clearly (Northern & Downs, 1991).

However, low-energy sounds (e.g., voiceless consonants) may be missed by children with a mild hearing loss (Northern & Downs, 1991). Since many grammatical morphemes in spoken English are carried by voiceless consonants, this problem may result in difficulties with language content-form interactions. For example, the regular plural is represented by the final *-s* morpheme (e.g., "boats"), as are the regular third-person singular verb form (e.g., "eats") and the regular possessive (e.g., "Kate's"). In addition, the *-ed* past-tense verb ending is often pronounced as the voiceless [t] (e.g., "coughed) and may be missed in the presence of mild hearing loss.

These low-energy sounds that carry significant meaning may result in confusions and misperceptions if missed auditorily. They may also be the source of production errors that lead to misunderstandings. The confusions caused by mildly reduced hearing are typically minor and can be overcome with a combination of production training, careful observation, and listening practice.

Moderate hearing loss is said to exist if the audiogram indicates a 30 to 50 dB reduction in hearing sensitivity (Figure 2–1). Without amplification, spoken conversation is difficult for the affected person to understand. For individuals with moderate hearing loss, vowels are heard more clearly than consonants, many speech sounds are not heard at all, and other speech sounds are heard inaccurately (Northern & Downs, 1991). In addition to word endings, short, unstressed words (e.g., prepositions, conjunctions, articles, auxiliaries, and relational words) are also frequently missed.

Without amplification, spoken language input is generally inaccurate or incomplete for the individual with moderately reduced hearing. Consequently, unless proper amplification is provided, spoken language is impaired across all three language dimensions.

Language form is affected in that many of the standard phonemes of the language are not perceived accurately and therefore, are not produced accurately. As a result, speech may be largely unintelligible to those who are not familiar with the individual's speaking pattern. Language prosody (i.e., pitch and inflection) may also be misunderstood or misrepresented by the person with moderate hearing loss. Various pitch and inflectional patterns that are represented by spoken language carry significant meaning, such as the sentence type (i.e., interrogative, imperative, exclamation, or statement) and the emotional tone of the speaker (e.g., angry, excited, or comforting). These patterns may not be heard accurately by the unaided individual with a moderately reduced hearing.

Language content-form is affected in that numerous grammatical markers are not heard by the language learner, and therefore, they are not produced or comprehended in spoken conversation. Moreover, the effect of moderate hearing loss on emerging vocabulary development may be significant. This, too, is the result of limited and inaccurate linguistic information received through the auditory mode (Northern & Downs, 1991). The individual with moderate hearing loss does not have adequate access to the standard linguistic information that represents concepts and experiences. Hence, vocabulary may be limited, word meanings may be confused, and in general, the person's ability to use spoken language for the purpose of expressing abstract and concrete ideas may be somewhat restricted.

The effect of unaided moderate hearing loss on language use is equally consequential. Due to the lack of hearing spoken language in conversation, individuals with moderately reduced hearing tend to lack interest in spoken communication. Inattention is a natural result (Northern & Downs, 1991). Having missed much of the auditory information that is used to demonstrate appropriate conversational strategies, an individual may be unaware of the most effective ways to interact with others for purposeful spoken communication.

Severe hearing loss occurs when the loss is measured at 50 to 70 dB (Figure 2–1). Without amplification, spoken language does not develop spontaneously for children with severely reduced hearing as they do not hear most conversational speech sounds. However, they do hear their own vocalizations, loud environmental sounds (e.g., lawn mower, ringing telephone, electric saw), and the speech of others if it is spoken very loud and at close range.

If unaided, the effect of severe hearing loss on spoken communication is universally critical. Language content-form is grossly misunderstood and misrepresented by the individual with severely reduced hearing, as the sounds that carry the phonological, morphological, syntactic, and prosodic systems are not accurately experienced by the language learner. Further, it is also by auditory information that the use of the language is typically learned by individuals acquiring spoken language. Hence, all three language dimensions are seriously affected by the condition of unaided severe hearing loss.

Profound hearing loss is indicated if the hearing loss is measured at 70 dB or more (Figure 2–1). Without amplification and training, spoken language is not accessible to individuals with profoundly reduced hearing, as the only sounds heard are their own vocalizations, some of the rhythm patterns of the speech of others, and extremely loud environmental sounds (e.g., airplane at close range, rock music band) (Northern & Downs, 1991)

Even with proper amplification, the person with profoundly reduced hearing may have extreme difficulty understanding and using spoken language. Intensive training is necessary in order for the individual to learn to understand and utilize the linguistic information that is received auditorily through a hearing aid.

Common problems in the language content and form of individuals with profound hearing loss include difficulties with articulation, resonance, voice, morphological, syntactic, and prosodic features of the language. It has been estimated that naive listeners are likely to understand only 20 to 25 percent of the speech produced by individuals with profoundly reduced hearing (Northern & Downs, 1991). Language use is similarly affected due to the limited and inaccurate auditory information that is received.

Age of Onset.   The age at which a person begins to experience reduced hearing has quite an impact on the effect of the hearing reduction on the development of spoken language. Clearly, for individuals whose hearing reduction begins **prelingually**, the impact is greater than for those who have the opportunity to hear and understand language prior to losing some of their hearing.

Therefore, whether hearing reduction is congenital or acquired, if the reduction manifests itself prior to the attainment of consistent understanding and use of spoken language for communication, it is considered to be a *prelingual hearing reduction*, the effects of which depend on the degree of sensitivity reduction, as described. In order for all dimensions of standard spoken language to be acquired, amplification *and* training are necessary.

Individuals with *adventitious hearing loss* (postlingually acquired) may also require amplification and training in order to maintain and continue to acquire new spoken-language skills. Training may be necessary to facilitate an adjustment to the loss of hearing sensitivity and to familiarize one's self with the use and maintenance of an amplification device.

Consistency of the Hearing Reduction.   Whether reduced hearing is experienced consistently or inconsistently may influence language development (Menyuk, 1986). For some children, a sensitivity reduction that is sporadic results in unstable or incomplete auditory input, which in turn results in confusions in any or all of the three language dimensions, and particularly, language content-form interactions.

Configuration of the Hearing Reduction.   The exact shape of the hearing loss, as shown on an audiogram, also influences language development. This includes which frequencies are affected, to what degree, and whether the sensitivity reduction is **unilateral** or **bilateral**. Specific frequency losses (i.e., mild, moderate, severe, or profound) and how they impact speech-language development were discussed in a previous section of this chapter.

In addition to frequency, whether hearing reduction is unilateral or bilateral is an important factor that is considered when determining the effect that the reduction in hearing has on spoken-language acquisition. Certainly, a unilateral loss has a less serious impact than a bilateral loss. In fact, children with unilateral hearing reduction typically develop language normally and perform at their age level on communication tasks.

Remediation is required for unilateral hearing-sensitivity reduction, primarily for the purpose of assisting the individual in developing compensatory strategies that can be used when encountering negative listening conditions (Maxon & Brackett, 1992). Seeking and accessing visual cues, requesting clarification, and arranging for preferential seating are very important tactics for individuals with unilateral hearing loss.

On the other hand, bilateral hearing reduction impacts communication with mild, moderate, severe, or profound consequences, depending on the degree of effect. Many people with either unilateral or bilateral hearing reduction are able to benefit from appropriate amplification depending on the degree of loss.

Further, the actual *pattern of the audiogram* (Figure 2–1) is important. For example, many individuals with sensorineural hearing loss show a distinct audiogram pattern with the most serious reductions in the higher frequencies. This occurs such that many hearing losses are classified by degree using more than one category. Severe-to-profound, moderate-to-severe, and mild-to-moderate are degree ratings that describe a hearing reduction that crosses over more than one category. Exactly which frequencies are affected and to what degree each is affected impacts spoken language acquisition, as it has a definite influence on the exact nature of the phonological and morphological difficulties experienced.

Type of Hearing Loss.   The three basic types of hearing loss that may be experienced are conductive hearing loss, sensorineural hearing loss, and mixed hearing loss (Northern & Downs, 1991). Conductive hearing loss occurs when there is interference, preventing the transmission of sound from the ear canal (Figure 1–7) to the cochlea (Figure 1–7). Although the inner ear (Figure 1–7) is capable of receiving sound from the middle ear and transmitting it to the acoustic nerve, the air conduction pathway (Figure 1–7) by which the sound normally reaches the inner ear is not fully usable, preventing the sound from reaching the inner ear (Figure 1–7) (Northern & Downs, 1991).

Conditions that impede the normal transmission of sound include foreign objects or excessive cerumen (i.e., ear wax) in the ear canal (Figure 1–7), fluid buildup in the middle ear preventing malleable movement of the ossicular chain (Figure 1–7), stenosis (i.e., stiffness) or discontinuity (i.e., separation) of the ossicular chain (Figure 1–7), and certain craniofacial malformations. In all these cases, sound is not heard because it does not reach the intact inner ear (Figure 1–7).

A conductive hearing loss is diagnosed if the audiologist is able to stimulate the inner ear directly by bone conduction via the skull or temporal bone (Figure 1–7). If bone conduction thresholds are within normal limits while air conduction thresholds indicate reduced hearing, then a conductive loss is diagnosed (see Figure 2–2). Most conductive hearing losses are correctable through medical treatment or surgery (Northern & Downs, 1991).

Sensorineural hearing loss occurs when either the cochlea (Figure 1–7) or cranial nerve VIII (Figure 1–7) does not function properly. It is difficult to differentiate between a sensory loss, which is caused by cochlear damage, and neural loss, which is caused by damage to the nerve. Therefore, these two types of hearing loss are typically discussed together as one type, described as sensori-neural (Northern & Downs, 1991).

An audiologist determines that a hearing loss is sensori-neural as opposed to conductive if an audiogram shows that the sound reaches the cochlea, through the outer and middle ear, but is not sent to the brain for processing, because either the cochlea or cranial nerve VIII is damaged. This situ-

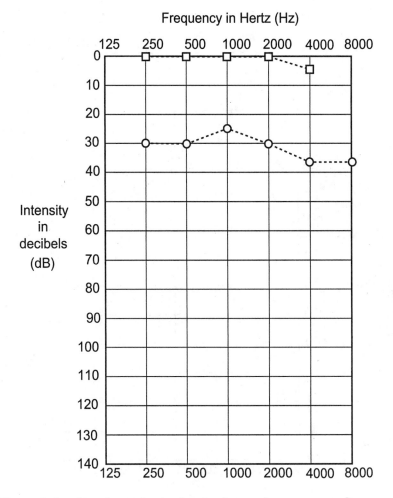

Figure 2-2. Sample conductive hearing loss as shown on an audiogram. Air conduction is reduced; bone conduction is near normal.

ation is determined to be the case if an audiogram shows that the air and bone conduction thresholds are reduced but at nearly the same level (see Figure 2–3).

Sensori-neural hearing loss may be the result of a number of different factors. Metabolic disease, bacterial or viral infection causing high fever, chromosomal disorders, and familial inheritance are a few etiologies. Sensori-neural hearing loss is nearly always irreversible (Northern & Downs, 1991).

Mixed hearing loss occurs when conductive and sensori-neural hearing losses are both present in the same individual. That is, the air conduction pathway is blocked by any of the obstructions mentioned, and either the cochlea

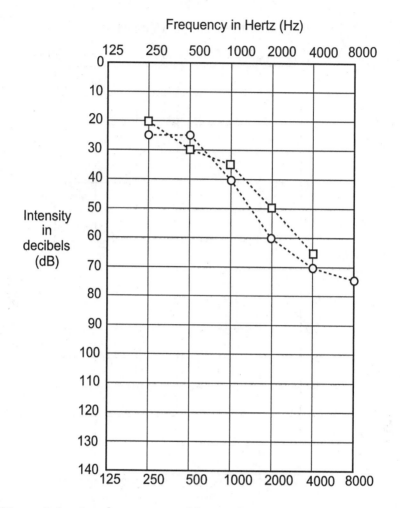

Figure 2-3.   Sample sensorineural hearing loss as shown on an audiogram. Air and bone conduction are reduced.

or the auditory nerve is also damaged. A mixed hearing loss is diagnosed by an audiologist if an audiogram indicates that neither air conduction nor bone conduction are within normal limits, bone conduction is closer to normal than air conduction, and a significant gap exists between air and bone conduction thresholds (Figure 2–4).

Causes of Reduced Hearing.   Hearing loss may be the result of a number of factors. Five common etiologies are discussed in this chapter. They are otitis media, prenatal factors, acquired disease, genetic disorders, and chromosomal disorders.

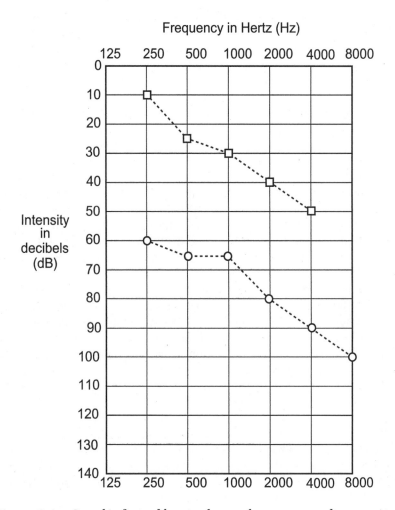

Figure 2-4.   Sample of mixed hearing loss as shown on an audiogram. Air and bone conduction are reduced; bone conduction is closer to normal limits.

Otitis media is an inflammation of the middle ear (Figure 1–7) and is nearly always due to poor eustachian tube function. The consequence is fluid in the middle ear that prevents the normal movement of the ossicular chain (malleus, incus, and stapes) (Figure 1–7) and results in some degree of conductive hearing loss (Northern & Downs, 1991).

Otitis media is the most common childhood illness and one of the most frequent reasons for a young child to need medical attention (Northern & Downs, 1991). Regarding the incidence of otitis media, it has been estimated that (1) on any given day, up to 30 percent of all children across the nation suffer from an ear infection, (2) before the age of six, a full 90 percent of the children in the United States have had at least one ear infection, (3) 50 percent of the children who experience a middle ear problem in the first year of life experience at least six more episodes before the third birthday, and (4) nearly 20 percent of all children who suffer with ear infections require surgery to correct the condition (Grundfast & Carney, 1987).

During an episode of otitis media, a child is likely to experience a hearing reduction of 20 to 30 dB in the affected ear (Fria, Cantekin, & Eichler, 1985). Hence, it is apparent that an inconsistent conductive mild-to-moderate hearing loss may be an etiological factor for children who have a history of chronic otitis media concomitant to language disorder. (Although some researchers disagree, there is data to suggest that recurring episodes of otitis media may have a potentially detrimental effect on speech and language development [Menyuk, 1986].) If this deleterious effect does indeed occur, it is probably because of the confusions caused by inconsistencies in the linguistic information that the child receives as a result of fluctuations in hearing sensitivity.

The most common of the prenatal diseases that is apt to cause severe-to-profound hearing loss is maternal rubella, a condition that is also potentially apt to result in visual handicap as well as mental retardation (Gerber, 1991). Maternal syphilis is a less common disease which, if it does not result in death of the infant, is likely to result in sensori-neural hearing loss, mental retardation, blindness, psychosis, skeletal anomalies, and abnormal teeth (Gerber, 1991). Apparently, these diseases interfere with the embryonic and fetal development of the ear, as well as other structures.

Meningitis, particularly the *diplococcus pneumoniae* type, is an acquired disease that is likely to result in severe-to-profound hearing loss. In years past, measles and mumps were also common etiological factors causing hearing loss in childhood. However, most children are now vaccinated against measles and mumps, thus minimizing their potentially damaging effects (Gerber, 1991). Theoretically, any disease that results in an excessively high fever for an extended period of time places a child at risk for hearing sensitivity reduction and a number of other potentially handicapping conditions (Northern & Downs, 1991).

Certain disorders of genetic origin may result in severe or profound hearing loss (Gerber, 1991). When we say that a condition is of genetic origin, we mean that the condition is inherited. The condition is transmitted through the individual's gene structure, and it may or may not appear congenitally (at birth). Severe or profound hearing loss can be inherited by either recessive or dominant factors.

It has been estimated that there are 5 to 10 gene locations for recessive hearing reduction. For the condition to be inherited recessively, both parents must carry the **recessive gene**. If both carry and pass along the concealed trait at different gene locations, there is a 25 percent chance that hearing reduction will occur in an offspring. If both parents carry and pass along the trait at the same gene location, then there is a 100 percent chance that each offspring will inherit reduced hearing sensitivity (Carrel, 1977). With recessive hearing reduction, it is not necessary for either parent to have reduced hearing in order for the child to inherit the condition, but both parents must carry the concealed recessive trait.

When reduced hearing is inherited by a **dominant gene type**, it is necessary for at least one parent to have reduced hearing in order for a child to inherit the condition. Dominant hearing reduction is inherited directly. If only one parent has the trait, and it is the result of one dominant gene, there is a 50 percent chance that a child will inherit reduced hearing sensitivity. If one parent has reduced hearing due to two dominant genes, there is a 100 percent chance that the offspring will inherit the trait, regardless of the condition of the other parent. If both parents have reduced hearing due to each having one gene for dominant hearing loss, there is a 75 percent chance of producing offspring with reduced hearing sensitivity.

Usher's syndrome is an example of hereditary deafness. Individuals who have it have both reduced hearing sensitivity and retinitis pigmentosa, a progressively degenerative condition of the eyes that leads to reduced visual field and blindness. The condition can be devastating because the person who has it faces a future of profound sensory deprivation. Counseling support services are critical to the successful management of individuals with Usher syndrome.

Some chromosomal disorders may also result in reduced hearing sensitivity. In both Trisomy 13 (Patau syndrome) and Trisomy 18 (Edwards syndrome), which were briefly addressed in the section on cognitive limitations, reduced hearing is a probable consequence, along with mental retardation and brief life expectancy. Children with both types of chromosomal disorders often are multiply handicapped and do not survive. If they do survive, communication management is a complicated venture.

Individuals with Turner syndrome often present with conductive, sensorineural, or mixed hearing loss. Turner syndrome (also called 45X0) is a relatively common syndrome in which chromosomal analysis shows that the individual has only a single X sex chromosome and lacks the second sex chromosome (X or Y), which generally determines the gender of the person. People with Turner syndrome are always female (as determined by the absence of a Y chromosome), and they are described as having reduced angle of the elbow, webbing of the neck, short stature, and sexual infantilism. Reduced hearing sensitivity is common. Intelligence is within normal limits. Additionally, patients are at risk for recurrent otitis media (Gerber, 1991).

When reduced hearing occurs secondary to Turner syndrome, early diagnosis and intervention are critical. Turner syndrome patients generally have normal verbal and intellectual abilities, so they are likely to benefit from amplification and training (Gerber, 1991). Those who suffer from recurrent otitis media are also likely to benefit from medical intervention.

Klinefelter syndrome (XXY) is another disorder of chromosome number that can result in reduced hearing sensitivity (Gerber, 1991). In all cases of

Klinefelter syndrome, the individual's chromosomal pattern include one Y sex chromosome and multiple X sex chromosomes. Patients with the disorder are always male (as determined by the presence of the Y chromosome). They typically have progressive mental retardation, about 20 percent have progressive hearing loss, and as many as 75 percent have language delay and phonological process disorder.

Klinefelter patients are likely to benefit from speech-language intervention. The treatment plan takes into account the exact nature of the language disorder, phonological disorder, and hearing sensitivity level.

Central Auditory Dysfunction.   Central auditory dysfunction is a type of reduced auditory input that is not necessarily characterized by a reduction in hearing sensitivity but instead by decreased ability to perceive and process auditory information. Under these circumstances, although spoken language may be heard, it is not recognized or interpreted accurately. This phenomenon is believed to be the result either of a breakdown at the level of the central nervous system (Northern & Downs, 1991), or of interference with the brain's ability to process auditory information (Boone & Plante, 1993).

One should always suspect central auditory dysfunction if a child behaves as if hearing is reduced yet has a normal audiogram. Further, as with any child for whom reduced hearing is suspected, always refer the child to an audiologist or ear, nose, and throat specialist for in-depth testing and a diagnosis.

Auditory-processing problems are often associated with language acquisition difficulties. For example, a child with a central auditory-processing problem is likely to develop language according to normal expectations for the first few years of life and then experience a sudden loss of language after that time. The language difficulties first manifest themselves in spoken-language reception. The child may begin to behave as if spoken language is not even heard, and subsequently, the development of expressive language begins to falter. Eventually the condition leads to disturbed receptive and expressive language development as well as long-term academic difficulties. The sudden change in performance is generally confined to language development, leaving motor and cognitive domains relatively intact (Boone & Plante, 1993).

Although associated with language-learning problems, it is not reasonable to assume that central auditory dysfunction is an undisputed cause of language disorder. Some researchers have suggested that instead, language-processing problems result in poor performance on auditory-processing tests (Rees, 1981). Others have argued that central auditory dysfunction is the causal factor when associated with language disorder, as normal language acquisition depends on normal auditory-processing skill (Elliot, Hammer, & School, 1989). Still others have shown evidence that central auditory-processing disorder may occur in the absence of any functional disorder of language acquisition (Ludlow, Cudahy, Bassich, & Brown, 1983), casting doubt on the existence of any relationship at all. Therefore, the evidence does not point clearly to problems with central auditory processing as a cause of language disorders, although the two frequently occur concomitantly. Further, the etiology of central auditory processing disorder remains undetermined.

Motor Skills Deficits

Motor skills deficits are likely to have a deleterious effect on certain specific aspects of language form—specifically, phonology, prosody, and some vocal characteristics. Deficits in motor skills do not directly affect the content and use of language, nor the morphological and syntactic aspects of language form.

However, depending on the severity of the disorder, the presence of a motor skills deficit may limit one's opportunities to practice expressive language skills and interact socially with others. Since these two activities are necessary for typical language acquisition, the limitations imposed by the motor skills deficit may indirectly have an adverse effect on the acquisition of all aspects of language.

Further, motor skills deficits result particularly from some degree of neurological involvement. Therefore, they are frequently accompanied by additional neurological disorders associated with the same or a coexisting neurological lesion. Some neurological disorders that may appear concomitant to motor skills deficit are mental retardation, behavioral disorders, and epilepsy. If mental retardation or a behavioral disorder accompany the motor skills deficit, then the direct and indirect limitations imposed by the disorder are complicated by the likelihood of coincidental language disorder.

Two motor skills deficits are addressed in this chapter. They are developmental **apraxia of speech** and the developmental **dysarthrias**.

Developmental Apraxia of Speech.   When apraxia of speech occurs in childhood, it is called developmental apraxia of speech (DAS) (Air, Wood, & Neils, 1989). By definition, apraxia of speech is a sensori-motor speech disorder that impairs one's ability to voluntarily produce phonemes and words (Darley, Aronson, & Brown, 1975). The effect that this has on speech is that the person may struggle in an attempt to produce speech-sound sequences. The struggle may be accompanied by audible or inaudible groping as the person attempts to find the desired combination of articulatory postures. Further, the manifestation of speech difficulty increases with increasing length and complexity of the utterances.

For children, certain characteristic speech behaviors are found to be typical of DAS (Aram & Glasson, 1979). They are (1) high incidence of accompanying oral apraxia (i.e., struggling and groping for volitional, nonspeech, oral movements), (2) marked struggle and groping when attempting to imitate oral or speech movements, (3) phoneme substitutions and distortions that cross over more than one distinctive feature (e.g., [m/s], [t/f]), and (4) more difficulty with multisyllabic words than with monosyllabic words.

Unlike apraxia of speech in adults, the exact cause of DAS is not clear and a precise site of neurological lesion is not typically identifiable. Patients may show "soft" signs indicating subtle neurological involvement. Soft signs include difficulty with fine motor skills or coordination. However, formal laboratory tests, such as computerized tomography (CT) scans, fail to reveal localized cortical lesions (Darley et al., 1975).

Linguistically, receptive skills are often normal while expressive language abilities are seriously delayed. Some children with DAS are unintelligible or even unable to speak. We may not assume that expressive language difficulties are secondary to the motor-programming limitations because in cases in which DAS begins to resolve in affected children, a concomitant expressive language disorder is sometimes identified (Air et al., 1989).

Evidence suggests that the apparent neurological breakdown that causes difficulties with selecting and sequencing phonemes may also cause difficulties with selecting and sequencing morphological and syntactic units as well. Some language disturbances accompanied by DAS are subtle and, in fact, do not emerge until the later elementary school years (Aram & Glasson, 1979). Further, the incidence of learning disabilities may be somewhat higher than average among children with DAS (Yoss & Darley, 1974).

Developmental Dysarthrias.   Manifestation of a developmental dysarthria is one of the primary speech characteristics of children with cerebral palsy, a population that frequently displays a number of coexisting motor, intellectual, and language difficulties as well. Here we concern ourselves only with the dysarthric aspect of cerebral palsy, in keeping with the topic of this section. Intellectual and language difficulties resulting from brain injury are discussed elsewhere in the chapter.

The dysarthrias are a heterogeneous group of communication disorders. They generally result in difficulties with coordinating and performing acts of respiration, phonation, articulation, resonance, and prosody. The severity and exact nature of the symptom complex depends on the location and extent of lesion. Individuals may experience difficulties so serious that they are unable to speak, or they may have a mild disorder with only a few insignificant differences in speech production. Three types of dysarthria are typically seen in children with cerebral palsy. They are dysarthrias of the spastic, athetoid, and ataxic types (Hegde, 1991).

Spastic Dysarthria.   Spastic dysarthria results from injury to the pyramidal motor pathways, which are the cortical centers of motor control. In spastic dysarthria, the muscles seem to be stiff and rigid, probably because muscle groups that normally work cooperatively work in opposition to one another.

As a result, the speech movements made by the person with spastic dysarthria are abrupt, jerky, rigid, slow, and labored. Each of these features is likely to have a detrimental effect on respiration for speech, voice production, ability to coordinate and complete articulatory movements, accomplishing velopharyngeal closure for coordinating oral and nasal resonance, and the production of speech that is prosodically meaningful and typical of the person's native language. Spastic symptoms are seen in approximately 60 percent of the children with cerebral palsy.

Athetoid Dysarthria. Athetosis is caused by an injury to the extrapyramidal motor pathways, particularly the basal ganglia. The lesion is not in the cerebral cortex but in the brainstem (Figure 1–12). The basal ganglia assist the cortex in planning physical movements by way of screening and modifying the impulses that are sent from the cortex to the muscle groups. When the basal ganglia are damaged, the cortical impulses reach the muscle groups without appropriate modification. This results in intentional movements accompanied by involuntary movements that are slow, writhing, and wormlike in nature and occur whenever the individual with athetosis attempts to move a muscle group.

Involuntary, athetoid movements interfere with speech production if certain muscle groups are involved. All aspects of speech production, including respiration, voice production, oral-nasal resonance, articulation, and prosody, may be affected by the slow, writhing movements of athetosis.

Ataxic Dysarthria. Ataxia is the result of injury to the cerebellum (Figure 1–12), which is the neurological organ that assists in balancing and coordinating the movements of all muscle groups. When the cerebellum is damaged, muscle coordination is impaired. Generally with ataxia, the person's movements are clumsy, awkward, and uncoordinated. Further, muscle weakness may be a symptom of ataxia.

All muscle groups responsible for coordinating speech production are potentially involved. Therefore, awkwardness may be noted in the movements required for respiration, phonation, oral-nasal resonance, articulation, and prosodic variation.

Deficient Social Relations

Language is a social phenomena, and it develops naturally in the context of social relations. Young children learn to use language for a number of social reasons. For example, language is a method for successfully communicating one's needs and desires to those who are able to satisfy them. Language is also a means for sharing ideas and learning the ideas of others, and can be used in initiating and developing social relationships. Further, language is one vehicle by which we learn to understand the people, things, and events that we encounter in the world around us.

Within the first year of life, most children begin to interface language stimulation and language learning with social events, and thus they discover how handy language is for accomplishing a variety of social and communicative purposes. Few individuals appear to miss the important connection between language and human relations. Children with elective mutism and autism are two examples of those who do.

Elective Mutism.   A child is considered to be electively mute if he or she is capable of speaking and yet consistently chooses not to speak in at least one frequently encountered social situation. The disorder usually begins between the ages of three and five years (Shvartzman et al., 1990). The electively mute child is *not* the shy child who hides behind his or her mother when introduced to new people or is reluctant to talk when encountering unfamiliar situations. This is the child who can, but consistently does *not*, talk whenever encountering a particular situation, regardless of the level of comfort and familiarity with the people and surroundings associated with the context.

Some electively mute children have only one situation that that causes them to manifest voluntary silence, such as home or school. However, others choose to remain silent the majority of the time, electing to speak only on rare occasions.

Such children may view silence as the most effective means for accomplishing a number of communication objectives. For some reason, the child may have learned that a need or desire is more apt to be met (even to excess) if caretakers are uncertain about its exact nature. For that reason, it may be to the child's perceived advantage to communicate only the fact that a need exists and to do this through a nonverbal strategy (e.g., crying, whining, throwing toys, standing near an item that contains many options for the caretaker to choose, such as the refrigerator or an out-of-reach toy shelf). By so doing, the child prompts the caretaker to try to guess the need or desire and to offer a number of options, some of which are far beyond the immediate need.

For example, if a child wants ice cream and indicates to the caretaker by means of crying and gesturing that a need exists, the sensitive caretaker is likely to make every attempt to identify the cause of crying. If the child does not directly request the ice cream, by the time the crying is discontinued he or she may have successfully accumulated a number of tasty treats, such as cookies, candy, Popsicles, and the like, in addition to the ice cream. This nonverbal routine may be found to be an especially effective method for a number of indulgences, including the appropriation of affection, activities, and toys and the satisfaction of needs and desires.

However, the motivation behind this pattern is not readily apparent. It may be that the child begins to use this nonverbal routine because language abilities are so low that it is the only viable communication option. Some may begin to use the nonverbal routine because they are embarrassed by a coexisting langauge difference or communication disorder. Traumatic experiences precipitate the disorder in a number of children, while a few may use the routine because, although they are able to speak clearly, they seem to prefer the outcome of the guessing game created by their silence.

Regarding language dimensions, elective mutism appears to be a disorder of language use that is either the result of, or has a significant impact on, generalized difficulties with language content and form. The language use aspect of the disorder is readily apparent because the child chooses not to use spoken language for either communication or social interaction. The degree to which the other dimensions are affected may be masked by the disorder itself. Moreover, the effect may be the result of lack of practice with spoken communication or may be attributable to some condition unrelated to the elective mutism.

Coexisting communication disorders are common with electively mute children, indicating that when the behavior is first initiated it may be an attempt to hide inadequate communication skills or an attempt to find some method for successful communication. However, when elective mutism becomes a habit, this may be because experience proves to the child that silence is more effective than spoken communication.

Autism.   When a child has autism, one should expect to observe significant impairments in reciprocal social interaction affecting both verbal and nonverbal communication (Ruter, 1983). The autistic child can be identified by four cardinal features. They are: (1) severe language comprehension deficit, (2) a notable preference for being alone, (3) stereotypical behaviors (e.g., hand flapping, rocking, spinning), and (4) remarkable ability in one area that does not coincide with overall ability or achievement (e.g., unusual command of mathematics, puzzles, memory, or visual-motor skills).

The communication impairment of autism is not an impairment of spoken-language production but an impairment in the social aspects of communication. In fact, autistic children do not generally use speech and language for the purpose of communication. Instead, autistic utterances have been described as "self-sufficient," "semantically and conversationally valueless," and consisting of "grossly distorted memory exercises" (Kanner, 1943).

No definite cause of autism has been determined (Fay & Schuler, 1980). Many years ago, it was believed and taught that autism was caused by parents who neglected to provide a caring, communicative environment for their child (Kanner & Eisenberg, 1955). Since that time, however, the "social deprivation" theory has lost credence and a number of alternative explanations have been suggested (Boone & Plante, 1993).

A series of studies provide sufficient indication of a probable neurological explanation for autism. A relatively clear pattern of abnormal brain development is apparent in autistic individuals (Brown, 1978; Courchesne, Yeung-Courchnese, Press, Hesselink, & Jernigan, 1988; Rimland, 1964). Further, the high incidence of autism among children with fra X (discussed previously in this chapter) may indicate a genetic etiology (Wolf-Schein et al., 1987).

Even though the cause of autism is probably neurological or genetic, and not social, the symptoms of autism continue to implicate a pattern of abnormal social development. For example, with regard to attention paid to social stimuli, children with autism are delayed or abnormal (Dawson & Lewy, 1989). Social eyegaze is atypical (Dawson, Hill, Spencer, Galpert, & Watson, 1990), motor imitation is delayed or aberrant (Curcio, 1978), the ability to establish and maintain joint attention is delayed or abnormal (Wetherby & Prutting, 1984), and the ability to communicate affectively is disturbed (Dawson et al., 1990). By way of contrast, children with autism display normal or superior skills in the development of nonsocial prerequisites to language learning (Klinger & Dawson, 1992), such as acquisition of the Piagetan concept of object permanence (Dawson & Adams, 1984) and of early categorization skills (Ungerer & Sigman, 1987). This pattern indicates that the neurogenic problem of autism that generally leads to language impairment is a problem with the language of human interaction and not a predicament with language in general.

With regard to language development, autistic children acquire language later and much more slowly than their peers. Initially, hearing loss may be suspected because autistic children may not respond to speech and human voices. However, hearing loss usually is ruled out early in the diagnostic process as autistic children generally respond to mechanical and other nonverbal sounds.

Once expressive language development begins, all dimensions of language and the way in which they interrelate are affected by autism. Language form, content, and use are all disrupted. The three dimensions do not interact well, and a separation exists between form, content, and use.

Regarding language form, telegraphic speech is common, with omissions of function words and grammatical morphemes. Word order may also be somewhat irregular (Hegde, 1991). Regarding language content, words referring to objects are learned more frequently than words referring to people, words expressing emotion are extremely difficult to learn, and the meanings of words may only be understood and used in a limited number of contexts. Pronoun reversal is also common with autistic children (Hegde, 1991), such that *I*, *me*, *my*, and *mine* are confused with *you*, *your*, and *yours*. Regarding language use, words are not necessarily used for the purpose of communication or social exchange (Hegde, 1991). Instead, one may hear an autistic child talking to him- or herself. Self-absorbed recitations and wordplay are some typical autistic language activities.

Language form, content, and use do not interact well for autistic children. This is evidenced by the contradictions that exist between the meaning of the message, the way in which the message is delivered, and the form that is used to carry the message. In other words, the ideas expressed are often inconsistent with actions, and comments are often inconsistent with the context or situation. The example of poor dimensional interaction at the beginning of this chapter may very well have been spoken by a child with autism. Recall that the child said, "Don't spank the baby. Be nice to the baby," while at the same time the child was hitting a doll.

Form, content, and use are also frequently separated for autistic language. This pattern is exemplified by echolalia, perseveration, repeated repetitions of phrases and sentences heard or used in an earlier context, and long recitations of announcements that have been heard with some regularity on the radio or television.

The prognosis for an autistic child benefiting from communication intervention is *not* particularly encouraging (Boone & Plante, 1993). An intervention program requires that the idiosyncratic behaviors of the child be identified and addressed, with periodic re-evaluations to determine whether continued treatment is ethically justified by the benefits to the client.

Lack of Linguistic Opportunity in the Environment

Since typically the linguistic environments of language-disordered children are *not* significantly different from the environments of their peers, there is little evidence to support the supposition that language disorders may be caused by environmental deprivation (Lahey, 1988). However, for certain children, difficulty with language acquisition may result from reduced or abnormal linguistic input, lack of proper reinforcement for communication efforts, and difficulties with the affective relationship established between the child and primary caretaker.

Extreme cases of social deprivation have been described (e.g., Itard's wild boy), and they demonstrate that in the absence of social and environmental opportunities, language learning, among other things, will suffer. Since complete lack of social stimulation is a rare occurrence, such children are not addressed specifically in this chapter.

Further, early intervention programs have been established throughout the nation based on the assumption that some children lack the environmental stimulation necessary for language learning and other preacademic skills. However, it may be speculated that this assumption is based on certain cultural expectations in the classroom and not on a true lack of socialization or environmental stimulation in the home environment. Therefore, this group of children is also not discussed in this chapter.

Twins and multiple births, however, present a very practical example of language development under unusual environmental conditions (Tomasello, Manle, & Kruger, 1986). In twins, environmental resources are compromised from the time of conception, and it is likely that the language problems often experienced by twins are the result of certain reductions in the linguistic opportunities that are available to them. Therefore, for the purposes of this chapter, the group that is chosen to represent those with reduced linguistic opportunity is twins and multiple births.

Twins and Multiple Births.   When two or more babies are born to the same mother at the same time, language disorder is common (Day, 1932), but not inevitable (McCormick & Dewart, 1986). In some cases, the difficulties with language acquisition can be attributed to physical cause such as brain injury or craniofacial anomaly. However, the incidence of physical cause does not fully account for the incidence of language disorder in this special population, and a number of unique environmental factors common to multiple births and twins are sometimes given at least partial credit (Bornstein & Ruddy, 1984). For example, nonsingletons begin to share their environmental resources even prenatally, such that two-thirds of monozygotic (i.e., identical) twins even share the same placenta. This pattern of sharing all resources with a same-age sibling continues throughout childhood for most nonsingleton children.

A few perinatal experiences present nonsingleton children with medical hazards not usually faced by singleton children. Perinatally, more nonsingletons present with breech delivery than do singletons, and all but the first-born face a greater risk at delivery because of having to wait in line to exit the womb. In multiple births, birth tends to take place after a shorter gestation period and the babies weigh in at a lower birth weight than do their singleton peers (Mogford, 1988). The resulting increased perinatal medical risks lead to increased risks for postnatal health problems, developmental difficulties, and communication disorders. Then, the **neonatal** period is often rife with medical and health concerns. However, more nonsingleton children experience difficulty with language development than can be explained by the physical risk factors.

Beyond the neonatal period, a pattern of environmental factors typically develops (Tomasello et al., 1986), and is suspect as a potential cause for language disorder in multiple births. Although prenatal and perinatal risks may pose a threat to the child's life and overall development, it may be that once a child is out of physical danger it is the postnatal risks that most threaten language development (Lytton, 1980).

For example, a minor environmental concern may be that the simultaneous arrival of more than one child substantially increases the family size rather quickly and therefore is likely to strain the financial resources available to the family for child rearing. This may place the children at a disadvantage for social and educational opportunity (Mogford, 1988).

Of greater concern is the possibility of reduced opportunities for verbal communicative interaction with adults as a result of two interacting variables (Mogford, 1988). First, the coexistence of more than one infant in the family creates a social situation in which the children become dependent on each other and develop a very close sibling relationship (Biale, 1989). They communicate with one another, play with one another, and stimulate one another, reducing the need for adult communication and social interaction.

Second, the adult caretaker has a group of babies to tend and no more time or energy than mothers of singleton infants (Biale, 1989). For that reason, maternal bonding may suffer (Ahern, 1990) and adult time and attention may be somewhat compromised (Mogford, 1988). This is likely to explain why it has been found that the mothers of twins are more apt to speak to their children in directives as opposed to comments and questions, a communication style that is associated with slower linguistic development (Tomasello et al., 1986). Further, it may explain why mothers of twins give fewer replies that serve to encourage the child's conversational topic as compared to mothers of singleton children (Tomasello et al., 1986).

To complicate this second factor, language facilitation activities of the primary caretaker (as described in Chapter 1) may be somewhat jeopardized. For example, when a mother of a singleton infant interacts with her baby, it is most often in the setting of a communication **dyad**. Only two people are involved, so social communication is relatively simple. In the case of twins, however, the mother and children develop their social communicative relationships in the context of a **triad**, a situation that is far more complex (Biale, 1989). Further, the complexity of the task increases when more infants needing care and socialization are added to the situation, as in triplets, quadruplets, and larger multiple births.

The dyad situation allows a mother to adapt all dimensions of language to the needs of her individual child, speaking directly to the child (facilitating language use), speaking about whatever the child is looking at or doing (facilitating language content) (Tomasello et al., 1986), and using simplified language for the benefit of the child (facilitating language content-form). In contrast, the triad (and quadrad, etc.) does not lend itself so easily to this pattern of language stimulation and, therefore, the caretaker's language facilitation opportunities may be somewhat compromised.

For example, one can only speak directly to one person at a time, so experiences with communication directed at the individual child may be cut approximately in half for twins, and even more drastically for greater numbers of children. Further, unless two or more children are looking at or doing the same thing, one is able to talk directly about what holds the child's interest to only one child at a time. Again, at a rate approximately proportionate to the number of children, this state of affairs decreases the amount of experience that a child has with language pertaining to an immediate interest.

The language of nonsingletons is often difficult to understand, even though many such children appear to communicate well with each other. Therefore, it has been postulated that some nonsingleton children develop a private language (Luria & Yudovich, 1959; Malmstrom & Silva, 1986). **Cryptophasia**, **idioglossia**, and **twin talk** are terms used to label the apparent phenomena. However, whether twins and other nonsingletons actually use a private language is yet to be proven (Savic & Jocic, 1975). If, in fact, they do, the phenomenon is definitely a nonenvironmental, social factor that has the potential to interfere with normal language development.

By way of disagreement with the supposition of cryptophasia, it appears that a number of the **neologisms** (unique "words") that twins generate are onomatopoeically, phonologically, or semantically motivated. That is, the words either sound like the object being named, represent persistence of a phonological pattern, or describe the concept without actually using the standard word form. For example, a set of twins was observed to consistently represent the word "horse" by saying "[iha]," "water" by alternating "[b]" and "[l]," and "airplane" by producing a low-frequency bilabial raspberry. These are all examples of onomatopoeically motivated neologisms.

Since many singleton children also create neologisms that are onomatopoeically, phonologically, or semantically motivated, it is difficult to establish the use of cryptophasia based on neologistic production alone. Neologisms are used by many young children, and they do not necessarily indicate the use of a private language. As an example of one singleton child, in her second and third years, my daughter remarked that she had "a schnoozer" (onomatopoeic) whenever she needed to blow her nose, always said "[kɛpətʃ]" for "catsup" (phonological metathesis), and consistently referred to any time that had already passed as "yesterschmorning" (semantic). She also made up names for pretend foods (e.g., "bigeetahs" and "pickahnses") and unfamiliar concepts (e.g., "chiff" for "beard").

In further dispute of the theory of cryptophasia, personal experience has been that when twins are said to use cryptophasia when conversing with one another, the phenomenon that parents identify as such is the combining of long strings of unintelligible syllables when the twins are socially engaged with each other. The twins observed have been 2-year-olds who, if using their parent's language, would presumably have created sentences of maybe five to eight morphemes. It is unlikely that these children, who have had no exposure to a linguistic model demonstrating their private language, are able to create and use a linguistic system that is more complicated than the one used by their same-age peers who pattern their sentences after the language of their parents. A more likely conjecture is that for this population, a social form of variegated babbling persists beyond the middle of the second year. If, in fact, twin language does occur, it may interfere with the development of the standard language, but so far, the evidence has not emerged to either definitively support or disprove the theory. Therefore, further research on the topic is needed.

Reduced intelligence has also been reported by those who have studied twins. If verified, this could possibly be considered as a nonenvironmental factor contributing to language disorder. However, since verbal intelligence scores are low for twins while performance scores are *not*, it is probable that the reduced intelligence scores are an artifact of reduced language performance and not due to some cognitive limitation commonly present in the group. Reduced intelligence is not a reasonable explanation for language delay in twins (Zazzo, 1978). Reduced experience with dyadic interchange and compromised direct maternal attention are factors that are more likely to explain the developmental lags in both the language and cognitive domains (Bornstein & Ruddy, 1984).

CONCLUDING REMARKS

This chapter identifies the domain of language disorders with regard to a number of specific populations that typically experience difficulty with the acquisition of spoken language. Etiological factors, general symptoms, language symptoms, and impact on development of the language dimensions are included. In the two chapters that immediately follow, you will read about some general techniques that can be used to assess and treat the language-disordered individuals encountered by professionals practicing in the mainstream of the field of speech-language pathology.

REFERENCES

Ahern, C. K. (1990). My Greatest Surprise? It's twins? *Twin Magazine,* Jan.-Feb. 28.

Air, D. H., Wood, A. S., & Neils, J. R. (1989). Considerations for organic disorders. In N. A. Creaghead, P. W. Newman, & W. A. Secord (Eds.), *Assessment and remediation of articulatory and phonological disorders.* Columbus, OH: Merrill.

Aram, D. M., Ekelman, B. L., Rose, D. F., & Whitaker, H. A. (1985). Verbal and cognitive sequelae following unilateral lesions acquired in early childhood. *Journal of Clinical and Experimental Neuropsychology, 7,* 55–78.

Aram, D. M., & Glasson, C. (1979). Developmental apraxia of speech. Miniseminar presented at the annual convention of the American Speech-Language-Hearing Association, Atlanta, GA.

Biale, R. (1989). Twins have unique development aspects. *Brown University Child Behavior and Development Letter, 5*(6), 1–3.

Boone, D. R., & Plante, E. (1993). *Human communication and its disorders.* Englewood Cliffs, NJ: Prentice-Hall.

Bornstein, M. H., & Ruddy, M. G. (1984). Infant attention and maternal stimulation: Prediction of cognitive and linguistic development in twins. In H. Bouma & G. Bouwhuis (Eds.), *Attention and human performance X: Control of language processes: Proceedings of the 10th international symposium on attention and performance.* London: Erlbaum.

Brown, J. L. (1978). Long-term follow-up of 100 "atypical" children of normal intelligence. In M. Rutter & E. Schopler (Eds.), *Autism: A reappraisal of concepts and treatment.* New York: Plenum Press.

Carmi, R., Meryash, D. L., Wood, J., & Gerald, P. S. (1984). Fragile-X syndrome ascertained by the presence of macro-orchidism in a 5-month-old infant. *Journal of Pediatrics, 74,* 883–86.

Carrel, R. E. (1977). Epidemiology of hearing loss. In S. E. Gerber (Ed.), *Audiometry in infancy.* New York: Grune & Stratton.

Courchesne, E., Yeung-Courchesne, R., Press, G., Hesselink, J. R., & Jernigan, T. L. (1988). Hypoplasia of the cerebellar verbal lobes VI and VII in infantile autism. *New England Journal of Medicine, 318,* 1349–54.

Cranberg, L. D., Filley, C. M., Hart, E. J., & Alexander, M. P. (1987). Acquired aphasia in childhood: Clinical and CT investigations. *Neurology, 37,* 1165–72.

Curcio, F. (1978). Sensorimotor functioning and communication in mute autistic children. *Journal of Autism and Childhood Schizophrenia, 8,* 281-292.

Darley, F., Aronson, A., & Brown, J. (1975). *Motor speech disorders*. Philadelphia: Saunders.

Dawson, G., & Adams, A. (1984). Imitation and social responsiveness in autistic children. *Journal of Abnormal Child Psychology, 12*, 209–26.

Dawson, G., Hill, D., Spencer, A., Galpert, L., & Watson, L (1990). Affective exchanges between young autistic children and their mothers. *Journal of Abnormal Child Psychology, 18*, 335–45.

Dawson, G., & Lewy, A. (1989). Arousal, attention, and the socioemotional impairments of individuals with autism. In G. Dawson (Ed.), *Autism: Nature, diagnosis and treatment*. New York: Guilford Press.

Day, E. J., (1932). The development of language in twins. *Child Development, 3*, 298–316.

Elliot, L. L., Hammer, M. A., & School, M. E. (1989). Fine-grained auditory discrimination in normal children and children with language-learning problems. *Journal of Speech and Hearing Research, 32*, 112–19.

Fay, W., & Schuler, A. (1980). *Emerging language in autistic children*. Baltimore, MD: University Park Press.

Fey, M. E. (1986). *Language intervention with young children*. Austin, TX: Pro-Ed.

Fria, T. J., Cantekin, E. I., & Eichler, J. A. (1985). Hearing acuity of children with otitis media with effusion. *Otolaryngology Head Neck Surgery, 111*, 10–16.

Gerber, S. E. (1991). *Prevention: The etiology of communicative disorders in children*. Englewood Cliffs, NJ: Prentice-Hall.

Grundfast, K., & Carney, C. J. (1987). *Ear infections in your child*. Hollywood, FL: Compact Books.

Hagerman, R. J. (1987). Fragile X syndrome. *Current Problems in Pediatrics, 25*, 621–74.

Hammill, D., Leigh, J. E., McNutt, G., & Larsen, S. C. (1981). A new definition of learning disabilities. *Learning Disability Quarterly, 4*, 336–42.

Hegde, M. N. (1991). *Introduction to communicative disorders*. Austin, TX: Pro-Ed.

Kahmi, A., & Catts, H. (1986). Toward an understanding of developmental language and reading disorders. *Journal of Speech and Hearing Disorders, 51*, 337–47.

Kaminski, M., Rumeau, C., & Schwartz, D. (1978). Alcohol consumption in pregnant women and the outcome of pregnancy. *Alcoholism: Clinical Experimental Research, 2*, 155–63.

Kanner, L. (1943). Autistic disturbance of affective contact. *Nervous Child, 2*, 217–50.

Kanner, L., & Eisenberg, L. (1955). Notes on the followup studies of autistic children. In P. H. Hoch & J. Zubin (Eds.), *Psychotherapy of childhood*. New York: Grune & Stratton.

Klinger, L. G., & Dawson, G. (1992). Facilitating early social and communicative development in children with autism. In S. F. Warren & J. Reichle

(Eds.), *Causes and effects in communication and language intervention.* Baltimore: Paul H. Brookes.

Lahey, M. (Ed.). (1988). *Language disorders and language development.* New York: Macmillan.

Lees, J., & Urwin, S. (1991). *Children with language disorders.* London: Whurr Publishers.

Ludlow, C. L., Cudahy, E. A., Bassich, C., & Brown, G. L. (1983). Auditory processing skills of hyperactive, language-impaired and reading disabled boys. In J. Katz & E. Lasky (Eds.), *Central auditory processing disorders: Problems of speech, language, and learning.* Baltimore, MD: University Park Press.

Luria, A. R., & Yudovich, F. (1959). *Speech and the development of mental processes in the child.* Harmondsworth, UK: Penguin.

Lytton, H. (1980). *Parent-child interaction: The socialization process observed in twin and singleton families.* New York: Plenum.

McCormick, K., Dewart H. (1986). Three's a crowd: Early language of a set of triplets. In *Proceedings of the Child Language Seminar 1986: Durham University Journal,* Old Shite Hall, Dunham, United Kingdom.

Malmstrom, P. M., & Silva, M. N. (1986). Twin talk: Manifestations of twin status in the speech of toddlers. *Journal of Child Language, 13,* 293–304.

Maxon, A. B., & Brackett, D. (1992). *The hearing-impaired child: Infancy through high school years.* Boston: Andover Medical Publishers.

Menyuk, P. (1986). Predicting speech and language problems with persistent otitis media. In J. Kavanagh (Ed.), *Otitis media and child development.* Parkton, MD: York Press.

Mogford, K. (1988). Language development in twins. In D. Bishop & K. Mogford (Eds.), *Language development in exceptional circumstances.* Edinburgh, UK: Churchill Livingstone.

Myers, E. N., & Stool, S. E. (1968). Cytomegalic inclusion disease of the inner ear. *Laryngoscope, 78,* 1904–14.

Nielson, K. B. (1983). Diagnosis of the fragile X syndrome (Martin-Bell syndrome): Clinical findings in 27 males with the fragile site at Xq28. *Journal of Mental Deficiencies Research, 27,* 211–26.

Northern, H. L., & Downs, M. P. (1991). *Hearing in children.* Baltimore, MD: Williams & Wilkins.

Prutting, C., & Kirchner, D. M. (1987). Pragmatic aspects of language. *Journal of Speech and Hearing Disorders, 52,* 105–19.

Rees, M. S. (1981). Saying more than we know: Is auditory processing disorder a meaningful concept? In R. W. Keith (Ed.), *Central auditory and language disorders in children.* San Diego, CA: College-Hill Press.

Rimland, B. (1964). *Infantile Autism.* New York: Appleton-Century-Crofts.

Rudel, R. (1985). The definition of dyslexia: Language and motor deficits. In F. Duffy & N. Geschwind (Eds.), *Dyslexia: A neuroscientific approach to clinical evaluation.* Boston: Little Brown.

Ruter, M. (1983). Cognitive deficits in the pathogenesis of autism. *Journal of Child Psychology and Psychiatry, 24,* 513–31.

Satz, P., & Bullard-Bates, C. (1981). Acquired aphasia in children. In M. T. Sarno (Ed.), *Acquired aphasia.* New York: Academic Press.

Savic, S., & Jocic, M. (1975). Some features of dialogue between twins. *International Journal of Psycholinguistics, 4,* 34–51.

Scharfenaker, S. K. (1990). The fragile X syndrome. *ASHA, 32,* 45–47.

Sever, J. L. (1983). Maternal infections. In C. C. Brown (Ed.), *Childhood learning disabilities and prenatal risk.* Skillman, NY: Johnson & Johnson Baby Products Co.

Shvarztman, P., Hornshtein, I., Klein, E., Yechezkel, A., Ziv, M., & Herman, J. (1990). Elective mutism in family practice. *Journal of Family Practice, 31,* 319–22.

Sparks, S. M. (1984). *Birth defects and speech-language disorders.* San Diego, CA: College-Hill Press.

Swisher, L. (1985). Language disorders in children. In J. K. Darby (Ed.), *Speech and language evaluation in neurology: Childhood disorders.* Orlando, FL: Grune & Stratton.

Tomasello, M., Mannle, S. & Kruger, A. C. (1986). Linguistic environment of 1- to 2-year-old twins. *Developmental Psychology, 22,* 169–76.

Ungerer, J., & Sigman, M. (1987). Categorization skills and receptive language development in autistic children. *Journal of Autism and Developmental Disorders, 17,* 3–16.

van Dongen, H. R. & Loonen, M. C. B. (1977). Factors related to prognosis of acquired aphasia in children. *Cortex, 13,* 131–36.

Wetherby, A., & Prutting, C. (1984). Profiles in communicative and cognitive-social abilities in autistic children. *Journal of Speech and Hearing Research, 27,* 364–77.

Wolf-Schein, E. G., Sudhalter, V., Cohen, I. L., Fisch, G. S., Hanson, D., Pfadt, A. G., Hagerman, R., Jenkins, E. C., & Brown, W. T. (1987). Speech-language and the fragile X syndrome: Initial findings. *ASHA, 29,* 35–38.

Yoss, A., & Darley, F. L. (1974). Developmental apraxia of speech in children with defective articulation. *Journal of Speech and Hearing Research, 17,* 399–416.

Young, P. (1987). *Drugs and pregnancy.* New York: Chelsea House.

Zazzo, R. (1978). Genesis and peculiarities of the personality of twins. In W. E. Nance, G. Allen, & P. Parisi (Eds.), *Twin research: Progress in clinical and biological research: Psychology and methodology.* New York: Liss.

STUDY GUIDE 2

1. Define the term *language disorder.*

2. Describe the relationship between the following terms. What assumption(s) can be made about each?
   a. language delay
   b. language disability

    c. language impairment
    d. deviant language
    e. specific language disability
    f. specific language impairment

3. Describe each of the following disorder patterns, giving examples of each.
    a. late or slow development of all three language dimensions
    b. disrupted language content
    c. disrupted language form
    d. disrupted interaction between form and content
    e. disrupted language use
    f. disrupted interaction between content, form, and use
    g. separation of content, form, and use

4. Define echolalia and perseveration. Give examples of each.

5. When there is a disparity between language production and language comprehension ability, what is the typical relationship between the two and why is this pattern likely to occur?

6. Define each of the following and describe its potential impact on language development.
    a. cognitive limitation
    b. sensory input reduction
    c. motor skills deficit
    d. deficient social relations
    e. lack of linguistic opportunity in the environment

7. What impact does mental retardation have on language acquisition?

8. Differentiate between mental retardation caused by each of the following.
    a. brain injury
    b. chromosomal disorder
    c. genetic disorder

9. Differentiate between the way in which each of the following occurs.
    a. chromosomal disorder
    b. genetic disorder

10. Give some examples of toxic chemicals that lead to brain injury.

11. Describe each of the following according to cause, symptoms, and speech-language characteristics.
    a. Fetal alcohol syndrome
    b. Fetal alcohol effect
    c. Trisomy 21
    d. *Cri du Chat* syndrome
    e. Fragile X syndrome

12. Define learning disability.

13. How does ability to identify handicapping conditions in general impact our ability to accurately diagnose a learning disability?

14. Compare and contrast learning disability and specific language impairment.

15. How should our knowledge of the relationship between learning disability and specific language impairment impact our treatment of preschool-age children with a language disorder?

16. What symptoms in language disorder may indicate that a preschool-age child is at risk for learning disability?

17. What are the language symptoms of acquired childhood aphasia? How do they relate to intervention?

18. What factors should influence prognostic decisions regarding a child with acquired childhood aphasia?

19. What are the symptoms of attention deficit disorder? Include language symptoms in your answer.

20. Define hearing loss.

21. Explain why the terms *hearing loss* and *reduced hearing* are preferred over *hearing impairment* and *hearing defect*.

22. Differentiate between the four levels of hearing reduction according to criteria for amount of reduced sensitivity, impact on perception and comprehension of spoken language, and impact on production of spoken language.

23. Differentiate between prelingual and adventitious hearing reduction according to the effect on spoken language acquisition.

24. How might an inconsistent reduction in hearing sensitivity impact spoken-language acquisition?

25. What is the speech-language pathologist's concern with the pattern of an audiogram?

26. Explain the phenomena of conductive hearing loss, sensori-neural hearing loss, and mixed hearing loss according to etiology, diagnosis, and clinical implications.

27. How is central auditory dysfunction different from reduced hearing sensitivity?

28. Describe the association between central auditory dysfunction and language disorder.

29. Describe how each of the following may cause reduced hearing sensitivity.
    a. otitis media
    b. prenatal factors
    c. acquired diseases
    d. genetic disorders
    e. chromosomal disorders

30. Describe the direct and indirect impacts that a motor skill deficit may have on language acquisition.

31. What are the characteristics of developmental apraxia of speech?

32. How is developmental apraxia of speech different from apraxia of speech in adults?

34. In a general way, describe each of the developmental dysarthrias. More specifically, how is spoken language affected by each?

35. Differentiate between spastic, athetoid, and ataxic dysarthrias according to the following variables.
    a. site of lesion
    b. symptoms
36. How are social relations related to the process of language acquisition?
37. Define elective mutism.
38. What are some of the common behaviors that distinguish the electively mute child from other children? What may be the explanation for this communication pattern?
39. How does elective mutism effect the three dimensions of language?
40. What is autism?
41. What is the probable cause of autism?
42. Describe the symptoms associated with autism.
43. How does autism affect the three dimensions of language?
44. Describe some of the unusual environmental conditions experienced by twins and other multiple births, beginning with the prenatal experience and including perinatal and postnatal factors.
45. Explain cryptophasia and how it may impact language acquisition. Explain the reasons for concern as to whether this phenomenon actually occurs.
46. Twins, as a group, have reduced language and cognitive abilities. Explain.

PART II

Introduction to Clinical Procedures

CHAPTER 3

An Introduction to Language Assessment

Guidelines for a Traditional
Client-Centered Approach

LEARNING OBJECTIVES

At the conclusion of this chapter, you should be prepared to:

- Discuss guidelines for clinical practice;
- Apply communication screening procedures;
- Apply principles, purposes, and procedures commonly used to guide language assessment;
- Prepare formal language assessment reports.

INTRODUCTION

As an individual who plans to build a career in the field of speech-language pathology, you may anticipate spending many hours of your professional life conducting assessments, so it is important that you take pride in the process of successfully evaluating the communication needs of the clients you serve. Further, the competence that you bring to the assessment process impacts the success of the intervention programs that you recommend and administer. This is because the assessment results become the foundation for all clinical services delivered to individual clients and intervention requires continual assessment of progress and performance.

Language assessment is a clinical service. Therefore, comments on language assessment are preceded by some general guidelines for clinical practice.

GUIDELINES FOR CLINICAL PRACTICE

Basic guidelines for clinical practice include adherence to the American Speech Language-Hearing Association (ASHA) Code of **Ethics**, the ASHA Certificate of Clinical Competence (CCC) as the minimum credential for independent service delivery (as well as state licensure in most states), and the client's right to **confidentiality** in the clinical relationship. These topics are addressed below.

Code of Ethics

As a student who provides clinical services under the direct supervision of a certified speech-language pathologist, you and your supervisor are ethically obliged to know and abide by the ASHA Code of Ethics. (The code is published annually in the March issue of ASHA magazine.) The responsibility to know and abide by the code applies to all individuals who practice speech-language pathology or audiology in the United States.

Since ASHA's Code of Ethics is periodically revised, you are further obligated to alter your professional behavior in order to comply with all changes as they occur throughout the years. Now, if you are a member of the National Student Speech-Language-Hearing Association (NSSLHA) (and later, as a certified member of ASHA) you will be eligible to receive the necessary ASHA publications so that any changes in expectations for professional conduct are readily accessible to you and your colleagues.

The consequences for failure to follow ASHA's Code of Ethics are serious. You and your colleagues are accountable to report any suspected violations to the Ethical Practices Board of ASHA. The board is under obligation to investigate all complaints and remove the CCC from those whose professional behavior fails to comply with the code.

Certificate of Clinical Competence and Licensure

The CCC is necessary because it is considered by ASHA to be the entry-level credential for independent delivery of clinical services. Without the CCC, individuals who practice in the fields of speech-language pathology and audiology are obligated to operate under the proper supervision of a person who holds the ASHA certificate in the appropriate profession.

In most states, a license to practice is required as well, and it is considered to be the entry-level credential for independent clinical service delivery in the state. However, the acquisition of a state license does not negate the national requirement for the CCC.

Client's Right to Confidentiality

In keeping with the Code of Ethics, people who seek professional help for communication problems have the right to expect that their concerns and your findings are maintained as private matters, so you must take every measure to protect that right from beginning to end of the process. The only circumstances that call for unauthorized sharing of information about clients are (1) when the law requires disclosure of records, and (2) when sharing information is necessary in order to protect the welfare of a client or the community. (These two circumstances rarely occur.) Otherwise, the unauthorized sharing of information about clients is inexcusable.

Simple oversights, such as a door left open and amplifying audio equipment left on during a parent interview, an overheard conversation with a colleague or fellow student in a semiprivate corridor, or a misplaced set of notes, may result in an unauthorized individual accessing private information about a client. Failure to protect clients from all errors that may result in breach of confidentiality are likely to lead to consequences that vary in degree of severity. At the very least, clients have reason to become angry with clinicians (and agencies) who carelessly allow information to leak. More serious consequences include public embarrassment, loss of reputation, legal action, loss of employment, and investigative or disciplinary action from the Ethical Practices Board of ASHA.

COMMUNICATION SCREENING

Speech-language pathologists are periodically requested to screen large numbers of children in order to identify those for whom a speech-language and/or audiological assessment is indicated. Usually the requests come from public and private schools that are in the process of **screening** large numbers of children annually or upon registration.

Preparing for the Screening

In arranging for the communication screening, it is necessary to obtain written parental permission for the child to participate. This is done by sending a form letter to each child's parents, with a permissions blank attached to the letter and instructions to return it before the day of the screening. You may screen children only with written permission from a parent or guardian. A sample screening letter and permission blank are shown in Appendix 3–1.

Screening Procedures

Since the purpose of the screening is only to identify those children who may need a comprehensive assessment, and *not* to conduct the assessment, the procedures are relatively simple. Standardized tools are available (Fluharty, 1974; Texas Department of Health, 1993).

Usually, the screening procedure includes articulation, language, and hearing components with planned observations of voice and fluency. The articulation component typically requires that the children pronounce a short list of words containing phonemes that are expected to be produced accurately at the age of screening. Picture or auditory stimuli may be used.

The language component is often somewhat more complicated. Typically, this includes (1) comprehension of oral commands and sentences that are typically understood by children of the same age, (2) opportunity to use age-appropriate expressive language in a structured format, such as responses to questions, describing pictorial stimuli, and participating briefly in conversation, and (3) perhaps a brief **conversational speech sample** that can be used to make a cursory judgment about voice, **fluency**, and intelligibility.

For the hearing component of the screening, a quiet environment is absolutely necessary. By using a portable audiometer, pure tones are tested across the speech frequencies at 20 dB of intensity. (This procedure is described in more detail in the section on hearing screenings that appears later in the chapter.)

Children who perform according to age expectations are said to "pass" the communication screening, and no further testing is planned. Children whose performance is below age expectations are referred to an ASHA-certified speech-language pathologist for a comprehensive speech-language assessment or to an ASHA-certified audiologist for a complete audiological evaluation.

Informing Parents of Screening Results

Following the screening, whether or not a complete assessment is recommended is communicated clearly to the parents in writing. Ordinarily this is accomplished by a form letter that specifies the areas screened, whether the child "passed" or "is referred," and some suggestions for **follow-up** if necessary. A sample letter appears in Appendix 3–2.

The next step for children who are referred is assessment. Specifically, the language component of that step is the topic of this chapter, and it is described in the following section.

LANGUAGE ASSESSMENT

Parents and clients seek assistance from speech-language pathologists in an attempt to address a plethora of communication concerns. Some examples include language disorders, articulation disorders, motor-speech disorders, voice disorders, disfluency, and reduced hearing sensitivity. Proficiency in assessing each area is critical to competent service delivery and to professional satisfaction and success.

The scope of this chapter is *limited to the assessment of language disorders in children.* Therefore, the following discussion is primarily limited to the principles, purposes, and procedures that apply specifically to childhood language assessment.

Initiating the Assessment Process

The assessment of a child's language is usually initiated by the child's parents because either behavior or an identified condition suggests that the communication domain requires professional attention. Regarding children with a preidentified condition, some present a congenital state known to potentially result in language acquisition difficulties. In many cases, these children are identified at birth as infants at risk. These include, but are not limited to, babies with craniofacial anomalies, cerebral palsy, Down syndrome (i.e., Trisomy 21) or other chromosomal disorders, reduced hearing sensitivity secondary to prenatal infection or heredity, diverse genetic conditions, and fetal alcohol syndrome (FAS). For infants and very young children who are identified as being at risk, a family-centered approach (Chapter 5) is the most effective way to assess communication potential and should be given first consideration whenever planning the assessment of any child below the age of four years.

In addition to infants at risk, many children with communication difficulties are identified for assessment not as a result of a predisposing condition, but because language does not develop as expected in the preschool and school-aged years. Either a traditional or family-centered approach may be applied when assessing such children.

Candidates who are likely to benefit from the traditional, client-centered approach are generally at least three years of age, separate well from their parents, participate in semistructured activities, and converse freely in the unfamiliar, clinical environment. Only the traditional, client-centered methods are discussed in this chapter, as family-centered assessment principles and procedures are introduced in Chapter 5.

Regardless of whether the approach to assessment is traditional or family-centered, the speech-language pathologist becomes involved after a parent becomes aware that a predisposing condition is likely to result in communication impairment or when a parent determines that a child's communication is inadequate. Therefore, a critical preliminary step to the assessment process is the contact made by concerned parents. Once they call attention to the fact that communication is a matter of concern, we begin the procedures that lead to assessment, diagnosis, and intervention.

At the time of the initial contact, the family representative (e.g., a parent) usually speaks to a clerical person whose job is to coordinate incoming requests for clinical services. This person supplies the parent with information about services provided at the center, fees, directions to the center, procedures for becoming eligible to receive services, and any additional information unique to the center or requested by the parent. Further, arrangements are made for the family to receive the required forms that are completed and returned before the assessment is scheduled. These forms typically include an agreement to receive services, **authorization** to seek and release information, and case history intake form. (See Appendices 3–3 through 3–5.) These forms are described in the following sections.

Obtaining Permissions

Prior to providing a service to any child or adult, written permission is required. Further, if any information is sought from, or provided to, anyone other than the client or legal guardian, written permission is required as well. The methods that are used to obtain such permissions are the topic of this section.

Agreement to Receive Services.   The fact that the parents agree to receive services at the agency is always verified by signature before scheduling any sessions. This is necessary because it is at the signing of the agreement that the client and parents enter into a business relationship with the agency. The signature on the agreement form indicates that the parents have been informed and understand all basic procedures and guidelines of the agency, along with the potential benefits, risks, or obligations. By this signature, the agency is protected against anyone's claim of misinformation, providing that all agency personnel abide by the guidelines established in the agreement.

Therefore, all information that the parents need in order to knowledgeably enroll in services appears on the agreement form. For example, if services are customarily provided or observed by students or if videotaping or audiotaping are standard procedures, the details are included in the agreement. Further, agreement to pay for services and attendance guidelines are included if appropriate. The exact information contained in the agreement varies from agency to agency. However, the purpose of the form is to document that the parents have been told and understand the terms, benefits, obligations, and potential risks (if any) of participating in clinical services at the agency. A sample agreement form can be found in Appendix 3–3.

Authorizations.   As mentioned, confidentiality is critical to all programs that offer clinical services to clients. The authorization procedure is one measure used to protect the clients' right to receive services in a confidential relationship. Many times, when serving clients a clinician needs to seek historical information from other professionals who have also served, or are concurrently serving, the same individuals. In addition, other service providers may require information about clients. Formal written authorization is required to follow through on these inquiries.

Upon scheduling the assessment, if one anticipates that information will be needed from an external agency, the authorization form is completed and signed at the onset. Additionally, whenever it becomes necessary to exchange information with an outside source, it is necessary to discuss this matter with the parents and verify in writing that they agree to each informational exchange.

A sample authorization form is found in Appendix 3–4. The sample is a single form that is used to authorize both the seeking and the releasing of information. (Some agencies use separate forms for each.)

Preparations for Assessment

Once the family notifies the center that they desire services and once they return all completed and signed forms that are required, preparations for assessment begin. The preparations include gathering initial case history information, planning the assessment session, and making final arrangements.

Gathering Initial Case History Information.   The case history intake form is part of the packet sent to the client's parents when they request services. Its purpose is to request identifying and historical information, and it must be completed and returned before scheduling an assessment. The completed case history form is required *without exception* because, if filled out according to instructions, it provides valuable information that is useful in determining the specific focus and procedures for the assessment. An example of a case history intake form can be found in Appendix 3–5.

Planning the Assessment Session.   Several steps are involved in planning an assessment session. They include reading and studying the case history intake form, identifying assessment objectives, determining questions to be asked during the interview, and selecting a test battery.

Reading and Studying the Completed Case-History Forms.   The first step to planning an assessment is to read and study the completed case history. If the parent has filled out the forms as directed, the information gives an historical sense of the child's performance in a number of domains, including language, speech, hearing, physical, cognitive, health and medical, social, family, and educational development. Further, it acquaints one with the concerns that caused the parents to initiate the assessment process.

If the case history form is not filled out according to instructions, the information that it contains is valuable nonetheless. For example, some case history forms arrive with illegible handwriting, numerous informational gaps, ambiguous grammar and spelling, misused or unfamiliar medical terms, or any number of characteristics that interfere with one's ability to understand exactly what the parent means. Although such an intake form may not provide the exact information that one hopes to receive, it is very useful in directing interview questions and adapting language to suit the needs of the interview informant.

Further, if case history intake provides inadequate or unclear **data**, placing a polite phone call to the parent in order to clarify information may be advisable for two purposes. Primarily you may clear up a confusing issue prior to the assessment interview, and thus facilitate a smooth and proficient assessment session. In addition, the call communicates to the parent that you are concerned about the child and interested in obtaining accurate information, thereby creating an atmosphere of cooperation that persists through the clinical relationship.

Identifying Assessment Objectives.   After reading the case history form carefully, the second step is to identify objectives that are to be addressed by the language assessment **protocol**. The fundamental purposes of assessment are (1) to identify whether a communication problem exists, (2) to accurately describe the problem and make appropriate **recommendations** if a communication problem is identified, and (3) if a communication problem is *not* detected, to identify the source of concern and make appropriate recommendations. These purposes are general, as they apply to most assessments. However, nearly all language assessments are driven by several more specific objectives. The specific objectives seek to provide accurate information that is useful in describing the condition and making appropriate recommendations, as suggested by the second fundamental objective listed here.

Specifically as a result of the session, (1) the foundation for a workable relationship is established with the client and (2) through interview and testing, each of the questions in Figure 3–1 is addressed. In addition, even more specific objectives may be developed individually as each assessment session is planned. These idiosyncratic objectives depend on the multifarious variables that characterize the presenting case history.

Determining Exact Interview Questions.   A third step is to determine the exact questions to ask during the assessment interview. The answers to the selected questions enable a very clear understanding of significant preceding events, why the family is seeking help, exactly how the client and family view

(a)   What are the communication concerns of the parents and client? What are the client's communication needs?

(b)   In general, how does the child's expressive and receptive language compare to that of same-age peers?

(c)   Regarding each dimension of language and the interactive relationships between the dimensions, how does this child's expressive and receptive command of language compare to same-age peers? This includes command of phonology, morphology, and syntax, expression of ideas, and purposeful use of contextual language.

(d)   If speech is intelligible, are articulation errors present? If so, what are they and how does the child's performance compare to that of same-age peers?

(e)   If speech is *not* intelligible, what are the simplification patterns (phonological processes) that contribute to speech-sound production difficulties and how do these patterns compare to those of same-age peers?

(f)   Can an anatomical or physiological cause for the communication difficulties be identified?

(g)   Is hearing within normal limits or is an audiological evaluation needed?

(h)   Do voice or fluency patterns indicate a need for further testing?

(i)   Is further testing needed in any area other than lanugage, speech, and audiology?

(j)   Is the client a candidate for intervention? If so, what objectives are recommended for the onset?

(k)   If intervention is being considered, how likely is it that the child will benefit from it (prognosis)?

Figure 3-1.   Questions that are addressed through assessment.

the condition, and what the family expects to gain from the assessment and potential intervention.

Certain questions are asked as a matter of routine. For example, many clinicians customarily ask the family to explain exactly why they are concerned about the client's communication, to describe the problem as they see it, to elaborate on exactly what they expect to gain from the assessment session, and to indicate the exact nature of the communication changes that they desire.

These issues are important to address because the answers help coordinate assessment activities with the family's purpose. For example, communication skills of children are sometimes reported inaccurately on case history intake forms. Some extreme examples include the child with seriously delayed language who is reported as having a mild intelligibility problem and the pragmatically disordered child who is reported as being disfluent.

When case history data is misleading, the preplanned assessment protocol is not apt to address the client's actual communication needs. However, by asking a few purpose-oriented questions at the time of the interview, one takes a precaution against discovering that the assessment protocol is inappropriate once it is in progress, or worse yet, once testing is complete. Nevertheless, knowing that the protocol may change as a result of the answers to these questions requires that one build flexibility into the assessment protocol.

In addition to the purpose-oriented questions, plan to ask the family to clarify and expand on selected parts of the case history intake data. This step is necessary when information on the form is missing, scanty, incomplete, or vague, or because case history data simply calls attention to a situation requiring elaboration. The exact questions asked are different for every client as each presents a different history and individual styles vary for completing the forms.

Selecting the Test Battery.   The fourth step is to select a battery of tests that is likely to answer pertinent questions about the client's language performance and reported communication difficulties. In the case of a child referred for language assessment, standardized and informal language testing, articulation or phonology testing, a hearing screening, and an oral mechanism exam are mandatory parts of the assessment procedure. Exactly which tests are selected and precisely how these procedures are performed depend on a number of client variables including chronological age or age equivalency, attention, related problems already identified, reported symptoms, cognitive skills, and social factors.

In addition, a few other areas may be tested or recommended for testing, depending on the client's needs. They include voice, fluency, and any other aspects of the communication domain identified by the case history as potential areas for concern.

In ordering the events of the assessment session, consider this suggested sequence. Begin with informal play or conversation for the purpose of establishing **rapport**. As soon as possible, initiate more structured, nonspeaking activities (e.g., standardized test of language comprehension), and follow them with structured tests that require verbal responding (e.g., standardized tests of articulation or phonology and of language expression). Less formal, less structured, interactive activities may be planned to occur next (e.g., conversational speech sample, **language sample**, and motor imitation). Finally, plan to carry out any activities that may be perceived by the child as invasive (e.g., oral mechanism exam, hearing screening).

Preparing to Begin the Assessment Session.

Preparing Materials.   A number of steps are taken prior to the assessment in order to increase the likelihood that it will proceed efficiently and effectively. Begin by preparing the materials for the session. This includes reviewing the chosen tests, collecting materials for testing, and organizing all tests and materials so that they are easily accessed by you and out of reach of the child.

Determining Activities to be Used with the Child during Parent Interview. Prior to the session, determine what is to be done with the child during the interview. Make arrangements for the child to be entertained or tested during the part of the session that you hope to use for collecting case history information. This is facilitated in some university clinics where teams of two or more clinicians are sometimes assigned to the same case. Working in teams makes it possible for one well-prepared clinician to establish rapport and administer a standardized test during the interview portion of the session. However, in most clinical settings, independent service delivery is more commonly practiced, making it necessary for a single person to occupy the child while simultaneously interviewing the parent.

Under these circumstances, regulating the child's behavior during the interview becomes somewhat more complicated. This objective may be accomplished by providing quiet toys and play materials for the child to use during the interview. The toys serve to acclimate the child to the clinical environment before the testing begins, while also providing a suitable diversion. Beware, however, that some children become rowdy at play even when alone and with quiet toys, making it difficult to concentrate on the interview or preventing a smooth transition to the testing format. Further, some children demand parental attention regardless of how interesting a diversion is provided. For these reasons, plan to closely monitor the child's behavior during the interview, even if the child is supposed to be preoccupied at play. Also keep in mind that the situation can be used to one's advantage. That is, if a skilled interviewer is able to earn the parent's trust during the interview and the child is present to observe the interaction, the task of establishing rapport with the child may be simplified. Moreover, the situation can be used to observe parent-child interaction and the child's independent play skills, particularly as they bear upon the opportunity for language learning.

Preparing the Assessment Room.   Immediately before the session, prepare the assessment room. Check the video- and audio-recording equipment and set it up so that it can be turned on quickly at the appropriate time. Organize the materials, placing them so that they are readily accessible to you and out of the child's reach. If selected materials are to be made available to the child during the interview, place them within reach and encourage the child to choose from them. These may include toys for quiet play, crayons and paper, modeling clay, blocks, and coloring books.

Place testing materials and other accouterments that you wish to control completely out of sight and reach. Such materials include tests, test manuals, stimulus items, materials for the language sample and informal testing, and all other items that you expect to use as part of the test protocol.

Some centers have a high shelf in each room which is an excellent place to store objects that you wish to control. In other clinical environments, it is necessary to be more creative in managing the testing materials. The far end of a table, between your chair and a wall or table, inside a closed box or sack, and just outside the door in a semiprivate corridor are some options that are often successful.

Arrange the environment so that it is comfortable for an interview. Use a room that is large enough for all the individuals who are expected to participate. Arrange the furniture so that people feel at ease and able to converse freely. Sitting around a table is desirable, as most people have a history of positive and comfortable experiences sitting around a table at mealtime. Further, the table serves as a place to write the information that the parents offer as well as providing a barrier that tends to minimize feelings of vulnerability.

Take measures to assure that the interview room is neat and orderly. Further, domestic effects such as flowers or decorations may be added because they sometimes help to relax the people being interviewed and enhance the physical atmosphere. Just prior to beginning the session, close all doors to observation rooms. Observation rooms are kept inaccessible to passers-by in order to protect confidentiality. Further, legitimate observers are not visible to the client and parents, as their conspicuous presence may be distracting even though the observers are present only with written permission from the parents.

Memorizing Names.   Take the time to commit the name of the client, names of significant family members, and major case history details to short-term memory. By the time that you meet the family and client, they have been anticipating the event for a number of weeks. They made a phone call initiating the process, received materials in the mail, completed the materials, and returned them to the center. Further, the clerical staff called to set up an appointment for the assessment. Therefore, interviewees often anticipate that you know who they are and are somewhat familiar with the nature of the problem. Regardless of how many clients are on your caseload or how busy you are on that particular day, you are obligated to readily recall the client's name, names of the persons significant to the client, nature of the complaint, and significant details of the case history report.

Ready Access to Protocol and Materials.   Finally, make sure that your written assessment protocol and materials are handy. The materials that should be readily available include the client's file (with a completed case history intake form), a list of the concerns that you hope to address through the assessment, specific and general interview questions, a list of tests sequenced according to the order of administration, and all test forms, similarly sequenced according to planned order of administration. Clipboards, folders, accordion files, and notebooks are some methods for keeping these items organized, accessible to you, and out of the child's immediate reach.

Client Absence.   If on the day of the assessment the client does not arrive within 15 minutes of the appointed time, call to determine whether attendance should be expected. If the parents have forgotten the appointment or have decided not to keep it, there is no reason to continue to wait. Further, a pattern of tardiness and poor attendance may be avoided if the parents are aware that someone will call. As a rule, continue to call an absent client until reaching the responsible adult so that absence does not become associated with avoidance.

If the parents have forgotten the appointment and it becomes necessary to call, be courteous and respectful in approaching the telephone contact. Having spent time in preparation and having waited needlessly, it may be tempting to communicate disapproval or inconvenience, especially if the call reveals that the parents forgot the appointment or decided to cancel without calling in. However, keep in mind that the purposes of the call are only (1) to verify that the appointment was missed and (2) to find out whether the responsible person wishes to reschedule. Communicating disapproval or personal inconvenience is inadmissible.

Introductory Procedures

Prior to beginning the interview and assessment procedures, the contact with the client and family is somewhat informal. However, the method used to make the transition from the waiting room to the ass sment session is consequential to the success of the overall procedure.

Meeting the Client and Family.   Meeting your first client for the first time is a somewhat stressful experience for most clinicians, and one that is not soon forgotten. As one gains experience handling introductions successfully, they become a familiar and amicable part of the professional experience. Introductions go very smoothly if one considers the following suggestions.

Being on Time.   Some centers have a receptionist to announce the client's arrival, whereas others do not. Regardless, it is important to be on time for the appointment. Check the designated waiting area at the appointed time. If the client has not yet arrived, check frequently for the next 10 to 15 minutes or until the client arrives. Meeting the client and family in the waiting area is preferred to asking them to find an office or cubicle; however, procedures vary in different settings.

Your Entrance.   When entering the waiting room, enter with confidence and with a smile on your face. Use a voice that is clear, audible, and confident. Demonstrate by your demeanor that you are pleased to meet them.

Introducing Yourself to Adults.   Introduce yourself by the name that you prefer that they use. Find out the name of each individual present and verify that person's relationship to the client. Introduce any members of a clinical team who may be present. Shake hands with adults, and accompany your handshake with suitable eye contact and a friendly smile.

Introducing Yourself to Children.   When meeting children, assess their behavior before deciding exactly how to greet them. Approach a reticent child with friendly caution and a gregarious child with cautious enthusiasm, gauging your manner according to the child's response to your attempts at initiating contact. Whatever you choose to say or do, in general children often accept professional adults who meet them at their physical level, call them by name, use sincere eye contact, smile, and interact briefly about something the child is doing. Some children are friendly upon an initial meeting, while others withdraw or hide behind a parent. Both extremes and all responses in between are possible and should be anticipated.

Never apply pressure to a child who hesitates to converse, especially at the initial meeting. Making comments on how well the child talks or otherwise calling attention to communication is inappropriate. Further, comments about evaluating the child's speech may only serve to delay achieving the desired level of comfort. Remember that a shy child often becomes comfortable after a reasonable period of acclimation without being forced.

Moving to the Assessment Room.   Once everyone has been introduced, a quick transition to the assessment room is expedient. Suggest that the assessment begin and then lead the individuals to the designated area. What you do or say en route may vary according to the distance from the waiting area. Small talk is fine. For example, the walk to the assessment room is a good time to ask about the trip to the center, the availability of parking, and the weather outside. Avoid questions about the client in the public and semipublic walkways to ensure that confidentiality is maintained.

Small Talk.   Upon reaching the room where the assessment interview is scheduled to take place, more specific discussion may ensue. Initially, you want to establish rapport, so continued small talk is fitting for a short time. However, the family is aware that they have come for a communication evaluation and they may become frustrated or impatient with extended chitchat.

Communicating Guidelines and Expectations.   As soon as possible, begin to let the family know about any guidelines they should observe during the session. For example, if you desire for the parents to be involved in managing the child, then identify reasonable behavioral expectations and clearly communicate their responsibilities to them.

Communicating the Assessment Plan.   Inform the family of the protocol of assessment activities. Let them know that you plan to ask them questions during the interview, that standardized and informal tests are to be expected, that a hearing screening is planned, that you plan to look inside the child's mouth, that you plan to partially inform them of the results before they leave the center, and that they may expect to receive a written assessment report in the mail within a few weeks.

More detailed information about what to expect may also be given during the introductory remarks if a parent seems uncomfortable or unsure. However, before providing a detailed account of the plan, the parents may be best served by asking if they have any questions about what to expect. Then, if they request, you may elaborate briefly on the types of interview questions or perhaps the general nature of some of the language tests.

The Opening Interview.   You have met your client and the concerned family members, you have given them some information about the procedures, and you are sitting in the room where the language-assessment interview is scheduled to take place. It is now time to begin. In so doing, remember that in keeping with the general assessment purposes, the objectives of the opening interview are (1) to obtain the necessary information efficiently and politely and (2) to begin to establish a clinical relationship. Although a number of questions are asked that are important to the outcome of the session, the overriding interview objective is *not* to ask your questions but rather to collect the information that the questions address. Further, productive interview behavior includes paying attention to posture, body language, prosody, and the language expressions that you use.

Posture.   Appropriate interview posture communicates approachability, comfort, professionalism, and confidence. Sitting naturally in a chair near the table is desired. Avoid rocking, reclining, swiveling, fidgeting, wiggling, shuffling, tapping, pen clicking, slouching, rigid body posture, and all extraneous movement.

Body Language.   Body language is important. Your physical demeanor communicates willingness to accept the information offered and inclination to use the information for the client's benefit. By maintaining natural eye contact, listening carefully, and taking notes as needed, you communicate a positive message while avoiding some of the negative nonverbal messages that are given by some interviewers. For example, an interviewer who does not listen carefully and neglects to take notes communicates to the parents a lack of interest in what they have to say—a message that sabotages all efforts to learn needed information. It is advisable to keep one's mind on the general and specific purposes, listen very carefully to what the informants say, think about how this information addresses the questions about the child's communication pattern, and avoid thinking about yourself and how you appear to them.

Prosody.   Prosody carries an important message, so use a tone of voice that is friendly, compassionate, and seriously interested. Use variations in pitch and loudness, speaking rate, and pauses that are within the normal range for formal conversational speech.

Verbal Language.   Select language carefully when phrasing questions or comments, wording questions and remarks as gently as possible. Use words and phrases that are socially acceptable, respectful, and easy to understand. Avoid professional jargon, as it can confuse or alienate lay people. Instead, know and understand the terminology well enough to explain it in plain, simple language.

Initiating the Opening Interview.   Initiating the opening interview can be done in a very natural way by beginning with a question that asks what the parents want the assessment to accomplish. Although elaboration may be needed, the answer to this question generally leads to a clear statement of the problem, description of the communication pattern, information about the exact direction to be taken in testing, and insight into expectations for intervention. The question also communicates genuine interest in meeting the parents' felt needs and addressing their idiosyncratic concerns. This facilitates establishing rapport and the comfort of the parents. Questions about current communication patterns, developmental milestones, and history flow easily once the parents' expectations and purposes for initiating the evaluation process are clearly established.

Ending the Interview.   Establishing a natural, yet definite, ending to the interview is also advantageous. Having asked the planned and spontaneous questions and being satisfied that you have accumulated all the information needed in order to proceed with testing, a natural way to indicate that the questions are over is to give the parents the opportunity to ask questions and make comments. When they indicate that all their questions have been addressed satisfactorily, it is expedient to suggest that the standardized and informal testing begin. Then you can move comfortably from the interview to the testing format.

The People Factor.

Anxiety Level.   When engaged in assessment interviews, one encounters a number of behavior patterns, which clinicians must learn to handle skillfully. For example, a degree of anxiety is naturally associated with the experience of providing information about one's child to strangers, even concerned professionals. How much stress an individual experiences and how the individual reacts to stress are different for each person. Some people clearly demonstrate a significant level of anxiety and concern over the situation, while others appear very comfortable and spontaneous. Adapt your style to suit the individual, taking whatever precautions are necessary to make certain that you get the needed information while at the same time establishing a workable clinical relationship.

If parents demonstrate concern or anxiety, it is up to you to make an attempt to put them at ease. In general, people who are uncomfortable can become somewhat more comfortable if they believe that they are speaking to a person who relates to them, listens to them, and is interested in their concerns. For that reason, use body language and a tone of voice that communicate acceptance; assume a posture that is similar to, but not exactly like, that of the parent informant; take on a facial expression that shows genuine compassion and concern; select friendly and nonthreatening words and phrases; and engage in a little extra small talk about some common interest or experience.

Conversely, some people appear quite relaxed at the time of the interview. If this is the case, rapport may be established quickly and the amount of energy to be invested in putting the informant at ease is markedly reduced. Even so, it is wise to demonstrate sensitivity in gathering information. It is also advisable to maintain a suitable level of professionalism even if the informant appears relaxed and comfortable. Regardless of how comfortable the clinical relationship, always think carefully before offering even the most innocent, spontaneous remark.

Willingness of Informant.   The amount of information that people offer and how willing they are to offer it varies greatly. Some people practically interview themselves, volunteering very appropriate information and anticipating questions before being asked, while others are extremely difficult to interview, offering minimal responses to questions and leaving one with the impression that information is being withheld. Most people fall between the two extremes in their styles of providing information.

When people hesitate to offer information, one may attempt to identify the reason for this response pattern. For example, a taciturn informant may behave in such a way because of an increased level of anxiety or distress, lack of trust, cultural orientation, unfamiliarity with the circumstances or surroundings, and any number of additional factors, in any combination. The likelihood of immediately identifying the exact cause of reserved behavior is low because there are so many possibilities and potential combinations of the possibilities. Further, many variables are difficult to change once the assessment is in progress (e.g., the identity of the assessing clinician).

However, most problems with informants who hesitate to inform can be resolved, at least in part, by remembering the purposes of the interview. That is, you are there to obtain needed information efficiently and politely and to begin to establish a clinical relationship. Therefore, ask the necessary questions with sensitivity and respect, carefully listen to the responses however minimal they may be, and gently ask more specific supplementary questions in an attempt to assist the parent in providing the data necessary for a successful outcome to the assessment session.

Further, you should develop sensitivity to the individual's limitations. If a parent becomes agitated, angry, or emotional with detailed inquiries, drop the issue, at least temporarily. You may return to difficult questions later if they are critical to the assessment and if the parent becomes more relaxed later in the session. Otherwise, important unanswered questions may be included in the recommendations section of the assessment report. Since individuals vary in the amount of prodding necessary to get them to provide information, exactly how you deal with each person has to be determined on a individual basis.

Emotions.   A communication assessment is an emotional time for many parents, and individual styles vary for dealing with the emotions. Again, although extremes exist, most people fall somewhere in the middle regarding how much emotion they experience and how they handle their emotions. For example, many people cry when they begin to discuss the communication difficulties that their offspring experience. Although crying is a completely natural response, the amount of crying and the degree of control vary greatly.

Since you cannot predict from the case history whether crying will occur, expect that it will and be prepared for it. At the very least, it is your responsibility to make sure that a box of facial tissues is both visible and accessible from the onset of the interview. Making tissues handy from the very beginning communicates, without words, that crying is normal and that you have seen it before.

More important, however, being prepared to handle crying involves mental preparation. Think about how you might feel if you cried in the presence of a stranger during a session that could not be terminated abruptly and consider what you would prefer that stranger to do for you. For example, the person who cries probably feels ugly, embarrassed, and out of control, at the very least. Although staring or looking away are somewhat instinctive responses, they are both undesirable as they increase the awkwardness experienced by the person crying. Do your best to maintain *natural* eye contact during the crying episode. Acknowledge the crying, and to the best of your honest ability, seriously assure the parent that you understand what it feels like to cry. Do *not* pretend to understand exactly how they feel or what they are going through, as such comments are rightfully interpreted as insincere. And do not laugh. Give the individual a few moments but continue the interview as soon as possible, perhaps moving temporarily to a less emotional topic. In general, the crucial communication to the parent who cries is that crying is natural in this circumstance, that you know what it feels like to cry, and that you are a compassionate person who cares about the concerns that bring on tears.

Other emotional responses may include excessive anger, inappropriate laughter, and extreme frustration. Regardless, when an immoderate or inapt emotional response is elicited by the interview, in most cases it is legitimate to suspect that the emotion is precipitated by the stress commonly associated with the circumstance. Therefore, focus on gathering the necessary information while acknowledging, yet making very little of, any emotional outbursts.

Staying on Topic.   Staying on the topic of the interview is difficult for some people. Your responsibility is to see to it that a minimum of time is wasted on topics unrelated to the communication problem, while still communicating to the parents that their concerns are important to you.

The topics that are likely to interfere with progress during an assessment interview are varied and unpredictable. Some parents have an uncanny knack for introducing and relentlessly pursuing unrelated topics. These may include detailed accounts of recent family arguments, illnesses or accidents of family members, explanations for having missed a session or for tardiness, marital disputes, personal dilemmas, and recent events that are apparently relayed for entertainment purposes.

In order to deal effectively with off-topic issues, it is necessary to first verify that an issue is unrelated to the communication needs of the child. Unfortunately, this takes some time as, in order to be sure that the issue is unrelated, one must first listen to a certain amount of rambling about the matter. However, such behavior must be brought under control as quickly as possible because if the habit is not checked, some individuals can go on indefinitely while providing very little clinically useful information.

One way to handle off-topic behavior is to verify the conversation's relationship to the interview. This can be accomplished by politely mentioning that you are not certain exactly how this part of the conversation relates to the issue. By doing this you (1) expedite the process of getting to the point if the topic is related, (2) pave the way for resuming the topic if it is unrelated, and (3) communicate to the person that you are truly interested in the communication needs of the client.

Further, with some parents, accounts of marital and family disputes often include an invitation for the professional to take sides. It is critical that one learn to effectively handle this particular type of off-topic behavior, as it not only wastes time unnecessarily but also opens the door to the possibility of alienating at least one family member (and probably two or more).

One way to manage invitations to become involved in disputes is to briefly recapitulate all sides of the issue and point out the redeeming features of each perspective. By doing this, you communicate (1) that you are a good listener who heard all sides equally and (2) that you appreciate the value of each point of view. Never handle disagreements by taking sides.

Separating the Child from the Parents

If you are using a traditional client-oriented approach to assessment, in most cases it is desirable for the child to separate from the parents in order to accomplish testing with a minimum of distractions. If separation is desired, there are two probable times for initiating the transition to separate accommodations. If two clinicians work on the assessment cooperatively, separation from the parents can take place prior to the interview as one clinician will be able to take the child to different quarters for preliminary activities and testing while the other clinician conducts the parent interview. Typically, however, only one clinician orchestrates the assessment and when that happens, separation is often scheduled to take place immediately following the interview.

For a traditional assessment, many clinicians expect the child to separate from the parents for a number of reasons. For one, establishing a pattern of attending the sessions independently may be desired so that the clinician can establish a working relationship with the child and the child can form a habit of independent activity at the center. Moreover, standardized test administration is not enhanced by *unplanned* parental presence. That is, if not instructed properly, parents often provide the child with information that contaminates the standardized test results and can inadvertently serve to distract their child from the task.

Children vary in their responses to separation from parents. Some make the transition quite easily, while others panic and experience serious separation anxiety as well as stranger anxiety. For many children aged 3 and older, separation concerns are overcome almost automatically by curiosity. That is, the transition from the interview to the testing format can be facilitated by making accessible some alluring toy or activity, emphasizing the opportunity to do this interesting work independently, informing the child of the exact location of the parent, and allowing an anxious child to be accompanied by some familiar toy, object, or even one of the parent's possessions (e.g., car keys).

Nevertheless, certain young children persist with tears and other symptoms of anxiety, so that some parents may decide to separate without the child's permission or even not to separate at all. If the decision is made not to separate, then a skilled clinician can use parental involvement to facilitate cooperation and gather information about the communication patterns of the home environment. (See Chapter 5 for specific information on collaborating with families.)

If, however, the decision is made to separate even with continued anxiety, the child's crying often stops during a period of acclimation. However, some very young children do not adjust to unfamiliar surroundings, regardless of how attractive the enticement. Consequently, in determining whether separation is crucial to the success of the assessment, keep in mind that forcing an unwilling child to separate can work against the purposes of gaining information about language performance and establishing a positive clinical relationship. For example, panic-stricken, frightened children who are beside themselves with tears generally provide very few representative examples of their language skills. Further, forcing a child to separate may serve to establish several nonproductive patterns in the clinical relationship that will be difficult to change. The act of attempting to coerce a child to separate sets up an adversarial relationship between the client and clinician. Moreover, the emotions of fear and anxiety become strongly associated with the experience of attending the center, a pattern that, if allowed to continue, will interfere with the acquisition of work habits that are expedient for participating in a productive assessment session and intervention program.

For these reasons, if it becomes obvious that a child is not willing to separate, the decision to include a parent in the assessment probably benefits the long-term interests of the child. Although the standardized information that is obtained may be somewhat compromised, valuable information will be gained about the child's spontaneous communication patterns with parents and the clinician. Moreover, once the child enters the testing environment, even with the parents in tow, a wealth of standardized and informal data can be accumulated by a careful clinician who is a skilled observer, provided the dynamics of the familial relationships are monitored carefully. (See Chapter 5 for specific suggestions.)

Establishing Rapport with the Child

Whether or not the child separates from the parents, it is necessary to establish a friendly, workable relationship with the child before beginning the testing. Therefore, for the first several minutes of the session, you may decide to participate in **parallel play** (described in Chapter 4) until reaching a level of trust and comfort that allows for friendly social interaction with the child.

The age and experience of the child heavily influence the amount of time and type of interaction needed to achieve a suitable level of trust. As a rule, adolescents require a short, relaxed conversation, perhaps in the context of culturally salient paraphernalia. School-age children often become reasonably relaxed following a brief conversation, guessing game, or an introduction to a puppet or cartoon character, again taking cultural orientation into account. Some preschool children, however, require extended informal play at their level with interesting and familiar stimuli before becoming comfortable. This need is sometimes exacerbated if a child has a history of negative experience with strangers or with clinical, medical, or educational settings.

In general, establishing rapport requires that one engage the child in some activity that is unstructured, fun, nonthreatening, culturally relevant, and client-oriented. Although the purpose of the activity is simply to help the child become comfortable with you and the clinical setting, information about communication and social skills can be learned while establishing rapport. In fact, important observations of play skills, motor coordination, and sociability can be made while at the same time building the foundations for trust and for social interaction.

Further, if conversation is a part of the rapport-building activity, the conversational speech sample can be collected while establishing rapport. The conversational speech sample is different from the language sample that is collected and analyzed as part of the formal testing (to be discussed later in this chapter). By contrast, it is simply the act of engaging the client in conversation for the purpose of informally judging intelligibility, language performance level, voice, fluency, prosody, and pragmatics. Although the conversational speech sample is not formally analyzed, taping it is advised so that it may be used later to confirm judgments about these parameters of communication.

The Testing Situation

Once the child is relatively comfortable in the clinical environment, standardized and informal testing can begin. A host of specific tests are available to formally assess language from birth through adolescence. You are encouraged to familiarize yourself with them so that you can choose appropriately. Since new tests become available all the time and since we assume that one's preparatory curriculum includes specific instruction and practice in the use of available tests, this chapter does not include a detailed description of discrete tests. Instead, the chapter addresses specific assessment objectives and general procedures for accomplishing the objectives.

Where to Begin.   Once the child is comfortable in the testing situation, it is still important to continue to nurture his or her confidence and trust, keeping in mind that this is the child's first encounter with you and the testing situation. For that reason, it is advisable to begin with a test that allows the child to perceive a reasonable degree of success, requires little or no verbal responding, and presents little or no perceived threat to the child. A reasonable place to start may be with an evaluation of motor imitation or play skills or a test of receptive language. Moreover, unless speech intelligibility is seriously reduced, a test of articulation may be a suitable icebreaker for some young children, especially if using a test with colorful pictures, since the activity is not verbally challenging and it gives the child the opportunity to succeed at the very onset of the clinical interaction.

Some activities that are *not* suitable for initiating the testing are the oral mechanism examination and language sampling. This is because both activities require a significant level of rapport before they can be executed successfully. Specifically, the oral mechanism exam is perceived by many children as invasive, and therefore threatening. Further, difficulties with the oral mechanism exam can serve to undermine cooperation for the remainder of a session. For that reason, the oral mechanism exam is not a good starting activity and rather is best left until the end of an assessment session.

Encouraging Continued Responding.   Standardized tests of language are important parts of the assessment. However, they can take considerable time and can be somewhat tedious for both you and the child. For that reason it is important to plan to incorporate some strategies that encourage the child to continue participating and responding after the interest level associated with the novelty of the test has worn down. The type of feedback that you give is important to that end. Most children continue to respond if success is experienced. Therefore, appropriate feedback is used to communicate success to the child. If the child is responding, whether the answers are right or wrong he or she is nonetheless succeeding, so you should *reinforce participation only*. Compliment the child for working so hard and praise the child for cooperating well. Avoid any comments that indicate the accuracy of responses and avoid changing to a neutral or negative tone when an incorrect response is given.

Another way to encourage a child to continue to respond is to provide some sort of *tangible reinforcement* that is scheduled to be given at fixed or variable intervals, regardless of accuracy. For example, a child may receive a star or a sticker on a chart (or picture) for every 5 to 10 responses on a language test, 5 to 10 pages on a test of articulation, or for 3 to 5 minutes of cooperation. Children are idiosyncratic in what motivates them, so the decision to provide tangible reinforcers should be made on an individual basis. When the more commonplace stars and stickers lack appeal, alternative options are available. Some children enjoy reinforcers such as earning ice chips, opportunities to blow bubbles, periodic peaks out the window, or permission to push a toy car for a few seconds after several responses. Regardless of the method of reinforcement, the important thing is that the child perceive success, remain interested in the activity, and complete the task.

Managing the Child's Behavior.

Cooperation.   Successfully managing the child's behavior is critical to childhood language assessment. That is, you are best able to learn what you need to know about the child if he or she cooperates and interacts socially. Successful behavior management is essential to achieving cooperation and positive social interaction for many children.

Cooperation can be achieved by a number of strategies. Primarily, to achieve cooperation the child has to sense your *genuine interest* or positive attitude. On the other hand, if the child senses dislike, frustration, or any other negative attitude, cooperation is unlikely. People often make an extra effort for people who like them and whom they like, and children are no exception.

Second, the child needs to *experience success*. People like to succeed, and experiencing success often causes one to anticipate more success. By communicating that the child's work meets your expectations, you enhance the chances of having the child "play on your team" during the assessment and during subsequent clinical sessions.

Further, a child is likely to cooperate if presented with some *sense of choice or limited control*. For example, when administering a standardized test to a young child, plan to provide tangible reinforcers for specified intervals of cooperation; then, give the child a sense of control by providing a choice of tangible reinforcers. In order to present this choice, before even beginning the test, show it to the child and briefly summarize the expectations according to the procedures described in the test manual. Then show the child the method that will be used to collect the tangible reinforcements (e.g., a chart or picture for stickers, a racetrack for playing with a car), and present the child with two choices for reinforcers by asking which the child prefers (e.g., animal stickers or colored stars, the red car or the blue car). By providing a choice of reinforcer, one allows the child to control some aspect of the activity while at the same time controlling the aspects that are critical to acquiring the needed information.

Choices are also very useful for distracting a child from noncompliant behavior. For example, if a child refuses to point to test stimuli, you may provide a choice as to how the responses are to be indicated (e.g., puppet points to pictures or child puts a token on the picture). Further, by way of example, if a child refuses to go to the assessment room, you may provide a choice as to how the child will walk to the destination (e.g., walking in front of an adult or holding the adult's hand). When given two choices on how to perform the act, many children forget to refuse and take the opportunity to make a choice.

Sometimes when a child refuses to cooperate, it is easy for a clinician to fall into the trap of begging and negotiating. Avoid this pattern at all costs, as it puts the child in control. There is a difference between offering choices and allowing the child to control the session. For example, if the child refuses to participate in an activity, you give up all authority by offering one alternative after another. By so doing, you put yourself in the position of being refused and the child in the position of waiting for the best offer and perhaps even enjoying a sense of power.

If the child refuses to participate in the activity, a more suitable course of action is to present only two choices as to *how* the activity is to be done (not whether it is to be done). In this way, you remain in control while allowing both yourself and the child to preserve a sense of dignity.

Making Behavioral Observations.   One part of the language assessment that is critical to the success of the diagnosis and recommendations is the act of making behavioral observations when interacting with, and watching, the child. These are not necessarily a part of any standardized test, although they may be observed informally while administering one.

Some behavioral parameters that come under scrutiny include, but are not limited to, attention span, distractibility, frustration, compliance, willingness to participate, ability to focus and complete a task, play skills, motor imitation skills, social skills, and use of gestures or alternate means of communication. When a child does not readily participate in standardized testing, the list may become quite lengthy as it may be necessary to gather nearly all assessment data through observation.

Assessment Protocol and Objectives for Specific Testing

The language assessment protocol typically includes each of the following parts: (1) detailed testing of expressive and receptive language, including all three dimensions, (2) articulation or phonology testing, (3) oral mechanism examination, (4) hearing screening, and (5) ancillary testing if necessary (voice or fluency). Each part of this protocol is driven by a set of objectives in that area.

Language Testing.   For each young child who is referred for language assessment, the protocol usually includes standardized tests of language, language sampling, and observations of spontaneous language performance apart from testing and sampling. Each aspect of language assessment provides unique and valuable information.

Standardized Testing.   Standardized tests are administered whenever possible because they provide a means by which the child's performance may be quantifiably compared to the performance of large groups of children in a similar age category. This is valuable information because it quantifies a level of functioning for the individual child. In addition, specific information is learned regarding performance on all dimensions of language from both expressive and receptive perspectives. (Tests and subtests exist to measure overall language performance, semantics, syntax, morphology, and pragmatics, all from both expressive and receptive points of view. Further, standardized instruments are available for testing language learners from birth through adulthood.)

Precise administration of the standardized test is critical to the outcome of the language assessment. Before attempting to administer a test, always read the manual carefully, practice the test format as suggested in the manual, and seek clarification to avoid any potential trouble spots in test administration.

These steps are necessary because tests are standardized under a specific set of conditions. If you unintentionally or unsystematically alter the conditions under which the test is given, you may find yourself in the situation where the test results are not usable. Some examples that may result in this circumstance are inadvertently selecting a test that is inappropriate for the child's chronological age, inaccurate use of instructions and carrier phrases, neglecting to allow for a specified response time, and recording the wrong information on the response form.

It is not always possible to achieve standardized administration of standardized tests for every client. For example, when no standardized test is available in the child's dominant language or dialect, alternatives to standardized testing are explored. (Some alternatives are described in Chapter 6.)

Other circumstances that may interfere with standardized administration of tests include, but are not limited to, lack of voluntary participation, excessive distractibility, and sensory impairment. For example, a child who refuses to participate in standardized tests leaves you with no choice but to assess language through less formal methods. A highly distractible child may require that the standardized test be administered in a number of short sessions or with an excessive use of reinforcers, while a child with reduced vision may require that the test stimuli be enlarged or altered so that they can be perceived either visually or tactilely.

Despite the justification behind altering a standard procedure, the **ratio-nale**, a clear description of the alternate procedures, and the exact outcome must be clearly documented on the test form and in the written assessment report whenever a standardized test is altered in any way. Further, when informal procedures are used instead of standardized tests, regardless of the rationale, the details must be explicitly documented in the assessment report. The reason for choosing an informal format, the exact nature of the informal procedures, and the information obtained by the informal procedures are all important to the clinician who next sees the child for further assessment or intervention.

Collecting a Spontaneous Language Sample.   Language assessment often includes a spontaneous language sample, especially for preschool and younger school-age children. Unlike the conversational speech sample taken early in the assessment session, the spontaneous language sample is taken with the understanding that the child's utterances are to be transcribed and analyzed in detail immediately following the assessment, and the sample conversation does not commence until the child is relatively comfortable in the clinical setting.

A number of methods are available for analyzing the samples (Crystal, Fletcher, & Garman, 1976; Lee, 1980; Miller, 1981: Prutting & Kirchner, 1987; Shriberg & Kwiatkowski, 1986; Tyack & Gottsleben, 1974), so you must follow the specific guidelines of the protocol that you select. In addition, some general guidelines seem to apply for most language sampling analyses. For example, in general, the purpose of collecting the sample is to make a representative portion of the child's speech accessible for analysis. Therefore, the child is engaged in a spontaneous, informal conversation under conditions that are believed to elicit a representative sample of the child's language, and measures are taken to preserve the conversation on videotape and, perhaps, audiotape. In order to increase the probability of collecting for analysis a sample that is representative, a number of steps are taken as a matter of routine. These include collecting the sample in a familiar (or at least comfortable) setting, engaging a conversational partner who is familiar to the child (or at least giving the child time to become accustomed to the examiner before engaging in conversation), providing interesting and familiar materials that are age-appropriate and culturally relevant, avoiding all stimuli and materials that either structure the session or limit response options, asking few if any direct questions, avoiding questions to which one already knows the answer, listening carefully to the child, and attempting to look at the conversation from the child's perspective.

The conversation is preserved on video- and/or audiotape so that it can be transcribed according to the format recommended by the selected analysis procedure. Videotape is preferred to audiotape since it maintains the visual as well as the auditory context. However, reel-to-reel audiotaping results in clearer auditory reproduction. Therefore, many professionals recommend using both media. Audio cassette recording also has its advantages in that it can be done less conspicuously than reel-to-reel, and if high-quality tape is used, the auditory reproduction is usually suitable for assessment purposes.

Measures may need to be taken to further preserve contextual cues, especially when a child's intelligibility is compromised. When you are directly involved in collecting the language sample, the objects and events are clear because they occur in context. However, when you are reviewing the tape, even soon after the session, the context may escape your immediate recollection. For that reason, make the effort to add audible comments that will serve to enhance your ability to remember the conversational context at a later time. (For example, repeat what you think the child has said and then comment.) Once recorded, the sample is analyzed according to one of the available formats. All aspects of each dimension of language are of interest in the analysis of the language sample data.

The spontaneous, *expressive language form* is assessed in several steps. First, the most obvious aspect of language form, which is perhaps the least complicated to measure, is the utterance length, called the mean length of utterance (MLU).

When calculating MLU, it is first important to determine whether the sample is truly representative of the child's spontaneous, connected speech (Miller, 1981). In order to be considered representative, the conversation must not contain a high rate of imitative responses (not exceeding 20 percent), frequent self-repetitions, high proportion of answers to questions (not exceeding 30–40 percent), memorized routines (e.g., ABCs, counting, rhymes), or high proportion of conjoined clauses (e.g., clauses joined by *and* or another conjunction). If it is determined that the sample is not representative, no further analysis takes place and the procedure of collecting a spontaneous conversation for analysis must be repeated.

The calculation of the MLU is a simple procedure (Miller, 1981), requiring that one count all morphemes in a selected series of consecutive utterances and then divide by the total number of utterances counted. The result is the average number of morphemes for each of the speaker's utterances, or mean length of utterance (MLU). Guidelines are available for counting morphemes and calculating MLU (Miller, 1981).

$$\text{MLU} = \frac{\text{number of morphemes}}{\text{number of utterances}}$$

Beware that MLU can only be reliably interpreted when it is between 1.01 and 4.49 (Miller, 1981), and that at best, it is only a general indicator of structural development. Once MLU has been calculated, it is possible to calculate an approximate MLU age equivalent for utterance length by using the following formula (Miller, 1981):

Age in months = 11.99 + 7.857 (MLU)

A comparison of the age equivalent to the child's chronological age can be used to partially determine whether language structure is age-appropriate or delayed. However, MLU is never the only determining factor for defining the age-appropriateness of language structure, and calculating MLU is never substituted for a detailed analysis of the spontaneous language sample.

The average number of morphemes that a child uses in each utterance is largely influenced by the number of morphemes in the child's expressive repertoire. This is a mathematical artifact because MLU is based on a count of morphemes in each utterance and therefore is dependent on morphological development. For example, children who do not yet have command of the -*ing* verb ending, regular past-tense -*ed* ending, possessive -*s*, and regular third-person -*s* ending tend to have shorter MLUs than children who do have a command of these morphemes.

An analysis of 14 grammatical morphemes that are spread across Brown's stages II through V+ is suggested (de Villiers & de Villiers, 1973; Miller, 1981) so that a more elaborate (than MLU) structural analysis may be obtained. By making this analysis, mastery level is determined for a number of morphemes. This mastery data, combined with MLU, enables one to define the child's structural language development according to one of Brown's stages, which then permits a detailed analysis of the language structures that are expected at the child's stage of language performance. Specific instructions for accomplishing a complete morphological and syntactic analysis are available (Miller, 1981).

Finally, regarding language form, a language sample can be used to analyze phonological development (Ingram, 1981; Shriberg & Kwiatkowski, 1986; Weiner, 1979). However, if phonological development becomes a matter of concern, it is because speech-sound production is so aberrant that the words and sentences are highly unintelligible. Therefore, it is unlikely that the same language sample used to identify phonological processes is also usable for an accurate analysis of morphology, syntax, and content. The purposes and general procedures of phonological assessment are discussed in the upcoming section on assessing unintelligible children.

Language content is another dimension of language that can be examined by subjecting a transcribed conversation to specific analysis. For language-sample analysis, content is often divided into two parts—referential meaning and relational meaning (de Villiers & de Villiers, 1978).

Referential meaning concerns the one-to-one link between words and the concepts or ideas that they represent. Two methods are used for analyzing referential meaning. The first, the type-token ratio (TTR), measures lexical diversity, or the variety of different words at the expressive command of the child. Basically, the TTR is a ratio calculated as follows (Templin, 1957):

$$\text{TTR} = \frac{\text{number of different words in the sample}}{\text{total number of words in the sample}}$$

That is, in evaluating the language sample for TTR, one first counts all words in the sample. If the same word (e.g., *dog*) occurs more than once in the sample, it is counted each time it occurs. This number becomes the denominator in the TTR equation. Then, the clinician counts each different word that occurs in the sample. For example, if the word *dog* appears five times in the sample, it is only counted once. The number of different words becomes the numerator in the TTR equation.

For children ages 3 through 8 years, the type-token ratio is typically 1:2 (or .5) (Miller, 1981). That is, the total number of words spoken by the child during the language sample is usually about twice the number of different words in the sample. Specific procedures for calculating TTR are available (Miller, 1981).

Semantic field analysis is another way of measuring the relationship between the words and concepts or ideas that they represent. This measure is used to identify the total number of meaning categories and the number of words that are expressed in each meaning category. Completing a semantic field analysis is a complicated process, which is done when the sample is relatively simple or if semantic deficiencies are suspected. The 21 semantic categories used for the analysis are shown in Figure 1–1. Procedures are available for conducting a semantic field analysis (Miller, 1981).

Relational meaning is the other side of language content that can be subjected to analysis by language-sampling procedures. Relational meaning concerns the semantic connections between concepts, words, and sentences (de Villiers & de Villiers, 1978). Three levels of analysis are described (Miller, 1981). They are intrasentencial relations, or relations between the words in a sentence; intersentencial relations, or relations between sentences; and nonlinguistic relations, or relations between the context and the content. Procedures for analyzing relational meaning are available (Miller, 1981).

Language use is the third dimension of language, and parts of the language sample can be used to analyze this dimension as well (Prutting & Kirchner, 1987). The pragmatic protocol (Prutting, 1982) provides a framework for evaluating 30 pragmatic aspects of language as obtained from an observed conversation.

Making Observations.   Finally, as part of the language assessment protocol, observations of language performance are made. Although informal, this part of the assessment can provide some useful information about the practical way in which the person uses language. The observations begin when the child is met in the waiting room, with attention paid to the child's interactions with family members, clinicians, and others.

Observations continue throughout the evaluation, whether or not the child participates in planned activities. When a child does not comply with standardized testing, informal observations of language performance become a critical portion of the assessment protocol. In this case, each and every sentence, social exchange, or attempt at human interaction becomes an essential part of the assessment data and is potentially usable for informally estimating level of function and identifying performance patterns.

Articulation or Phonology Testing.   The testing of speech-sound production is part of every language assessment. Articulation testing is one option for evaluating speech-sound production, and it is selected when the client is relatively easy to understand. The purpose of articulation testing is to identify speech-sound production errors that potentially require intervention or to rule out speech-sound production as a matter of concern for the client.

Conversely, phonological testing is selected for clients whose speech is highly unintelligible. The purpose is to identify phonological processes, or speech-sound production patterns, that are different from those of the standard adult model and have persisted beyond the age at which they normally occur. Processes (simplification patterns) are identified so that they can be targeted in intervention. More information on this topic appears in the section on evaluating unintelligible children, later in this chapter.

Hearing Screening.   A hearing screening is part of every language assessment. Several key frequencies across the audiogram are tested at 20 dB of intensity. With a compliant client, if responses are achieved for all tones, reduced hearing sensitivity can be ruled out.

However, if responses are not achieved for all frequencies and if the client is compliant, then behavioral observations are made and a complete hearing evaluation is recommended. The hearing screening is not used to identify a hearing loss but only to identify individuals who require a complete audiological evaluation, to be conducted by an ASHA-certified audiologist.

Some clients do not comply with the hearing screening. In that case, it is important to document that the hearing screening was attempted and to make plans to prepare the child to participate in an audiological evaluation in the near future. Many very young clients require that **behavioral audiometry** training be incorporated into an intervention plan in order to prepare for an accurate hearing screening or hearing evaluation.

Oral Mechanism Examination.   For every language assessment, an oral mechanism exam is completed in order to rule out or seek to identify any anatomical or physiological causes for the communication disorder. This requires examining the oral mechanism in order to determine whether structure and function are adequate for the production of speech sounds in connected speech. The anatomical structures that must be intact and operational and can be examined by visual inspection include the lips, teeth, tongue, palate, velum, and uvula (Figure 1–3). On visual inspection, examine each structure for symmetry, completeness, lack of tremor or involuntary motion, and lack of malformation. Further, each movable part should move symmetrically, smoothly, precisely, and accurately. Velopharyngeal competence can be informally evaluated by visual inspection and auditory perception. Laryngeal function is evaluated by acoustic perception. Specific testing formats are available (see, e.g., Dworkin & Culatta, 1980). If anatomical or physiological differences are identified, then a medical **referral** is usually in order. This is especially true if a relationship is suspected between the communication disorder and the physical difference.

Additional Testing.   Specific additional testing depends on case history data and the outcome of the conversational speech sample. If the voice is aberrant for the age or gender, then *voice testing* is an important part of the complete assessment. Likewise, if fluency is affected, *fluency testing* becomes consequential to the complete assessment. If one becomes aware that either of these is a matter of concern prior to the language assessment session, voice or fluency testing may be included. However, the presence of a voice or fluency problem often becomes apparent only after the language assessment has begun. In this case, a detailed assessment of fluency or voice may either be done extemporaneously or may become part of the recommendations rather than becoming an ancillary part of the assessment itself.

Modifications to the Protocol for Use with Unintelligible and Taciturn Children

The effective assessment of unintelligible and noncommunicative children often requires a thoughtfully adjusted protocol. Therefore, the protocol suggested in the previous section can be modified to meet the needs of some children. Suggested modifications follow.

Assessing Unintelligible Children.

Language Testing. Undoubtedly, as a speech-language pathologist, you will have the opportunity to assess the language performance of children who are difficult to understand. This situation presents a considerable challenge because when a child's words are not understood, it is difficult, if not impossible, to evaluate many aspects of the expressive side of each of the three language dimensions.

For example, expressive language content cannot be surmised accurately when the phonological or articulatory form of the language is so distorted that the content of the message escapes the listener. Further, with regard to the evaluation of expressive language use, the appropriateness of the language generated by the child is difficult to evaluate if it is carried by an unintelligible emissary. Expressive language content and use are subservient to speech-sound production in this way.

Language form is even more dependent on speech-sound production. That is, when morphemes are omitted or distorted in the context of numerous phonological errors, one may be unable to determine whether the morphological errors are due to a language disorder or a problem with speech-sound production. Further, when considering language form, if the message is unclear as a result of serious speech-sound production errors, then word order, lexical selection, and relations between **lexical items** are also difficult to ascertain, making the evaluation of expressive semantics, morphology, and syntax impracticable.

Therefore, in order to definitively assess all three dimensions of expressive language performance, most of the client's language has to be reasonably comprehensible. For that reason, when a child's language is unintelligible, formally assessing most aspects of expression may be tabled until the necessary levels of intelligibility have been achieved.

Poor intelligibility does not prevent one from obtaining limited information about language expression and extensive information about language comprehension. For example, the mere fact that the child is unintelligible suggests that phonological testing is required and that the possibilities of phonological process disorder, developmental apraxia of speech, and developmental dysarthria should be explored.

For the unintelligible child, a specific assessment objective ought to be to identify the persistent *phonological processes* (simplification patterns) that interfere with intelligible speech-sound production in connected speech. This can be done by a standardized test of phonology (Hodson, 1986; Kahn & Lewis, 1986; Weiner, 1979) or by transcribing and phonologically analyzing the child's utterances in connected speech (Ingram, 1981; Shriberg & Kwiatkowski, 1986). In general, these procedures require the identification of phonetic patterns in words that the child apparently intends to say and the identification of the phonetic patterns actually produced by the child. By this analysis, the phonological patterns that differentiate the child's speech-sound production from the adult model are identified. In addition, phonological testing may include a phonetic inventory (inventory of phonemes used or mastered), syllable structure analysis (frequency of words having a particular syllable structure such as CV, VC, CVC, CCVC, CVCC, and CCVCC), and measures of homonymy (frequencies of similar-sounding word approximations that represent different meanings such as *no/snow* and *no/nose*) in spontaneous speech (Ingram, 1981).

Another aspect of language that is assessed carefully in the unintelligible child is *receptive language*. Although expressive language may not be understood, receptive scores often reveal many clues about the knowledge of language as compared to that of same-age peers. Therefore, another goal of language assessment for the unintelligible child is to completely assess receptive language skills.

Standardized tests may be used to determine whether language reception approaches age expectations. If it does, one may cautiously presume that the apparent expressive language delay is secondary to the speech-sound production difficulties. In this case, a resulting intervention objective is likely to be directed at achieving substantial improvement in intelligibility, followed by a complete reassessment of language expression and comprehension.

If standardized receptive language testing indicates that language comprehension is low compared to that of children in the same age range, then it becomes necessary to conduct a more detailed analysis of language reception to identify specific aberrant characteristics. The results of standardized testing may be used to guide a detailed analysis of receptive skills.

For example, if the standardized tests show that the child has an unaccountable difficulty comprehending certain parts of speech (e.g., adjectives, adverbs, or verbs), certain morphological markers (e.g., -ed endings, -s plural endings, or -ing verb endings), or certain sentence structures (e.g., subject-verb-object, agent-action-object), then the clinician may create a series of informal tasks designed to estimate the client's level of comprehension for each identified area of difficulty.

The specific reception difficulties can be appropriately addressed in intervention even when poor intelligibility interferes with the comprehensive assessment of language expression. As with children who display no comprehension difficulties, substantial improvement in intelligibility is an intervention objective and is followed by a complete reassessment of language expression and reception.

Further, when speech is unintelligible, the oral-mechanism exam becomes critical as the unintelligible speech-sound production may be the result of anatomical or physiological differences. Sluggish or uncoordinated oral movements, velopharyngeal incompetence, palatal insufficiency, or other anatomical or physiological differences may be responsible for the distorted speech-sound production. Therefore, a third goal of the language assessment for the unintelligible child is to search for any evidence of physical differences that may account for speech-sound production errors.

The hearing of the unintelligible child is screened as a part of the assessment, in the same way as it is routinely screened for every child who undergoes a speech-language assessment. Hearing loss may be the cause of unintelligible speech. It is particularly suspect as a cause if receptive language skills are also depressed, nonverbal intelligence approaches or exceeds average, and speech production is characterized by hollow resonance, monopitch, prolonged vowels, and the omission of high-frequency, low-energy consonant sounds. For that reason, a goal of the assessment for an unintelligible child is either to rule out reduced hearing sensitivity or to refer him or her for a complete audiological evaluation.

Voice and fluency can be judged informally when the child's speech is unintelligible. This is done while taking a conversational speech sample at the beginning of the assessment session. If either is judged to be questionable or inappropriate, as is also the case with an intelligible child, specific voice and fluency testing can be attempted immediately or recommended for a subsequent session. Therefore, a final goal of the assessment for an unintelligible speaker is to identify whether voice or fluency testing is indicated.

Assessing Taciturn Children.   When a child's language performance is being assessed and that child hesitates to speak or speaks only rarely, a unique set of challenges is presented. The first objective is to determine whether the child is able to speak and chooses not to or whether the child is simply unable to speak.

If one determines that the child is able to but chooses not to speak, the second objective is to determine the factors that contribute to the child's decision to remain quiet. For example, a child who can speak but does not may opt for silence because of compromised intelligibility, voice disorder, foreign accent, dialect, discomfort in unfamiliar settings, or because nonverbal communication is more effective in achieving desired results. (See the section on elective mutism in Chapter 2.) With a taciturn child who can speak but does not, it is critical to include in the assessment objectives the identification of the child's reason for electing a silent life-style, since the child's rationale definitively influences the proper course of treatment.

If, on the contrary, one determines that the child is *unable* to speak, then it is important to identify the cause of the child's inability to use spoken language for communication and the level of competence for both receptive and expressive language performance. In order to accomplish this objective, refer to the general assessment guidelines that were delineated previously in this chapter.

In some cases, it may be determined that the child is unable to speak and also lacks motivation to learn to use language for social communication. If so, identify the cause of the language delay, the level of language competence, and the social pattern that prevents the child from becoming motivated to learn to use spoken language for communication. In most cases these three factors are interrelated, since a child who has difficulty learning language may consequently lack enthusiasm about social verbal communication.

In addition to these specific language assessment objectives, when assessing the language abilities of taciturn children it is important to include testing in each of the following areas: (1) expressive and receptive language performance with regard to content, form, and use, (2) examination of the oral mechanism to identify any physical cause for difficulty with learning spoken language, (3) hearing screening to identify or rule out the need for an audiological evaluation, (4) articulation testing for those whose speech production is somewhat intelligible, (5) phonological testing for those whose speech production is highly unintelligible, and (6) observations of voice and fluency to determine whether further voice or fluency testing is needed. Often, with taciturn children, some of these assessment objectives must be tabled with the intent of gathering more information at the onset of the intervention program.

Scoring Tests and Interpreting Results

When the interview, testing, and observations are completed, a primary objective is to organize and interpret all the information that has been amassed. Scoring and interpreting tests is a significant part of meeting this goal.

When scoring and interpreting standardized tests, the objectives are to (1) accurately and quantifiably compare the child's performance to age-matched peers for a variety of expressive and receptive language activities, (2) correctly identify specific areas of strength and weakness, and (3) make solid recommendations for language intervention, if appropriate. With these purposes in mind, carefully score the tests, abiding by the instructions printed in the manual and using the manual as a guide for interpreting test results. Additionally, in order to ensure that the standardized test data remains a part of the client's permanent record, take care to check that all identifying information has been provided in the appropriate spaces on the test form.

Informal tests and observations can be scored and interpreted as well. In order to do this, first identify the exact behavior that you wish to observe. Examples of observable behaviors include using speech to make requests, combining words to make short sentences, and amount of time spent in social interchange whether verbal or nonverbal. Then, during the session, either count the number of times that each behavior occurred or measure the amount of time that the child spent engaged in the behavior of interest. If appropriate, percentages or frequency counts are calculated. It is then possible to use this information to informally verify the mastery of identified behaviors so that a performance level may be cautiously estimated for the child.

Summarizing the Results

Once the tests and observations have been scored and interpreted, you should have a clear understanding of exactly how the client's language behavior is different from peers and some ideas as to what must change in order for the behavior to be brought closer to age expectations. In summarizing what has been accomplished in the assessment, answer each of the following questions: (1) Does a language disorder exist? (2) If so, what are the exact characteristics of the language disorder and what can be done to improve the client's language performance? (3) If a language disorder is not identified, what prompted the parents to request a language assessment and what can be done to reduce, eliminate, or otherwise address their concerns?

Communicating the Assessment Outcome to Client and Family

The closing interview is used to communicate the outcome of the language assessment to the parents. In general, the same guidelines apply as for the opening interview. However, the purpose of the closing interview is *not* to gather information (unless questions emerge through the assessment activities), but to address the concerns that the parents expressed during the opening interview and to share the findings of the assessment session.

Begin the closing interview by reviewing concerns that the parents have expressed about the child's communication pattern. Then review the tests administered, including each test's overall purpose and the child's performance. Finally, share the summary of findings. The parents have a right to know whether a language disorder has been identified, the characteristics of the language disorder, and the resulting recommendations. If a language disorder was not identified, they also have right to know how that was determined, why their concerns about language are unsubstantiated, and what can be done about the concerns that they expressed.

Before leaving the center, the parents are given the occasion to ask any questions. The end of the closing interview is an excellent time to provide them with that opportunity.

WRITING THE ASSESSMENT REPORT

Upon completing the assessment, begin writing the assessment report immediately. The recollection of the events and of the client's performance is best if pen is put to paper on the same day as the assessment is managed.

Report Writing

In approaching the issue of professional report writing, it is important to mention the report's fundamental purposes. As a student clinician, it may seem that the report is written because it is a **practicum** requirement. Although report writing *is* a requirement of practicum, the reason for writing the report is unrelated to whether the clinician is enrolled in practicum, as reports are required at every level of experience in the profession of speech-language pathology. Instead, the report is written because the significant background information and the procedures and findings of the assessment must be documented in an accurate, concise, clear, complete, orderly, and purposeful way. If you write reports that accomplish these objectives, the reports are useful to you, the client, **third-party payers**, other members of the medical and professional community, and members of your own profession who follow you in serving the client.

Accuracy. Writing accurate reports includes verifying any significant background information and faithfully representing the procedures used and behaviors observed during the assessment. Accuracy is always enhanced by selecting the most appropriate words to document all that is reported.

Always remember that the report goes out over your signature and that if it contains inaccuracies, your reputation will suffer. Therefore, report only what happened during the assessment, not what might have happened or what you wish had happened.

Word choices influence accuracy. One particular word selection error that is often committed by students is the use of the words *can* and *able* when, in fact, ability is difficult to verify by observation, especially when one says that the child is *not* able to do something. *Cannot, could not, is not able*, and *does not have the ability* are all potentially inaccurate word choices because the child may very well be able to do something but chooses not to. For the record, it is more accurate to describe exactly what the child does or does not do, leaving out the question of whether the child has the ability.

Brevity. Writing concise reports is important because the length of the report is often the factor that determines whether the report is read by professionals who receive it. In my general experience, physicians rarely have time to read any report that exceeds two or three pages. Insurance companies and other professionals may be somewhat more lenient, but no one is apt to read an excessively long report.

If what you write deserves to be read, make every effort to keep it short. Weigh your words carefully, omitting all unnecessary verbiage and insignificant details. Say what you have to say one time and in the most appropriate part of the report. Reports written by new clinicians are often lengthy because information is repeated unnecessarily. This is usually done if the clinician is unsure of exactly where the information belongs in the report. Upon careful proofreading, if you find that you repeat yourself, evaluate the topic carefully and decide on the one place to report each fact.

Clarity. Regardless of how accurate and concise the report, it must also be clear so that the people who read it can understand exactly what has happened and what is known about the client. This requires that you be specific, use impeccable grammar, include significant details, complete each topic before moving on to the next, make use of paragraph divisions, and select the most meaningful words to represent the concepts you wish to express. You should also define medical and professional terms. A person reading the report should not have to refer to a medical dictionary or handbook of speech-language pathology in order to understand the conditions described therein.

Clarity is further enhanced by choosing a tense and sticking to it consistently throughout the report, with only a few, meaningful exceptions. Tense switching causes confusions that are difficult for the reader to resolve. As a general rule, use the past tense for everything that has already taken place and the present tense for describing current status. Avoid the future tense, except in the **prognosis** and recommendations sections, and in general, avoid the past-tense modals (e.g., *would, could, should*).

Furthermore, a part of clarity is legibility. All reports should be typed or word-processed so that the print is easily read.

Completeness. Complete reports require including all significant details. To determine whether a particular detail is significant, evaluate whether it influences the assessment findings or recommendations. If it does, include it; if not, leave it out.

Organization.   Well-organized reports require a logical order. Using a pre-determined format is essential to producing orderly reports. A sample assessment report format is found in Appendix 3–6. In addition, within each section of the format, a chronological or sequential pattern is helpful. Furthermore, organization is facilitated when each topic is covered completely in one place and not revisited throughout the document.

Rationale.   Writing purposeful reports requires including a rationale for each clinical decision recorded in the report. Clinical decisions reported in assessment reports include the selection of specific tests, assigning diagnosis, determining prognosis, and making recommendations.

Every clinical decision has a rationale behind it. For example, you choose to administer certain tests because you believe they are able to provide needed information. The fact that the supervisor told you to give a particular test and that the test is the only one that you know how to administer are not reasonable rationales. In making independent clinical decisions, your thinking must go far beyond that. If you do not know why the supervisor suggested the test, find out why and document the rationale. If a test is needed that you have not given previously, learn how to give it and know why it is recommended as a suitable choice for the particular assessment.

The same applies to all diagnoses, prognoses, and recommendations. None of these decisions are made without weighing evidence such as background information, test scores, and observed patterns of behavior. Consequently, you should always provide the reader with the evidence.

Parts of the Report

A sample report format is provided in Appendix 3–6. Refer to it for an outline of the parts that are typically included in an assessment report.

Identifying Information.   The first part of most assessment reports, called the identifying information, provides basic information about the client. At the very least it includes the name, address, and phone number of the client; names of parents or guardians; client identification number; languages or dialects; referral source, date of report; date of assessment; and the names and qualifications of all students and professionals responsible for managing the case.

Statement of the Problem.   The statement of the problem usually appears near the beginning of the report. It is typically a brief quote taken from the case history intake form or parent interview, which explains the communication concern as expressed by those requesting the assessment. The source of the statement is then documented.

Background Information.   Significant background information is also reported near the beginning of the report. This data is taken from the case history intake form and parent interview, as well as from records received from other professionals who have served the child. Always document the source of any information not learned through testing and clinical observations (e.g., "According to the case history intake form completed by the parent . . . ," or "Dr. Garcia's medical report, dated 12/1/95, states . . .").

When including background information, it is important to pay attention to the fact that only *significant* background information is appropriately supplied in the report. That means that only information that directly impacts the findings or recommendations is to be included in the report as part of the background. All other information remains part of the record but is not necessarily included in the report.

Testing Procedures and Results.   The next section of the report focuses on testing procedures and results. This is where one documents the tests selected, rationale for selecting the tests, and outcome of the testing procedures. The bulk of the assessment report comprises this section, which is divided into a number of subsections that include (1) language testing, (2) articulation or phonology testing, (3) oral mechanism examination, (4) hearing screening, and (5) ancillary testing.

Behavioral Observations/Clinical Impressions.   The behavioral observations and clinical impressions section typically follows. It is here that you report any pertinent information learned through informal procedures such as observation and interaction.

Summary of Findings.   The summary of findings is where you briefly summarize what you learned about the client during the assessment. Incorporate only the most salient data from the standardized and informal findings.

Diagnosis.   The diagnosis is a very brief statement that describes the client's condition with regard to language performance only. The diagnosis is always backed up with evidence, or a rationale.

For example, the diagnosis may be "moderately delayed language secondary to fetal alcohol syndrome (FAS)." The rationale for this diagnosis states how you know that language is moderately delayed, and it may include a brief summary of standardized tests or observations that led to determining the diagnosis of moderate language delay. The rationale also includes how you know that the child has FAS, which is most likely by way of parental report or medical records.

Diagnoses of conditions that are indirectly related to speech-language status may sometimes be reported as well. Examples include, but are not limited to, a diagnosis of mental retardation or emotional disability, and physical or medical condition. If these types of diagnoses are included in the report, the appropriate diagnosing professional is cited as the source, along with a rationale for including this information in the language assessment report.

Prognosis.   A prognostic statement is a statement of opinion regarding whether the client is likely to benefit from intervention. It is not a statement of whether the person will eventually achieve age-appropriate skills and it is not a guarantee of any kind, as we cannot, and do not, guarantee our services. However, when a person is enrolled in intervention, the clinician is obligated to consider whether there is reasonable evidence to support potential benefit from such services. If the evidence indicates that benefits are likely to be gained by the client, then intervention is offered as an option. However, if the evidence is uncertain, the client has a right to know that the services may not achieve the desired results. Further, if the evidence suggests that the client is unlikely to benefit from intervention, enrolling that person in an intervention program is unethical, regardless of who referred the client for services.

For these reasons, speech-language pathologists are required to prognosticate. Further, we must provide the evidence, or rationale, on which the prognosis is based. Some variables that may be considered when weighing the evidence include motivation, willingness to participate in the program, family involvement, room for improvement, attendance patterns, complicating medical or social conditions, personal emotional stability, and progress in the intervention so far.

Clients may be divided into four prognostic categories. They are (1) clients who are likely to benefit from intervention (good prognosis), (2) clients who may benefit from intervention but present some variables that may interfere with progress (fair prognosis), (3) clients for whom a prognosis cannot be determined (uncertain or guarded prognosis), and (4) clients who are not likely to benefit from intervention (poor prognosis).

Recommendations.   The recommendations are usually the last content area included in the report, and they appear in list form so that they can be scanned with ease. The purposes of the recommendations section are to (1) bring closure to the assessment, (2) initiate a plan for addressing the identified communication problems, and (3) provide the next professional who meets the client with a direction in which to proceed.

The recommendations always include a statement indicating whether intervention is recommended. This decision is based on the prognosis, as discussed in the previous section. For example, for individuals in the first prognostic category, it is judged that the person is likely to benefit from intervention, so intervention is recommended.

For individuals in the second and third prognostic categories, some factors indicate that improvement may be expected as a result of intervention while other factors indicate that some variables are likely to interfere with progress. Since a definitive prognosis *cannot* be determined for individuals in these categories, intervention is reasonably recommended on a trial basis, or the parents may be given the option to make a decision based on available evidence as it is presented to them.

For individuals in the fourth prognostic category, since evidence suggests that intervention is not likely to benefit the client, intervention is not recommended. In fact, it is unethical to recommend intervention under such circumstances. However, when stating the evidence and reporting that intervention is not recommended, it is sensible to make a statement inviting the parents to seek a reassessment in the event that circumstances change.

The recommendation for or against initiating an intervention program is based on whether the evidence indicates that intervention is likely to benefit the client. It must never be based on whether there is room in the caseload for the client to receive services. Clients have the right to know whether they need services, regardless of whether the center that provided the assessment is able to follow through on the recommendation. If there is no room in the caseload, individuals who need services ethically must be referred to outside agencies so that their needs can be met.

Moreover, a recommendation for intervention is not based on whether someone has already assigned that person to receive services. Assignments for intervention are not ethically made by uncertified personnel, who may assign people to receive services without considering clinical evidence or without credentials qualifying them to make such a decision. Only a certified speech-language pathologist who has recently evaluated the client is equipped to recommend intervention. In contrast, secretaries, school principals, special education coordinators, rehabilitation directors, department heads and other administrators, and even those who hold political office are not authorized to make that decision unless they hold the appropriate certificate of clinical competence and have recently evaluated the client.

In addition to making a recommendation with regard to whether intervention is warranted, the recommendations may also include a few suggestions for specific intervention objectives. If these are included, the evidence leading up to the objectives is included as well. For example, if behavioral audiometry is recommended as a part of the intervention program in order to prepare the child to participate in an audiological screening, then one does not simply state that behavioral audiometry is recommended. The reason behind the recommendation is also stated, which in this example is to prepare for accomplishing the objective of a hearing screening.

Referrals may also be a part of the recommendations section. Any time an assessment indicates that the client needs further testing that is not incorporated in the intervention program, a referral to an outside professional is expedient. Some potential referrals include recommendations for educational testing, psychological testing, medical examination, or audiological examination.

Finally, questions that remain unanswered may be listed in the recommendations section. Because of time limitations or human factors, the interview and testing may not completely answer all questions about the child's language performance. Usually few, if any, questions remain, and they may be listed in the recommendations as issues to be addressed in the immediate future.

Signature Lines.   The very last section to appear on the assessment report displays the dated signatures and credentials of all professionals and students who participated in the assessment and in the preparation of the report. The signatures are not inscribed on a report until all revisions have been finalized. By placing your signature on the line, you certify that the information is true to the best of your knowledge and that you agree to the findings and recommendations contained therein.

Dissemination of the Report.   Clinical reports are ready for dissemination within a reasonable time after completion of the clinical service. Some centers require that reports be ready within 1 working day of completing the service, while others allow up to 10 or 15 working days.

When ready for dissemination, the completed report becomes part of the client's permanent file at the agency and a copy is often mailed to the parents as a matter of record. Copies of the report are sent to outside agencies upon request *only* if a signed authorization to release information is obtained from the parents and filed in the permanent record.

Upon completion of the assessment and assessment report, intervention is the next step for many clients. Therefore, the chapter that follows begins by explaining how assessment information may be used to plan an intervention program.

REFERENCES

Crystal, D., Fletcher, P., & Garman, M. (1976). *The grammatical analysis of language disability: A procedure for assessment and remediation.* New York: Elsevier–North Holland.

de Villiers, J., & de Villiers, P. (1973). A cross-sectional study of the acquisition of grammatical morphemes in child speech. *Journal of Psycholinguistic Research, 2,* 267–68.

de Villiers, J., & de Villiers, P. (1978). *Language acquisition.* Cambridge, MA: Harvard University Press.

Dworkin, J. P., & Culatta, R. A. (1980). *Dworkin-Culatta oral mechanism examination.* Nicholasville, KY: Edgewood Press.

Fluharty, N. (1974). Fluharty screening test for preschool children. *Journal of Speech and Hearing Disorders, 1,* 75–88.

Hodson, B. W. (1986). *The assessment of phonological processes*: Danville, IL: Interstate.

Ingram, D. (1981). *Procedures of the phonological analysis of children's language.* Baltimore, MD: University Park Press.

Kahn, L., & Lewis, N. (1986). *Phonological analysis.* Circle Pines, MN: American Guidance Service.

Lee, L. L. (1980). *Developmental sentence analysis: A grammatical assessment procedure for speech and language clinicians.* Evanston, IL: Northwestern University Press.

Miller, J. F. (1981). *Assessing language production in children: Experimental procedures.* Austin, TX: Pro-Ed.

Prutting, C. A. (1982). Observational protocol for pragmatic behaviors [Clinic Manual]. Developed for the University of California Speech and Hearing Clinic at Santa Barbara.

Prutting, C. A., & Kirchner, D. M. (1987). A clinical appraisal of the pragmatic aspects of language. *Journal of Speech and Hearing Disorders, 52,* 105–19.

Shriberg, L. D., & Kwiatkowski, J. (1986). *Natural process analysis (NPA): A procedure for phonological analysis of continuous speech samples.* New York: Macmillan.

Templin, M. C. (1957). *Certain language skills in children: Their development and interrelationships.* Child Welfare Monograph, 26. Minneapolis: University of Minnesota Press.

Texas Department of Health. (1993). *Davis observation checklist for Texas.* Austin: Texas Bureau of Maternal & Child Health.

Tyack, D., & Gottsleben, R. (1974). *Language sampling, analysis and training.* Palo Alto, CA: Consulting Psychologists Press.

Weiner, F. F. (1979). *Phonological process analysis.* Baltimore, MD: University Park Press.

STUDY GUIDE 3

1. What does the acronym ASHA stand for?
2. How does a speech-language pathologist know the minimum expectations for professional conduct?
3. What are some potential consequences for failure to comply with ASHA's Code of Ethics?
4. To whom should you report suspected violations of the Code of Ethics?
5. To whom does the Code of Ethics apply?
6. What are the only two circumstances that call for the unauthorized sharing of information about a client?
7. What are the purposes of a speech-language screening?
8. What is the procedure to follow if a child performs below age expectations on a speech-language screening?
9. For what reasons do parents usually initiate a speech-language assessment?
10. What is the purpose of the form called "Agreement to Receive Services"?

11. What is the purpose of obtaining written authorization to seek and release information?
12. Once all forms have been completed and returned to the center, describe the procedures that you follow in order to prepare to manage the child's language assessment.
13. What should you do if you receive a case history intake form that is incomplete or unclear?
14. What are the fundamental objectives of an assessment?
15. More specifically, exactly what is accomplished by the language assessment session?
16. What are the purposes of the assessment interview?
17. During the interview, which questions are asked as a matter of routine, and why?
18. What introductory procedures can you follow to facilitate a smooth introduction to the assessment session?
19. What do you do if your client is excessively late for an assessment session?
20. Considering the opening interview, describe the difference between asking your questions and collecting the information that the questions seek to address.
21. What question might facilitate the smooth initiation of the opening interview?
22. As a clinician, how might you handle each of the following human factors during an interview?
    a.   excessive anxiety on the part of the parent
    b.   a reluctant informant
    c.   excessive emotion on the part of the parent
    d.   frequent off-topic conversation
    e.   bids for taking sides in an argument
23. What can you do to facilitate the transition from the interview to the testing format?
24. What might you do if a child refuses to separate from the parents? Why do you choose that course of action?
25. How is rapport established with the child?
26. What clinical objective can be accomplished while building rapport?
27. What type of testing may be introduced at the beginning of the session?
28. Describe the type of feedback that is most likely to encourage a child to continue to respond to the requirements of testing.
29. What can you do to facilitate cooperation?
30. List some behavioral parameters that are observed during an assessment.
31. List and describe the parts of the language assessment.
32. For each part of the assessment protocol, list the specific objectives and how they may be accomplished.
33. Differentiate between a language sample and a conversational speech sample.

34. Differentiate between standardized and informal language testing.
35. What are the general purposes for collecting a language sample?
36. What measures are taken to ensure that the language sample is representative of the child's speech?
37. What is done with language sample data if it is determined to not be representative?
38. What is MLU and how is it calculated?
39. What type of information is gained from calculating MLU? What are the limitations of MLU?
40. For what purpose is MLU never used?
41. When a language sample is used to evaluate phonological development, what types of analysis are usually impractical?
42. What is TTR and how is it measured?
43. What information is obtained from measuring TTR?
44. Describe the purposes of conducting a semantic field analysis.
45. Describe how a language sample can be used to evaluate pragmatics.
46. Differentiate between the type of client for whom articulation testing is appropriate and the type of client for whom phonological testing is appropriate.
47. Describe the purposes of a hearing screening.
48. Describe the purposes of an oral mechanism examination.
49. Describe the objectives and procedures used to guide a language assessment when a child is unintelligible.
50. Describe the objectives used to guide a language assessment when a child is taciturn.
51. What are the fundamental objectives for scoring and interpreting tests?
52. What questions are answered when summarizing the accomplishments of an assessment session?
53. Exactly what is accomplished during the closing interview of an assessment?
54. What are the fundamental purposes of the assessment report?
55. What is a clinical decision? What is a rationale? Why should all clinical decisions be substantiated by a rationale?
56. What is a prognostic statement and why is it included in the assessment report?
57. Describe the four prognostic categories and how they influence whether intervention is recommended.
58. In addition to intervention, what types of recommendations may be included in the report?
59. Who signs the assessment report and when is the report signed? What do the signatures at the bottom of the report mean?
60. What becomes of the assessment report once it has been approved and signed?

CHAPTER 4

An Introduction to Language Intervention

Guidelines for a Client-Centered Approach

LEARNING OBJECTIVES

At the conclusion of this chapter, you should be prepared to:

- Plan a language intervention program;
- Implement a language intervention plan;
- Regularly evaluate progress achieved in language intervention;
- Determine when discharge from language intervention is appropriate and plan applicable follow-up procedures.

INTRODUCTION

In the profession of speech-language pathology, a significant portion of time is spent planning and administering intervention programs. This is true for most speech-language pathologists, including those in private practice, public and private schools, hospitals, rehabilitation agencies, university clinics, and for those connected with special projects.

Career choices that do *not* traditionally require a great deal of applied intervention are occupied by fewer people, and they may include the positions of researcher, administrator, academician, and diagnostician. However, even diagnosticians are often intimately involved in planning intervention. Further, academicians and administrators are most effective if they are experienced service providers who are capable of planning and implementing intervention. Moreover, the researcher's ability to identify and solve practical problems faced by clinicians is greatly enhanced by firsthand knowledge and experience with identifying and treating individuals having communication disorders. Therefore, the content of this chapter is critical to every student who plans a career in the profession of speech-language pathology, regardless of any intention to specialize.

Enhancing language development in children is a distinguished goal. Language is a domain that enables people to make their needs and desires known, establish meaningful relationships, and succeed academically. Without adequate language skills, quality of life is almost invariably compromised. For that reason, the changes that a competent speech-language pathologist can facilitate in a young child's life and in the lives of that child's family members are often profound. Although our efforts may at times go unrecognized, it is important to take satisfaction in knowing that our contributions usually can, and do, make a difference.

Language intervention, like assessment, is a clinical service, so similar attention is paid to ethics and confidentiality. These issues are covered in detail in Chapter 3, and although not repeated here, they apply equally. Accordingly, refer to the annual March issue of *ASHA* magazine for a copy of ASHA's current Code of Ethics. If you have not done so already, read it and make a decision to comply, both in intent and in practice. Also review the section in Chapter 3 of this volume, called "Guidelines for Clinical Practice," for some elaboration on ethics, qualifications for service delivery, and the confidential clinical relationship.

PLANNING LANGUAGE INTERVENTION

Once a language assessment has been completed, a speech-language pathologist often determines that an individual child uses language that is different from, but not exceeding, age expectations. In other words, according to definition (Chapter 2), the tested child is found to have a language disorder. If that is the case, language intervention is often one of the recommendations resulting from assessment. Further, as described in Chapter 3, a productive assessment identifies some general and some very specific areas of strength and weakness. This general and specific information is extremely useful in guiding the initial planning for language intervention.

All recommendations and critical information about strengths and weaknesses should appear in the language assessment report. Although the final report may not be available at the time intervention begins, the information contained therein is accessible through communication with the diagnosing clinician. It is important to obtain this information prior to initiating any intervention program.

Following Up on Recommendations

When beginning to plan intervention, one first reviews the assessment report in order to identify any recommendations that require follow-up. In addition to the recommendation for language intervention, one may find that further testing is advised, that a referral was made to an outside service provider (e.g., audiologist, physician, physical therapist, psychologist), or specific **long-term objectives** have been identified by the person conducting the assessment. Therefore, prior to beginning to plan an intervention program, the managing clinician first develops a plan for following up on the existing set of recommendations.

Using General Assessment Data

Once the clinician has identified the recommendations and is in the process of planning follow-up, the assessment report is carefully reviewed so that the initial sessions of the intervention program can be planned. In general, the reported assessment results enable one to specify the dimensions of language that are disturbed. These may include any of the dimensional disturbances described in Chapter 2. Further, in a general way, the assessment report provides enough information to define the language disorder in terms of the balance between performance criteria in both comprehension and production.

For demonstration purposes, an example follows which will be referenced throughout the chapter. This example is presented for illustration only and is *not* to be interpreted as a model program. The sample procedures are only presented in order to demonstrate how the explicitly stated principles may be interpreted and applied. In order to facilitate a separation of the specific example from the generic principles, the example appears in italics throughout the chapter.

By using the general assessment data the disturbed dimensions of language are identified, and perhaps some details are described in a limited way. *For the example, assume that the child in the example is male, that his name is*

John, and that he is 52 months of age (4 years, 4 months). Furthermore, suppose that standardized testing (specifically, the standardized test called Test of Language Development–Primary, *or the* TOLD-P*) identified the language disturbance as generally characterized by a delay in expressive vocabulary (a disturbance of the content-form interaction). Table 4–1 summarizes the results of John's sample language assessment.*

Using Specific Assessment Data

In addition to an identification of the general dimensional disturbances, the successful assessment session produces some very tangible evidence about discrete performances, and this information is used to definitively describe the characteristics of the language disorder. It is this distinct information that is useful for planning the intervention program.

In the example (Table 4–1), since a standardized test indicates low performance in expressive vocabulary, more specific testing follows. For John, a type-token ratio (TTR) is calculated, which shows his vocabulary lacks diversity (Table 4–1). (TTR is described in Chapter 3.) Further, a semantic field analysis is then applied to determine those semantic categories (types of words) used by John and those lacking in his spontaneous conversation. (See Figure 1–1 for complete descriptions of semantic categories, and see Chapter 3 for a description of the semantic field analysis.)

The semantic field analysis for this sample client (Table 4–1) shows that words are used consistently to represent existence, recurrence, nonexistence-disappearance, rejection, denial, and attribution. It also shows that words are used to represent first-person possession but not second- and third-person possession, and rarely to indicate locative action, action, or locative state. Furthermore, no additional semantic categories are observed in the child's spontaneous speech.

Moreover, specific idiosyncratic needs of the child that may impact the course of intervention are identified by the language assessment. In many cases these needs relate to the etiology of the language disorder, age and sociability of the child, cognitive level, social and cultural orientations, family support, and concomitant conditions that directly or indirectly impact communication development and intervention. *For the sake of the example, assume that the etiology of the language disorder is unclear, intelligence is within normal limits, social skills are age-appropriate, family support is reasonable, and the child resides in the Midwest and identifies with a segment of Euro-American culture. In addition, the child is diagnosed as having attention deficit disorder in addition to the language delay (Table 4–1).*

Using all this information, a clinician establishes goals that begin to address the idiosyncratic needs of the child. From the evidence, the intervention program of the example case logically begins by addressing those aspects of language that are used inconsistently and those that are likely to interfere with

Table 4-1. Clinical Example

Summary of Assessment Results

Client's Name:	John
Client's Age:	52 months (4 years, 4 months)
Diagnosis:	Expressive language delay, primarily limited to delayed expressive vocabulary (a content-form interaction). This was determined by standardized testing, type-token ratio, and semantic field analysis.
Etiology:	Uncertain
Concomitant Symptoms:	Attention Deficit Disorder (ADD)

Standardized Test Results:	*Subtest*	*Standard Score*	*Percentile*
	Picture Vocabulary	10	50
	Oral Vocabulary	5°	5°
	Grammatic Understanding	10	50
	Sentence Imitation	9	37
	Grammatic Completion	8	25
	Word Discrimination	11	63
	Word Articulation	12	75
Informal Test Results:	*Type-token ratio* (TTR) of .32 indicates that vocabulary lacks diversity.		

Semantic field analysis indicates: Semantic categories used consistently are existence, recurrence, nonexistence-disappearance, rejection, denial, and attribution.

Semantic categories used inconsistently are possession (used to represent first-person possession, but not second- and third-person), locative action, action, and locative state.

Semantic categories not used at all are state, quantity, notice, dative, additive, temporal, causal, adversative, epistemic, specification, and communication.

(See Figure 1–1 for description of semantic categories.)

°Significantly below age expectations.

the client's ability to benefit from intervention and/or succeed academically. Those aspects of language that are used consistently are not addressed because apparently they have been mastered by the child. Those aspects of language that are not used at all are not addressed directly because the child may not be developmentally ready to comprehend and use them. (However, they may be brought to the child's immediate attention in preparation for later work.)

It is, however, the aspects of language that are used inconsistently that are likely to be chosen as targets (1) because they have *not* yet been mastered, and (2) because inconsistent use suggests that the child is somewhat aware of them and therefore may be developmentally ready to begin to include them in the expressive repertoire. *More specifically, with reference to the example, the semantic categories of possession, locative action, action, and locative state are selected to be addressed in intervention because these are the categories that are used inconsistently. (See Figure 4–1.)*

In addition, the example intervention program addresses the sample child's need to learn to focus attention and manage distractions (Table 4–1). This direction is pursued in an attempt to provide the child with strategies to compensate for the concomitant condition of attention deficit disorder because it is likely to impede clinical intervention and eventually academic progress. By learning to make the most of incoming stimuli, language acquisition can be facilitated, potential efficiency of language intervention is increased, and preparations are made to improve the likelihood of academic success.

Writing Language Intervention Objectives

Once you have determined what you want to accomplish in intervention and why, you are ready to begin writing the intervention objectives. Long-term

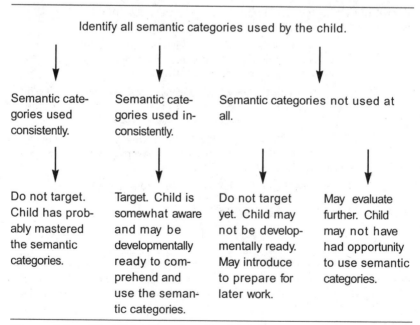

Figure 4-1. Identifying lexical targets through semantic field analysis.

and **short-term objectives** are both critical parts of the process of planning language intervention, so they are both discussed below.

Long-Term Objectives. Long-term objectives are written first in order to define the expected communication status of the client at the time of **discharge**. For that reason long-term objectives are often called terminal objectives or **discharge objectives**. Long-term objectives are usually somewhat general and are established by examining the overall findings of the assessment.

In the example, the child is identified as having attention deficit disorder and a delay in expressive vocabulary (an aspect of language content-form interaction). Assuming that no cognitive barriers prevent, the accomplishments that are rightly expected at discharge, are (1) achievement of age-appropriate expressive and receptive vocabulary, (2) managing distractions so that they do not interfere with performance, and (3) focusing attention to complete tasks (Table 4–2).

Exactly how these long-term objectives are documented is important. Although somewhat general, the written long-term objectives must be clear to anyone who has access to them, including parents, teachers, social workers, psychologists, physicians, audiologists, ancillary professionals, and other speech-language pathologists. The reason why the objectives must be clear to individuals outside the profession is that their input is often very valuable in evaluating progress toward achieving the objectives, and also because those who care enough to read the written intervention plan deserve to understand what it says.

The reason the objectives must be absolutely clear to other members of the profession of speech-language pathology is because the case may be picked up by someone else with little or no advance notice, and the next professional who sees the client may need to apply the objectives with minimal opportunity for detailed discussion. Family emergencies, medical emergencies, sudden or serious illness, and change of employment are all reasons that may result in an abrupt change of clinician, requiring that an unfamiliar speech-language pathologist implement the objectives you write.

Table 4-2. Clinical Example

Expected Status at Time of Discharge

Problem Identified	Expected Intervention Outcome
Delayed language, specifically expressive vocabulary.	Achievement of age-appropriate expressive vocabulary.
Attention deficit disorder.	(1) Focusing attention to complete tasks.
	(2) Managing distractions so that they do not interfere with performance.

It is often the case that unclear written objectives are not completely understood by the one who writes them. That is how they come to be written in a way that is not lucidly clear to others. For that reason, it is essential that the clinician have a firm grasp of what is to be accomplished in intervention before committing these intentions to paper.

In order to be clear, the long-term objectives explicitly state (1) who (2) will do what, (3) to what degree of mastery and (4) under what circumstances. *Consequently, a primary long-term objective for the client in the example may read something like this: "John will perform within age expectations on the Oral Vocabulary subtest of the TOLD-P (given at assessment) and will achieve a TTR of 0.5 as measured by a spontaneous language sample." (See Table 4–3.)*

In addition to being clear, an objective must be associated with a clearly stated rationale, the rationale being the tangible evidence on which the objective is based. *For the example, the evidence is the standardized test results that led to the identification of a delay in expressive vocabulary. Thus, the stated rationale in the example may be "because standardized testing and TTR indicate delayed performance in language content-form and the delay is specifically characterized by an expressive vocabulary that lacks diversity." (See Table 4–3.)*

Short-Term Objectives.   Short-term objectives clearly define the immediate steps to be achieved while working toward a particular long-term objective. These are taken from the more specific assessment data that is used

Table 4-3.   Clinical Example

Anatomy of a Long-Term Objective

Long-Term Objectives Explicitly Stated	A Long-Term Objective for the Example	
	(Part I)	*(Part II)*
(1) Who?	John	
(2) Will do what?	will perform	will achieve
(3) To what degree of mastery?	within age expectations	TTR of .5
(4) Under what circumstances?	on the Oral Vocabulary subtest of the TOLD-P	as measured by a spontaneous sample
(5) Why? (Rationale)	because standardized testing indicated delayed performance in the interactions between language content and form, specifically characterized by an expressive vocabulary that lacks diversity.	

Table 4-4. Clinical Example

Baseline Frequency of Occurrence of the Proposed Targets When Obligated by Context

Proposed Target		Baseline Frequency
A	Second-person possessive production	30%
B	Third-person possessive production	30%
C	Locative action production	35%
D	Action production	35%
E	Locative state production	20%

to define the particular weaknesses of the child. *In the example, the specific testing includes a semantic field analysis which identifies four semantic categories that the child uses inconsistently. Thus the short-term goals seek to facilitate the emergence of these apparently deficient semantic categories.*

Before actually beginning to write the short-term objectives, it is important to obtain **quantified** baseline data describing performance in the target area. *Since in the example we wish to facilitate the emergence of words that represent second- and third-person possession, locative action, action, and locative state, baseline data is collected to estimate the frequency of occurrence of these targets when obligated by context.*

For example, since we are interested in targeting words that represent third-person possessives (his, hers, her, their, Joe's, Mary's), we obtain a baseline for expression of the semantic category by associating items with a particular person, puppet, or doll, and then asking the child to identify to whom each item belongs (e.g., "Whose boat is this?" "Whose book is this?").

For the sake of the example, assume baseline data indicates that the child produces 3 of 10 expressive opportunities (30 percent) for that particular target. The procedure is repeated for all proposed targets (Table 4–4).

As with long-term objectives, the short-term objectives follow the format of defining exactly (1) who (2) will do what, (3) with what degree of mastery and (4) under what circumstances (Table 4–5). The short-term objectives are very specific. Each can be accomplished within a few weeks or months and, if accomplished, will bring the client closer to reaching one of the discharge objectives (Table 4–2). Further, as with long-term objectives, a rationale clearly defines the evidence on which the objective is based (Table 4–5). The following set of short-term objectives corresponds to the long-term objective in the example.

Table 4-5.   Clinical Example

Anatomy of a Short-Term Objective

Who	Will Do What	To What Degree of Mastery	Under What Circumstances	Why
(A) John	will use words representing second-person possessive	for 8 of 10 opportunities	in a spontaneous conversation.	This objective was selected as a result of semantic field analysis and standardized testing.
(B) John	will use words representing third-person possessive	for 8 of 10 opportunities	in a spontaneous conversation.	This objective was selected as a result of semantic field analysis and standardized testing.
(C) John	will use words representing locative action	for 8 of 10 opportunities	in a spontaneous conversation.	This objective was selected as a result of semantic field analysis and standardized testing.
(D) John	will use words representing action	for 8 of 10 opportunities	in a spontaneous conversation.	This objective was selected as a result of semantic field analysis and standardized testing.
(E) John	will use words representing locative state	for 8 of 10 opportunities	in a spontaneous conversation.	This objective was selected as a result of semantic field analysis and standardized testing.

A. John will use second-person possessives (e.g., your, yours) for 8 out of 10 opportunities in a spontaneous conversation. This objective is selected as a result of semantic field analysis and standardized testing.

B. John will use third-person possessives (e.g., his, hers, its, their, theirs, Sam's, Tina's) for 8 out of 10 opportunities in a spontaneous conversation. This objective is selected as a result of semantic field analysis and standardized testing.

C. John will use words representing locative action (e.g., going in, coming out, going up, coming down, putting on, taking off) for 8 out of 10 opportunities in a spontaneous conversation. This objective is selected as a result of semantic field analysis and standardized testing.

D. John will use words representing action (e.g., run, jump, walk, roll, throw, eat, drink) for 8 out of 10 opportunities in a spontaneous conversation. This objective is selected as a result of semantic field analysis and standardized testing.

E. John will use words representing locative state (e.g., in, out, on, under, next to, beside, between) for 8 out of 10 opportunities in a spontaneous conversation. This objective is selected as a result of semantic field analysis and standardized testing.

Developing Procedures That Address Short-Term Objectives

Procedures address the short-term objectives directly and the long-term objectives indirectly. Written procedures clearly define the activities that are to be completed by the client and clinician in order to achieve the short-term objectives. Anyone reading the description of the procedure or observing it in process must be able to see clearly how the procedure relates to and serves to accomplish the objective. Further, the evidence on which the procedure is based (rationale) is included in the description so there will be no question as to how the procedure is intended to accomplish its purpose.

The written description of the procedure describes the clinical activities and lists the materials needed in order to accomplish the activities. *Using the same example, let us develop two procedures that may be used to accomplish short-term objective B (as proposed in Table 4–5). The objective states that John will use third-person possessives (e.g., his, her, hers, their, theirs, Sam's, Tina's) for 8 out of 10 opportunities in a spontaneous conversation (80 percent). Baseline data shows that John used the forms at approximately 30 percent accuracy prior to initiating the intervention program (Table 4–4).*

In order to accomplish this objective, it is important to present John with opportunities to hear third-person possessives being used in simple contextual speech and for these words to be clearly and systematically associated with the possessive relationship between a third person and an object. It is also important for John to have the opportunity to attempt to label the third-person possessive relationship as it occurs in a natural context. The example proce-dures described in Figures 4–2 and 4–3 may be used to accomplish that end.

The Language Intervention Plan

The intervention plan—also called the individualized educational plan (IEP)—is a document that is written at the initiation of the intervention program. The purpose of the written plan is to formally document baseline informa-tion and the intervention proposal and to communicate this data to appro-priate family members and professionals. The exact form, length, and amount of detail vary according to setting. For demonstration purposes, two sample intervention plan formats appear in Appendices 4–1 and 4–2.

All the general report-writing guidelines delineated in Chapter 3 apply to intervention plans. The plan typically includes the following parts: (1) identi-

---

Materials: boy doll (Sam), girl doll (Tina), cookies, juice, four napkins, four cups, tea party set for four, small table, and four small chairs.

Location and Set-Up: Room 6. Place Sam and Tina (dolls) in chairs and set the table.

Time: 10–15 minutes.

Activities: The clinician gives a cookie to Sam and says: "I give Sam a cookie. That cookie is *Sam's*. It is *his* cookie." Each time the clinician says a word representing the third-person possessive relationship (in italics here), the clinician emphasizes the word slightly and gestures toward the posses-sive relationship. Each time the clinician gives Sam a cookie, the sentences or variations of them are systematically repeated, using a conversational tone. Similar sentences and gestures are repeated to describe the posses-sive relationship between Sam and his cup, napkin, chair, and spoon. The same procedure is also executed to clearly describe Tina's possessive re-lationship to her cookie, cup, napkin, chair, and spoon. (John and the clin-ician's possessive relationships with the same items are defined for John in objective A.) Small talk related to the tea party is expected in addition.

Rationale: By experience with hearing and using the third-person posses-sive in the appropriate contexts, John will begin to use the semantic rela-tionships in conversational speech.

Evaluation: The clinician evaluates John's expressive command of third-per-son possessive by asking him to express to whom each item belongs. (Probes include: "Whose cookie is this?" "Whose chair is this?" etc.).

Figure 4–2. Clinical Example: Procedure 1 may be used to accomplish short-term objective B (*Tea Party*).

Materials: boy doll (Sam), girl doll (Tina), boy and girl doll clothes (boots, shoes, socks, slacks, shirts, bow tie, hats, skirts, dresses, blouses, jewelry, play makeup, etc.), mirror.

Location & Set Up: Room 6. Sam and Tina (dolls) are sitting on top of a box full of doll clothes beside a doll-length mirror.

Time: 10–15 minutes.

Activities: Clinician identifies each clothing item as Sam's (*his*) or Tina's (*hers*). John is encouraged to undress and dress the rag dolls, and is encouraged to match the clothes with the appropriate doll. The clinician continues to verbally label the items according to owner and encourages John to do the same. The mirror is used to allow each doll to visually examine his or her self. Informal conversation is expected in addition.

Rationale: By experience with hearing and using third-person possessive in the appropriate contexts, John will begin to use the semantic relationships in conversational speech.

Evaluation: The clinician evaluates John's expressive command of third-person possessive by asking him to express to whom each item belongs. (Probes include: "Whose boot is this?" "Whose makeup is this?" etc.).

Figure 4–3.   Clinical Example: Procedure 2 May be Used to Accomplish Short-Term Objective *B* (*Dress Up*).

fying information, (2) diagnosis, (3) significant background information, (4) objectives and procedures, (5) prognosis, (6) recommendations, and (7) dated signatures with credentials. The first three sections are very similar to the information that appears in the most recent assessment report for the same client, as *identifying information, diagnosis,* and *significant background information* do not usually change between assessments. Having been described previously, they will not be revisited in this section.

Objectives and Procedures.   The objectives and procedures section is written in order to document the long-term objectives, short-term objectives, and procedures for the particular client. *Strategies for developing this aspect of the intervention plan, and some pertinent examples, appear in Tables 4–1 through 4–5 and Figures 4–2 and 4–3.*

In the plan, more than one long-term objective may be presented as, even in our simple example, it is possible to write a number of long-term objectives. (See proposed targets of Table 4–2.) Further, several short-term objectives appear under each long-term objective, a number of procedures may coincide with each short-term objective, and some procedures may be used to address several short-term objectives simultaneously. Therefore, a few options exist for recording objectives and procedures. Some clinicians prefer to outline them according to Appendix 4–3. However, an alternative way in which to report objectives and procedures is to report corresponding long- and short-term objectives together, separating the procedures section and taking care to refer to the appropriate short-term objectives when describing each procedure. This method may be selected if certain procedures address more than one objective. In this case, the format that appears in Appendix 4–4 may be a more useful guide.

Prognosis.   It is likely that the prognosis section of the plan is very similar to the prognosis that appears in the most recent assessment report. However, if additional evidence emerges, it is considered and the prognosis is revised as needed. Some evidence that may emerge, if a client is in intervention, is response to treatment and details about behavioral patterns that become apparent as a result of continued and regular contact with the child. In determining prognosis, one considers these and all the variables suggested in the prognosis section of Chapter 3.

As with the prognosis described in Chapter 3, if the evidence gives adequate reason to suspect that the client is likely to benefit from intervention, then the intervention plan is legitimately carried out. If such reasonable evidence is not available, then the client is discharged or admitted to intervention for a brief *trial period* to determine whether the client is likely to benefit from intervention.

Recommendations.   The recommendations section usually follows the prognosis. Since writing the intervention plan indicates that treatment is about to begin or is in progress, it is unnecessary to write a recommendation for or against treatment. However, if intervention is being conducted on a trial basis, then one of the recommendations specifies the length of trial and proposed method for evaluating whether treatment continues beyond the trial period. Further, the recommendations include any referrals not yet carried out (e.g., medical, educational, psychological), formal communication to be initiated (e.g., seeking information from parents or professionals), activities that are preparatory for an upcoming clinical event (e.g., behavioral audiometry in preparation for hearing evaluation), and testing scheduled to take place while the intervention plan is in effect.

Signatures.   As with the assessment report, the very last section of the plan is composed of the dated signatures and credentials of all professionals and students who participated in the writing of the report and are in the process of contributing to planning and executing of the intervention program. Your signature on the plan indicates that you have read it, that you agree to its contents, and that you take responsibility for executing it. For that reason, no one signs the report until all revisions are complete.

The signature of a family representative may also be included in this section. If included, the family member's signature indicates that the person has had the opportunity to read, question, and comment on the report. However, it does not necessarily mean that the family member has participated in the preparation of the report in any way.

Using Results of Intervention to Establish New Targets

Sometimes it is necessary to establish or revise a plan after a child has received intervention for a period of time. Some possible reasons for this may be that (1) the intervention plan has expired, (2) the short-term objectives have been achieved, or (3) the certified speech-language pathologist managing the case determines that the plan is no longer appropriate. When this happens, the process of establishing targets is somewhat modified in that one takes into account, not only the available assessment data, but also the achievements resulting from intervention.

When revising a plan, always refer back to the most recent assessment in order to identify the diagnosis and supporting evidence. *For the example, this information appears in Table 4–1.* Then refer to the previously identified long-term objectives that are documented in the client's previous intervention plan(s) (Tables 4–2 and 4–3). Since long-term objectives rightfully reflect the client's expected status at the time of discharge, plans are made to continue to systematically address each discharge objective, unless you suspect that the client has reached a long-term objective or unless the long-term objectives are no longer appropriate due to some significant change in status.

In order to address each long-term objective, one must first obtain definitive information about the client's current performance status with regard to each. *For the purpose of demonstration, our discussion elaborates only on the one long-term objective that appears in Table 4–3.*

For the sake of the example, suppose that the reason for revising the plan is that John has reached criterion on all of the short-term objectives (Table 4–5) that were initially developed. In order to continue to move in the direction of the long-term objective (Table 4–3), it is now necessary to establish a new set of short-term objectives. Therefore, the next step is to identify the short-term objectives that are most appropriate for the client's current performance level.

Since the example intervention program (Tables 4–3 and 4–5) targets semantic categories in order to achieve age-appropriate vocabulary and increase lexical diversity, we return to the results of the sample semantic field analysis as reported in Table 4–1. Further informal assessment then takes place in order to identify the semantic categories that are appropriate for continued intervention.

The targets (in the case of the example, semantic categories) not previously mastered and not recently targeted are probed according to the criteria presented in Figure 4–1. From that probe, the semantic categories that are found to be used consistently and those that are not used at all are not considered for targeting, for the reasons outlined in the figure. However, those used inconsistently are considered as potential targets.

Next, baseline data are collected and short-term objectives and corresponding procedures are developed in order to facilitate the development of the new targets. Methods for collecting specific baseline data and for developing short-term objectives and corresponding procedures are described earlier in this chapter. *Examples appear in Tables 4–4 through 4–7 and Figures 4–2 and 4–3.*

Reporting Progress

In university speech and hearing centers, progress is typically reported at the end of each academic term, and a progress report that is separate from the intervention plan is used to record the accomplishments of the program. The reason that separate reports are used to record planning and progress in university settings is that each case is closed at the end of term and then picked up by a new clinician, and perhaps even a new supervisor, when the next term begins.

A sample progress report format is shown in Appendix 4–5. The significant difference between it and the Intervention Plan (Appendices 4–1 through 4–4) is in section 4, "Objectives and Progress." In this section, each long-term objective is written with its corresponding series of short-term objectives. In a progress report, progress toward criterion is described and/or quantified under each short-term objective.

Further, section 5 of the Progress Report ("Clinical Impressions"), is similar to the same section in the Assessment Report (Appendix 3–5). The clinical impressions section puts forth any pertinent information that is not included elsewhere in the report and is likely to benefit the next managing clinician.

Settings other than university clinics follow a similar procedure for reporting progress. However, since it is not usually necessary to close each case at the end of the academic term, each revised intervention plan is likely to include a section on reporting progress.

The frequency with which progress reports are written varies depending on setting. For example, in university speech and hearing centers, the reports coincide with academic terms; and in schools, the reports coincide with state guidelines and perhaps the academic year. Hospitals, private agencies, rehabilitation centers, and other settings vary in their requirements for documenting progress. In general, progress reporting is done on a regular basis, it coincides with revision of intervention plans, and there should always be a current intervention plan on file with progress reports that correspond to all expired or completed plans.

IMPLEMENTING A LANGUAGE INTERVENTION PLAN

Although developing and writing clear and accurate plans is essential to the success of the intervention program, it does not ensure attainment of the desired results. The plan has to be carried out effectively and must be adapted as needed in order to suit the changing needs of the client.

Preparing and Organizing the Language Program

Effective administration of the intervention program begins with preparation for each session. Several suggestions for assessment preparation are detailed in Chapter 3 and, in essence, they apply to preparation for intervention as well. These suggestions include familiarizing one's self with the plan and materials, collecting and organizing the materials, rehearsing some of the activities (especially as a new clinician), and preparing the setting prior to beginning the session.

Lesson Plans.   As a student clinician, a detailed weekly (or daily) lesson plan is an important part of planning and administering the intervention program. These plans are necessary for a number of reasons: (1) The weekly lesson plan forces the inexperienced clinician to consciously address the changing needs and progress of the client on a frequent and regular basis; (2) It provides the clinical supervisor with information about the student clinician's problem-solving skills, ability to identify and address the changing needs of the client, and practical grasp of the clinical situation overall; (3) It provides the supervisor with an opportunity to evaluate and comment on the plan before it is carried out; (4) It provides the supervisor with an outline that can be referenced while observing the clinical activities in progress.

Weekly lesson plans come in a variety of formats. Usually they include a minimum of identifying information, a brief statement of diagnosis, long-term objectives, short-term objectives to be addressed in the sessions, procedures corresponding to each short-term goal (as outlined in Figures 4–2 and 4–3), a list of materials needed to carry out each procedure, and an evaluation of progress achieved during the previous lesson plan period.

For student clinicians, lesson plans are submitted to the supervisor in advance, revised as necessary, and administered once approved by the clinical supervisor. Revisions and suggestions are made by the supervisor so that the student clinician may benefit from the experience of the certified professional who is ultimately responsible for overseeing the management of the case.

Establishing Rapport

All that was said about establishing rapport in Chapter 3 (on assessment) applies to intervention as well. The notable exception is that in an intervention program you have access to more time for the development of the clinical relationship since the child returns for two or three sessions each week.

General Suggestions for Facilitating Change in Behavior

The concept of providing what is called "intervention" implies by its very name that someone (i.e., a clinician) does something to or for someone else (i.e., a client) in an attempt to intercept (i.e., intervene in) an identified behavior pattern and change it in some way. Generally, in language intervention, it is a new communication behavior that is to be acquired by the client. In many cases, an old behavior is suppressed at the same time.

In an effort to demonstrate how this may be applied, let us continue with the example (Tables 4–1 through 4–5 and Figures 4–2 and 4–3). The new behaviors that are to emerge in the demonstration are expressive use of words representing second- and third-person possessive, locative action, action, and locative state. Since the example targets third-person possession, let the example continue with that objective and say that specifically, words representing third-person possession will be acquired according to short-term objective B of Table 4–5. In order to acquire this new pattern, it may be necessary to suppress an old pattern, depending on what the child is already doing to represent the target forms. *For example, if the child is not representing third-person possession at all, then only a new pattern is presented and learned and no old patterns are suppressed. However, if the child is substituting the third-person objective case (e.g., him/his, them/theirs) or omitting the -s possessive morphological marker (e.g., Mary/Mary's), then the old pattern must be suppressed as the new pattern emerges.* From a clinical perspective, it is important to understand exactly how these changes in the client's behavior may be systematically orchestrated.

The A-R-C Paradigm.

Antecedents.   In attempting to change a person's behavior, one often follows a fairly simple three-step process that is referred to as the A-R-C paradigm. In this paradigm, the *A* stands for **antecedent**, or the event that elicits the **target behavior**. It is called the antecedent because it generally happens immediately before the target. Some call it an **antecedent stimulus** or a **stimulus**, which makes sense because it not only happens before the target, it is what is done to stimulate the client to produce the target.

Responses.   The *R* of the *A-R-C* paradigm stands for **response**, meaning the client's response to the antecedent stimulus. This is also called the target behavior, and its exact nature is driven by a short-term objective.

Consequences.   The letter *C* represents **consequence**, which is also called a **consequent stimulus**, stimulus, or **reinforcer.** The consequence is what occurs immediately after the response to the antecedent stimulus. A carefully selected consequence serves to either increase, maintain, decrease, or extinguish the client's response behavior. Logically, increasing or maintaining the response is the desired effect for language patterns that we hope to strengthen. However, a carefully selected consequence can be effective for decreasing and extinguishing undesired behaviors that may need to be suppressed in order to manage behavior or in order to allow desired behaviors to emerge.

Controlling Response by Controlling Antecedents and Consequences.   Using the A-R-C paradigm requires that one carefully identify and control all three aspects: the antecedent, the response, and the consequence. The first to be identified and controlled is the desired response, or target behavior, which is controlled through the antecedent and consequence. *For the example (Tables 4–5 and 4–6), the responses are identified as production of words representing third-person possession.*

Then, it is important to plan circumstances or procedures under which the target is likely to occur. These circumstances are the antecedent stimuli. Planning the antecedent is an important step because it is critical that the clinician select antecedents that are likely to elicit the desired response or target. A poorly planned antecedent may result in a response but not the one that is targeted, yielding the plan ineffectual for accomplishing its purposes. *For the example, some suggested antecedents are described in the tea party and dress-up procedures (Figures 4–2 and 4–3, and Table 4–6).*

Finally, it is important to plan a consequence that is likely to have the desired effect on the client's responsive behavior. If the response is a behavior that we hope to strengthen or develop, then the consequence is designed to increase or maintain the behavior (Table 4–6). If it is a behavior that we hope to suppress, then the consequence is designed to decrease or extinguish the behavior.

Hierarchy of Reinforcers.   A variety of consequences can be used to strengthen a response pattern. However, they range in effectiveness and in potential for facilitating **carry-over** to natural communication. A hierarchy of reinforcers that includes four types has been identified (Cole & Cole, 1989) (Table 4–6). For that reason, one carefully selects the consequences in order to maximize the desired effect.

Primary reinforcers are at the lowest end of the reinforcer hierarchy (Table 4–6). That is, they are the least effective and they are not particularly apt to facilitate carry-over to natural communicative contexts. Primary reinforcers are reinforcers that fulfill a physical need, such as hunger or thirst. They may include frosted cereal, chips, candy, food of any kind, and beverages as a reward for language behavior. Primary reinforcers (e.g., food and beverages) are recommended with reservation because (1) their presence in the mouth interferes with the child's ability to participate in activities requiring speaking, (2) they increase salivation, causing further interference, (3) they often present a distraction from the language-learning activity, and (4) unless used at mealtime, they usually require that one introduce a consequence that is not related to either the response or the activity at hand.

The second level of reinforcer is the *activity reinforcer* (Table 4–6). Activity reinforcers are exercises that the child is allowed to do as rewards for per-

Table 4-6. Clinical Example

The A-R-C Paradigm

Situation. The procedure is the dress-up example that appears in Figure 4–3. The clinician has identified each article of clothing according to its owner. John has taken the footwear off both rag dolls and appears to be interested in replacing Sam's with a pair of boots.

Antecedent. Clinician shows John Sam's boots and Tina's boots and says: "Whose boots do you want? His or hers?"

Response. John says, "his boots."

| Level | Consequence Options | | |
	Reinforcer	Potential Problems	Suggested Use
(1) *Primary*	Clinician puts a treat in John's mouth and then hands him the requested boots.	(A) Food in mouth interferes with speech production. (B) Salivation interferes with speech production. (C) Demonstrates to the child an unnatural and apragmatic response to a verbal request for boots.	(a) Use only if child is not motivated by higher levels. (b) Combine with higher levels, with the goal of decreasing and eventually eliminating the lower-level reinforcer.
(2) *Activity*	Clinician provides an opportunity for John to put a piece in a puzzle and then hands him the requested boots.	(A) Activity may detract from the procedure. (B) Activity takes time from the procedure. (C) Demonstrates to child an unnatural and apragmatic response to a verbal request.	(a) Use only if child is not motivated by higher levels. (b) Combine with higher levels, with the goal of decreasing and eventually eliminating the lower-level reinforcer.
(3) *Social*	Clinician says, "Good speech," and then hands John the requested boots.	(A) Demonstrates to child an unnatural and apragmatic response to a verbal request.	(a) Combine with higher level, with the goal of decreasing and eventually eliminating the lower level reinforcer.
(4) *Communication Success*	Clinician hands John the requested boots and then continues with the procedure.	Some children need lower levels in order to maintain interest.	Use whenever possible.

formance. Although more effective than primary reinforcers, they do not necessarily facilitate carry-over to natural communication. For that reason, they are used sparingly and usually for the purpose of encouraging continued participation in an activity or test. Examples of activity reinforcers include games, opportunities to manipulate a toy or desired object, coloring, building and constructing things, and crafts.

Some problems often occur with activity reinforcers. For example, many inexperienced clinicians have been observed to build intervention session around activities rather than around the objectives and procedures. Further, even if the language objectives are being addressed, it seems that the activities consume entirely too much time during the session. Hence, if an activity reinforcer is selected, one must see to it that the activity takes up a minimum of time, and that the objectives, and *not the activities*, are clearly the focus of the session.

At the third level are *social reinforcers* (Table 4–6). This is the second to highest level, so these types of reinforcers may be used with some degree of confidence. Keep in mind that social reinforcers are surpassed by another level with regard to effectiveness and facilitating carry-over. Examples of social reinforcers are comments and gestures directed at the child, communicating that the clinician is pleased. Verbal praise (e.g., "Good work," "Excellent," "Exactly!") and encouraging gestures (e.g., thumbs up, reassuring smile, handshake, high five) are included.

Unlike activity reinforcers, social reinforcers can be administered instantaneously and therefore do not distract from the intervention objectives. They are also useful to encourage continued responding. However, the noteworthy weakness of social reinforcers is that they may call attention to themselves because they are a somewhat unnatural response to the child's attempts at communication. For example, it is unnatural to respond to the child's verbal request with a comment such as, "I like the way you said that." A more natural response is to comply with the request, either verbally or nonverbally.

This brings us to the highest-level reinforcer, which is *communication success* (Table 4–6). The child's attempt at communication successfully accomplishes the intended purpose. If your response to the child communicates that what the child says accomplishes its purpose, then you are using a level of **reinforcement** that is effective and likely to facilitate carry-over to natural communication.

Regarding the hierarchy of reinforcers, please note that some children do not readily maintain satisfactory interest when only the higher levels of reinforcement are used. The lower levels are therefore useful and important for children who require them for motivational purposes. When this happens, (1) take care to ensure that the reinforcer does not become the focus of the session, (2) minimize the time spent delivering the reinforcer, and (3) whenever possible pair the lower-level reinforcer with a higher-level reinforcer, gradually replacing the lower with the higher as the child becomes self-motivated. For example, if the child requires an activity reinforcer (level 2), include verbal praise (level 3). Then, gradually decrease the frequency of the activity reinforcer and increase the frequency of the verbal praise. Moreover, gradually introduce communication success (level 4) as a reinforcer and increase its frequency as the child begins to respond to it.

Planning for Generalization.   If a language intervention program is necessary for a child, it is because of real-life communication needs. Therefore, clinical objectives never end with achieving specified goals in the clinical environment alone. Instead we always expect that the intervention gains eventually become incorporated into the child's everyday communication repertoire. Unfortunately, this takes place only if we plan from the beginning for **generalization**.

Therefore, the time to begin thinking about generalization and carry-over is not as each objective is achieved. Instead, it is during the initial planning for achieving the objective. The following suggestions, if applied throughout the intervention program, can be used to facilitate generalization.

Meaningful Context.   Always practice targets in contexts that are meaningful to the child. That is, create situations that the child is likely to encounter in the context of the familiar social and cultural sphere and where each target can be practiced purposefully. Repeating sentences and labeling picture cards are not particularly meaningful to most children. However, the sample procedures of Figures 4–2 and 4–3 are examples of contexts that can be modified so as to make them meaningful to children from a variety of backgrounds.

Real Communication.   Always practice targets in a context in which real communication occurs. This means provide the child with opportunity to communicate new information. For example, in Figures 4–2 and 4–3, the client has to tell the clinician which item is desired. Since the clinician does not know in advance the desires of the client, new information is communicated.

Conversational Cohesion.   Always promote conversational cohesion by practicing targets in conversations for which a number of turns are maintained on the same topic. One mistake that is easy to make when practicing a target is to direct the child to produce a series of unrelated sentences with similar grammatical form, rather than requiring the child to participate in an ongoing, cohesive conversation. In the real word, conversations are cohesive and the grammatical form of adjacent utterances varies. So the child needs experience with cohesive and varied utterances. Therefore, introducing a topic and sticking to it for a number of turns is advised. This also is demonstrated in Figures 4–2 and 4–3.

Motivation to Communicate.   Always practice targets in a context for which the motivation to communicate is high. Select topics that are interesting to the child. Keep your manner animated, so that you are seen as a person with whom the child wants to converse.

Variety of Speech Acts.   Practice all types of speech acts, not just repetitions and recitations. Every type of speech act is needed for communication outside of the clinical environment. So introduce all of them when in the clinical environment. (See categories of language function, Figure 1–2, for descriptions of a variety of speech acts.)

The Real World.   As much as possible, talk about real things. These are the topics that are socially and culturally relevant to the child, are of interest to the child, and involve things that the child is likely to encounter when outside the clinic.

Find ways to take the events of the intervention room out into the world. For example, if you can create an aura of the desired target around something that the child takes outside of clinic, do so. An example may be a sticker or prize that has "witnessed" all the child's work over a period of time. By emphasizing the object's association with the language work, and then by giving the object to the child, you create a constant reminder for the child with regard to a language pattern that you want to generalize.

Moreover, you should find ways to take the real world into the intervention room. For example, allow the child to bring a favorite toy or game to be used in intervention, as long as it does not become a distraction. You can also allow a family member to attend. Make sure that discussions revolve around the real experiences in the child's life.

Brief field trips are another way to facilitate the marriage between the real world and the therapy room. In nice weather, conducting a session or part of a session outdoors is possible. A walk to the vending machines for a soft drink is another possible way to take intervention out into the real world. However, frequent and extended field trips are rarely practical, and they may tend to dilute the effect of the intervention program.

Managing Environment and Behavioral Events

In managing the intervention session, it is of considerable importance to control certain environmental and behavioral factors. That is, when you skillfully manage the physical environment, the linguistic environment, and the child's behavior, you clear the way for carrying out your objectives effectively and efficiently.

The Physical Environment.   The physical environment that surrounds clinical interaction includes the room itself and all the furniture, decorations, materials, and effects contained therein. The proficiency with which intervention is carried out is enhanced by taking charge of all these accouterments.

The room ideally contains only the furniture and materials needed for the session. However, in practice it often occurs that an intervention room also serves as an office, a materials room, or all three. If this is the case, arrange the room so that the part used for clinical service is somewhat separated.

Minimize visual and auditory distractions as much as possible. Arrange the work table so that the toys, materials, and office equipment are out of view and especially out of reach. If you decorate the room, decorate only one or two walls, which permits you to arrange the table so that it does not directly face a host of opportunities for distraction. Further, do whatever you can to eliminate and minimize ambient noise.

In preparation for the session, organize the work area so that it contains only the materials needed for that session. Do not allow materials to pile up from one session to the next. During the session, keep materials organized, within your reach, and out of the immediate reach of the child.

The Linguistic Environment.   The linguistic environment is somewhat more abstract than the physical environment and is therefore somewhat more difficult to control. However, planning and controlling the linguistic environment are essential to successful intervention. Since one general objective of intervention is to clearly associate linguistic targets with objects, events, and relations, careful planning is required. The scenario is carefully set up, the words are carefully selected, and the timing has to be close to perfect so that the object, event, or relation coincides with the linguistic representation of it.

For example, in the demonstration (Figure 4–2), a tea party is used to facilitate the emergence of third-person possessives (e.g., his, her, hers, their, theirs, Sam's, Tina's). In managing the linguistic environment, it is important then to time the labeling of the possessive relationship with the occurrence of demonstrating the possessive relationship, such that it is absolutely clear to the child that the words represent the relationship between the object and its owner. That is, the words "Sam's cup" are spoken at a time in which the relationship between Sam and his cup is clearly illustrated.

Managing Behavior Problems.   Behavior management is important to the intervention program because the successful outcome depends on the child's ongoing cooperation and participation. Further, when guiding intervention, the clinician sees the child week after week for extended periods, providing ample opportunity for the child to challenge authority in the clinical environment, thus making it essential that the child understand and abide by the rules.

Cooperation. Cooperation is one fundamental ingredient for successful intervention, and it must be present if behavior is to be managed efficiently. A number of suggestions for enlisting a child's cooperation are discussed in Chapter 3 and therefore, are not repeated in this section.

Applying the A-R-C Paradigm.   The A-R-C paradigm can be applied in order to facilitate harmony with children who do not typically comply with the guidelines established by the clinician in charge. In making this A-R-C application, first identify the antecedent, response, and consequence according to the guidelines presented previously. When dealing with a negative behavior that you want to eliminate or redirect, the R of the A-R-C, or response, is the negative behavior. The event that precipitates the negative behavior is the antecedent (A), and the event that immediately follows is the consequence (C).

With recurring negative responses, if the antecedent is identified and suitably changed, the negative behavior often discontinues. For example, suppose a client repeatedly threatens the clinician by stating she is about to vomit. As a result, an inexperienced clinician may become visibly concerned, allow periodic trips to the rest room, and virtually beg the child to continue to work. Then, when it becomes apparent that the child is only making the claim in order to avoid work, the same clinician may no longer allow trips to the rest room and may begin to insist that the child work, ignoring any complaints of a stomachache. At this juncture, the child may voluntarily follow through on the threat and vomit, causing the clinician considerable distress. The neophyte clinician is left with no confidence for dealing with the situation in the event that it recurs.

In an attempt to intercept the antecedent and discontinue the recurring negative behavior rather than "playing the child's game," the more experienced clinician might consider allowing no trips to the rest room and making no attempt to insist that the child continue working with a sick stomach. Instead, at the first suggestion of the impending disaster, the clinician might consider providing the child with a suitable receptacle and instructing the child, in a matter-of-fact way, to go ahead and vomit in it (or keep it handy) so that work can continue (Table 4–7). By doing this, the clinician gives credence to the child's claim and at the same time establishes the fact that the planned activities are a very high priority and, therefore, cannot readily be manipulated or put aside.

For recurring behaviors such as the one in the Table 4–7, antecedents are often identified and changed so that the behavior is not likely to be repeated. However, some behaviors are difficult to predict and some antecedents are difficult or inconvenient to alter. In these cases, it is advisable to identify the event that immediately follows the negative behavior (the consequence) because in many cases it is the consequence that serves to keep the undesirable act alive.

The most effective consequence for maintaining or increasing a behavior is one that results in successfully achieving some personal objective. This is consistent with the levels of reinforcers described in Table 4–6. In many cases, the personal objective of the child who engages in a negative behavior is to gain attention, usurp control or authority, or become amused. If the child achieves any of these by engaging in the negative behavior, it is very likely that the same negative act will occur again in order to accomplish the same goal.

Table 4-7. Clinical Example.

Using the Antecedent to Decrease or Eliminate a Recurring Negative Behavior Pattern

Antecedent	*Response*
Child claims to need to vomit. Clinician becomes concerned. Many trips are made to the rest room. When convinced that the child is using the threat to manipulate the situation to her advantage, the clinician insists that the child do her work.	Child voluntarily vomits.

Alternative Antecedent	*Response*
Child claims to need to vomit. Clinician offers child a suitable receptacle and matter-of-factly informs the child that work will continue when she is through.	Child loses interest in vomiting and reluctantly returns to work.

Consequently, if manipulating the antecedent is not an option, it is important to identify the immediate consequence, determine whether it achieves a personal objective for the child, and substitute a different consequence that does not accomplish the child's objective. For example, a young child might repeatedly attempt to abuse clinic materials, only to receive a lecture (attention) from the clinician. In order to intercept the ineffective consequence, the clinician must cease lecturing the child and replace lecturing with a different consequence that does not provide the child with the desired attention or diversion from work. One possible alternative consequence that might decrease the frequency of the destructive behavior is for the clinician to immediately and matter-of-factly remove the materials from the child's reach, inform the child that the privilege of using the materials has been lost for the remainder of the session, and then immediately, and temporarily, replace the materials with something less interesting (Table 4–8).

When selecting a consequence, it is desirable to choose one that is a natural result of the negative behavior. For example, in the previous example, the mistreated materials are removed from the child's access. That is a natural consequence. Further, it is best if the consequence that is applied is fully understood by the child. This is partially accomplished by explaining to the child the relationship between the offense and the consequence. For example, you may say, "You lost the privilege of using these materials today because you are breaking them." However, just because the consequence is explained does not guarantee that the child understands, so follow through by asking him or her to explain why the materials were removed from access.

Disciplinary Action. In rare cases, it may eventually become apparent in working with some children that cooperation has not been achieved, even to the extent of deliberate defiance. When this takes place, suitable disciplinary action may be necessary in order to maintain control of the situation and accomplish the objectives of the session.

Before applying any disciplinary action, it is important to identify that the undesirable behavior is, in fact, a deliberate attempt to challenge authority. It is unacceptable to discipline a child for a behavior that occurs as a result of forgetfulness, fear, anxiety, or any other source that can be attributed to being a child in an unfamiliar situation. Discipline a child only if you are certain that he or she is aware of the expectations, has been reminded, and clearly has *chosen* to defy authority.

Even if you are certain that discipline is an appropriate action, you are limited to certain disciplinary options. For example, *you have no authority to punish* in any way. Punishment includes, but is not limited to, corporal (i.e., physical) punishment, which includes spanking, hitting, shaking, arm twisting, hand squeezing, roughly putting a child down in a chair or rough handling of any kind, and any touch that is more restrictive than what is required to accomplish the act of bringing the child's behavior under control.

Punishment also includes nonphysical punishment, which covers criticism of the child or the child's work, insults and labels (e.g., "naughty," "not good," "bad"), withdrawal of affection, influencing other people to respond negatively toward the child, and any consequence that has not been explained adequately. Further, nonphysical punishment covers any consequence that is unreasonable in relation to the offense or in relation to the child's age such as an extended **time-out** (i.e., more than 1 minute for each year of age), carrying a consequence over from one activity to the next or one day to the next, ap-

Table 4-8. Clinical Example.

Using Consequence to Decrease or Eliminate a Negative Behavior Pattern

Antecedent	Response	Consequence	Result
Clinician presents a deck of picture cards to be used for a language activity.	Client bends the cards.	Clinician lectures the client.	Client accomplished the objective of getting attention. Negative behavior was strengthened and will probably recur.

Antecedent	Response	Alternate Consequence	Result
Same	Same	Clinician removes client's access to the cards and replaces them with a less interesting activity.	Client did not accomplish the objective. Negative behavior was not strengthened, so it may decrease in frequency of occurrence.

plying the consequence to only one child when two or more are involved, and any disciplinary action that causes the child to feel badly about him- or herself.

Commonly, if natural consequences are exhausted, acceptable disciplinary action involves temporarily removing the child from the situation. Traditionally this procedure is called time-out, although some have found different names for it. If you need to use a time-out procedure, what you call it is important because its name becomes clearly associated with punitive action. For example, one teacher insisted on calling time-out "the thinking chair," whereupon some children in her class came to regard thinking as something that is done as a result of having broken a rule. Another teacher called it "the library" because of its location in the classroom, causing some children to associate a visit to the library with having broken a rule. These are unfortunate, but real, examples. If you choose to use a term other than *time-out*, make sure that it is neutral, does not encourage a negative thinking pattern, and does not cause the child to feel badly about him- or herself.

Time-out is accomplished by removing the child from all stimulation and opportunity for a short period of time. All materials may be removed from the child or the child may be sent to a specified location for a few moments of solitary time. Further, the reason for the time-out must be clearly and precisely explained to the child.

The duration of time-out is important to control. Once the child has been in time-out for more than 1 minute for each year of age, he or she has probably lost sight of the offense, rendering time-out ineffective as a consequence. Furthermore, leaving a child in time-out for an extended period of time is unreasonable. Even less than 1 minute for each year of age can be very effective if it is the child's decision to return to the work situation and to cooperate.

In general, the following guidelines may be helpful in determining and administering disciplinary action. Appropriate discipline always communicates to the child that the behavior is inappropriate and not that the child is bad, and it never compromises the child's self-image. The consequence is always clearly associated with the offense. Natural consequences are always tried before time-out or other unnatural consequences. Characteristically, appropriate discipline is fair, appropriate for the child's age, proportionate to the offense, and always applied with the express purpose of helping the child bring behavior under an internal locus of control.

Managing Groups.   In some settings, a clinician does not have the luxury of managing only one child at a time. Particularly in the public schools, most intervention is done in groups of two or more.

Selecting the *composition of a language group* is one important step toward successfully managing the children in it. Ideally, the children are of similar age and cognitive level and are working on similar short-term objectives, or at least short-term objectives that can be readily coordinated procedurally, moreover, their combined behavior patterns should be reasonably manageable for the clinician.

For example, the child in the demonstration model is working on expanding expressive semantic categories (Table 4–5). Although it is possible that several children exist in the same grade with a similar problem, it is unlikely. Thus, in order to provide a group program that benefits all children concerned, John may be placed in a group of children whose diverse language deficiencies can all be addressed using similar props and setups.

A number of content-form interactions can be addressed using scenarios such as those described in Figures 4–2 and 4–3. These may include children working on a number of morphological markers and grammatical forms. The difference between John and his cohorts may be that, although John is working on acquiring third-person possessive forms, his group members may, at the same time, use the tea party (Figure 4–2) and dress-up (Figure 4–3) experiences to hear and practice such forms as past tense -ed, present progressive -ing, and plural -s word endings. Other children may be in the group to hear and practice sentence structures, such as noun phrase elaboration, verb phrase elaboration, or subject-verb-object sentence composition. Regardless of the combination of objectives within the group, make it a priority to select children who can all experience and practice their targets through similar scenarios.

Once the children arrive for their group session, it is important to *maintain control of the situation* so that each child is able to gain the maximum benefit. In order to achieve this, a first suggestion is for the clinician to be intimately acquainted with each child's long- and short-term objectives and have a firm grasp of how each planned procedure can be used to accomplish them. Time spent during the session trying to recall or look up these matters is not only time wasted, it is also an invitation for the children to usurp control.

Second, the clinician must be well organized and impeccably prepared for the group session. Especially with younger children, it is important to keep them occupied and to move swiftly from one procedure to the next so that they do not become bored or distracted.

Third, the clinician must establish the rules and take a hard line on requiring that all individuals comply. Suggestions in Chapter 3 on soliciting cooperation and suggestions about behavior management are very helpful to anyone who is interested in monitoring an established set of rules in groups.

Finally, it is critical that the clinician remain keenly aware of the dynamics of the individual group members throughout the session. Action must be taken at the first indication that even only one child is becoming distracted. Remember that if you lose control, even momentarily, it will be difficult to regain any sense of dignity or authority. Consequently, if you are sensitive to the warning signs that control may be lost and if you intercept the challenging behaviors before they become a problem, you will be free to carry out your procedures as planned. However, if you do not take charge, you may spend the entire session attempting to regain your ability to guide constructive behavior. This is a situation that prevents you from carrying out your plan, and it also prevents the children from benefiting from the program as designed.

SYMPTOM-SPECIFIC SUGGESTIONS FOR LANGUAGE INTERVENTION

The preceding section includes a general outline and corresponding suggestions for implementing an ordinary language intervention program. The suggestions are meant to be applied aptly as a matter of course. In this section, more specific suggestions are provided with regard to the language intervention programs for children with a selection of specific language-learning needs. The suggestions that follow are for the language programs of **preverbal** children, children with deficient content-form interactions, children with disrupted language content and use, children for whom the language dimensions are separated, and children for whom the language dimensions do not interact well. They also apply to children with attention deficit disorder, children with central auditory dysfunction, children who are electively mute, children with reduced hearing sensitivity, and children who experience language difficulties that are concomitant with difficulties in learning to read and write.

Intervention Options for Preverbal Children

In order to move from being a preverbal child to being a child who uses even minimal language meaningfully, certain social, phonological, and cognitive milestones must be met. Some children who are preverbal have nonetheless already achieved some of these milestones. Therefore, it is important to determine exactly which milestones have been reached and which still need to be accomplished in order to move successfully from the preverbal to the verbal realm. Behaviors that are critical to first-word production and some corresponding facilitation suggestions are described in the remainder of this section.

Social Milestones.   Social milestones that are prerequisite to first words promote the development of the dimension of language use. In order to begin to use language meaningfully, a child must (1) desire social interaction and see language as a vehicle for social interaction and the development of social relationships, (2) see language as a means for communicating needs and desires (e.g., regulating the behavior of others), (3) take conversational turns, (4) initiate concrete topics, either verbally or nonverbally, and (5) maintain topics, verbally or nonverbally, for at least one or two conversational turns.

Social Interaction.   Social interaction may be facilitated through a number of play activities. Reciprocal gaze (i.e., looking at one another) and joint attention (i.e., paying attention to the same object) are fundamental to social interaction, and they may be facilitated by songs, nursery rhymes, finger plays, and games such as peek-a-boo and pat-a-cake. Further, they are very useful in helping a child to learn to enjoy verbal types of social interaction.

Communicating Needs and Desires.   Language as a means for communicating needs and desires is accomplished nonverbally first, and then, later, verbally. Pointing, gesturing, crying, and other nonverbal methods can be used by the child to successfully accomplish a personal goal. For example, if a child points at a ball and then an adult gives the ball to the child, the child may come to associate pointing at an object with being given the object. Initially, the clinician may physically manipulate a child's hand for pointing and then give the object to the child.

Alternately, if the child is capable of pointing, the A-R-C paradigm may be carefully applied in order to help him or her mentally associate the act of pointing with the accomplishment of controlling adult behavior. For example, suppose the desired response (R) is the act of pointing at the object. Then, the antecedent (A) is carefully planned to provide a motivation for the child to point. A possible antecedent may be to arrange the room so that several very attractive options are within the child's view but out of reach. If this antecedent alone does not precipitate the desired pointing response, then the environment may be further manipulated to encourage responding. For example, an adult may model the pointing response for the child. When the desired response (R) is elicited by the carefully planned antecedent (A), then the consequence (C) is applied immediately, with the most effective consequence being to comply with the child's request for the desired object.

Turn Taking.   Turn taking is learned preverbally through a number of experiences. Peek-a-boo, immediate verbal or nonverbal imitation, motor imitation, and vocal play are only a few examples of informal games that are used to preverbally facilitate turn taking.

Topic Initiation and Topic Maintenance.   Topic initiation and topic maintenance can be encouraged by making interesting items visible so that the child can point them out to the adult, either verbally or nonverbally. This may be enhanced by making the items visible but not accessible to the child. For example, a child who wants to use a visible jar of soap-bubble solution to blow bubbles but cannot reach it is likely to point it out in order to gain your assistance. Further, a number of additional conversational turns on the same topic, once the bubbles have been acquired, encourages topic maintenance. On the contrary, if the child can reach the bubbles, calling them to the attention of an adult seems unnecessary to the child. Keep in mind that placing any coveted object out of reach has the potential to encourage the child to initiate a topic.

In addition to making an enticement visible but not accessible, several other strategies are usually successful in encouraging a reticent child to initiate a topic and take a subsequent conversational turn. These may include providing an activity for which some of the necessary materials are missing. For example, a clinician may prepare a child for finger painting by providing a smock, easel, and paper, but deliberately neglect to provide the paint. If the child is interested in painting, he or she has a reason to find a way to request the paint.

Another strategy that often encourages preverbal children to initiate a topic is the transgression of a known rule. For example, most children know that when dressing a doll, the shoes go on the feet. If, instead, the clinician places the shoes on the doll's hands or head, then the child will have reason to initiate a topic in order to help the clinician dress the doll according to standard conventions.

One last strategy that may encourage a quiet child to initiate a turn and perhaps maintain the topic is to give the child two options for activities that may be performed. For example, by showing the child that both the ball and the modeling clay are the options, the child may be encouraged to indicate which one is desired.

Phonological Milestones.   The dimension of language form is promoted, in part, by developing the phonological aspect of language. In order to achieve phonological proficiency adequate for first-word production, the child must (1) produce a few recognizable consonants and vowels, and (2) consistently combine these phonemes to generate identifiable CV or VC syllables.

Producing Recognizable Vowels and Consonants.   In order to encourage the production of the recognizable vowels and consonants, the clinician systematically and clearly presents CV or VC syllables in a meaningful context, using consonants with the stop-manner feature ([k], [g], [t], [d], [p], and [b]) or bilabial-place feature ([p], [b], [m]), along with back or neutral vowels ([ʌ], [ɔ], and [u]). Some CV or VC combinations that may be considered for this purpose include [ʌp] (*up*), [aʊt] (*out*), [bɔ] (*ball*), [bʌbʌ] (*bubble*), and [bu] (*boo*, as in peek-a-boo].

Once produced, the syllables may be practiced in succession, as if practicing reduplicated babbling. However, reduplicating the syllables is not so much the objective as is working toward *producing the syllables consistently and in a meaningful context.*

Cognitive Milestones.   By achieving certain cognitive milestones, development of language content can be promoted. In order to produce meaningful words in context, the child must (1) mentally associate a combination of phonemes with an object, event, or relation and (2) consistently say the same CV or VC combination in order to represent the particular object, event, or relation.

Mental Associations.   Mental associations between a word and what the word represents emerge through repeated experience. That is, an adult consistently labels the same object, event, or relation by using the exact same combination of phonemes, and the child comes to associate that word with the concept that it represents. For example, the event of going up is always represented by the word *up*, the event of going out is always represented by the word *out*, and the object that is a ball is always called *ball*.

Therefore, in order to plan for the cognitive milestones to be met, a clinician selects objects, events, and relations that can be represented by simple CV, VC, or CVC combinations. Then, the clinician sets up situations in which he or she carefully and systematically labels each object, event, or relation in a meaningful context. By so doing, comprehension of the selected concepts is facilitated.

Regarding objects, in order for the first word to be produced, a child must be able to visually track objects, look for a moving object's reappearance after it disappears behind a screen, gaze at a partially hidden object and actively search when it fails to reappear, and actively search for an object that was recently the focus of attention (Lahey, 1988).

Regarding events, a child must be able to act on objects in prescribed ways, such as causing objects to disappear and reappear, imitating the actions of another person, performing appropriate actions on an object when the actions have not been seen before, and increasing the variety of actions and objects that are acted upon (Lahey, 1988).

Regarding relations, the preverbal child must understand certain object-to-object relations. These may be demonstrated by separating objects that have been joined in some way (taking a simple puzzle apart); rejoining objects that have been taken apart (putting the simple puzzle back together); joining objects that have not been joined previously, not necessarily taking into account how the objects may or may not relate (putting a toy cow into a play house); and joining objects in a way that shows an appreciation for the relationship between the objects (covering the doll with a blanket) (Lahey, 1988).

Consistent Representations. The other cognitive step necessary for first-word production is the *association between the object, event, or relation and the physical act of consistently producing the syllable that represents it.* For example, the child may be able to say [ʌp] consistently and even repeat the VC syllable again and again. However, in order to use the syllable as a meaningful word, the child has to clearly associate saying *up* with the event of going up.

This association is promoted by encouraging the child to express a known desire. For example, if the clinician becomes aware that the child wants to be picked up because the child's arms are outstretched in an upward direction, then the clinician might encourage the child to approximate the word *up* before actually picking up the child. Some ways to encourage the child to attempt to say the word might include saying, "Up? What do you want? Up?" or by saying, "Up?" while stretching one's arms out to the child. If the child can be encouraged to say *up*, if the clinician picks the child up immediately thereafter, and if this event is repeated a number of times, then a mental association will be formed between the production of the VC syllable *up* and the event of going up.

Talking With Preverbal Children.

Simplifying Linguistic Complexity. One principle that can be applied when modeling linguistic structures to preverbal children is the act of simplifying linguistic complexity (Fey, 1986). For example, when speaking to a preverbal child, you may use very short, simple sentences that include only key words (e.g., "Want up?" instead of "Do you want to go up?" or "More cookie," instead of "Here's another cookie"). This is done in order to provide a linguistic model that is within the child's grasp of both comprehension and production.

However, some controversy surrounds this procedure (Fey, 1986). Drastically reducing the length and complexity of utterances when facilitating language comprehension and production is not necessarily essential, as many children learn to comprehend and produce language when adult-language models are only minimally reduced. Further, modeling only utterances that are grammatically incomplete is not always desirable because it may deny the child the benefit of hearing longer, grammatically complete utterances in contextual speech.

Nevertheless, for the purpose of demonstrating with absolute clarity how words can be combined or how morphological markers can be used meaningfully, it is acceptable to model very short, simple, even telegraphic sentences to preverbal children and to children who primarily use single-word utterances. Still, once the simplified sentence has been clearly modeled in an appropriate context, it is wise then to present a similar sentence that is simple yet grammatically complete (e.g., while reaching out to the child, the adult says: "Want up? Do you want up?").

Self-Talk. Self-talk (Fey, 1986) is a very innocuous method for facilitating an interaction with a child who hesitates to communicate verbally. When engaging in self-talk, one verbalizes whatever one sees, hears, does, or feels. Self-talk is talk produced by the adult about what he or she is experiencing. It is always produced with a great deal of enthusiasm and the adult's activities are highly animated, so that the child is likely to be motivated to join in.

Self-talk is enhanced if the adult mimics the activities of the child and then uses the same enthusiasm and animation to describe the imitations. By this modification to self-talk, the adult enables the child to hear an account of ongoing, firsthand experiences. Further, the adult communicates a positive message about the child's choice of activities.

Several objectives may be accomplished during self-talk. For the reticent child, it provides a nonthreatening environment that places no demands to either speak or listen. Further, it provides a communication model that demonstrates spoken language at any level the clinician chooses. For example, if the objective is for the child to begin to increase utterance length to two words, then the clinician models two-word sentences, while if the objective is to facilitate certain morphological markers, then the clinician creates short sentences modeling the specific markers that are targeted.

Parallel-Talk. **Parallel-talk** (Fey, 1986) is similar to self-talk in that it is the clinician who does the talking. However, it is different from self-talk in that in parallel-talk, instead of talking about one's own experiences, the clinician makes comments about the actions of the child and the objects that appear to hold the child's attention.

Parallel-talk has far greater potential than self-talk for facilitating language development in children who hesitate to speak because, in addition to that which is accomplished by self-talk, parallel-talk accomplishes at least three important objectives: (1) parallel-talk communicates to the child that the adult appreciates the object or event that is of interest; (2) it provides a clear linguistic label describing exactly what is of apparent interest to the child at that moment; and (3) by talking about objects and events that are of interest, one increases the probability of the child producing a spontaneous utterance in response.

Facilitating Interaction between Language Content and Form

Content-form interactions, as defined in Chapter 2, are the linguistic occasions whereby the context of the utterance obligates a particular language form. When content-form interactions are disrupted, the context obligates the form but the form is *not* used. Because of the powerful interdependency and interrelation between language content and language form, this type of deficiency describes many of the disruptions of both language form and content.

For example, the vocabulary deficiency described in the demonstration sample (Tables 4–1 through 4–5 and Figure 4–2) may at first glance appear to reflect a disruption of language content alone. However, the content, or meaning, is represented by very specific words and other morphological markers, each having a particular and identifiable form. Therefore, it is not content alone that is disrupted, but the representation of content by form, or the interaction between content and form.

Furthermore, by way of example, any morphology errors are the result, not just of difficulties with language form but also with the way in which that form is used to represent content. For example, the *-ed* past-tense marker is an aspect of language form that carries a great deal of meaning. By leaving it out, the entire idea of a sentence is altered (e.g., "I love you" is very different from "I loved you"). The same holds for nearly all morphological markers, including, but not limited to, *-s* (plural), *-s* (possessive), *-s* (third-person singular verb form), *-ing* (present progressive), *-ing* (gerund), copula *be*, auxiliaries, modals, and prepositions.

Syntactic structure is also an aspect of form that is mutually dependent with content. Word order, for example, is clearly important to meaning, as is demonstrated by changing the order of the words in a simple sentence such as, "The *boy* chased the *dog*" to "The *dog* chased the *boy*," which conveys an entirely different idea.

Toddlers and Preschoolers Who Talk.   Once the child uses single-word utterances with some degree of regularity, he or she is no longer considered preverbal. However, once language intervention is initiated, it usually continues until reaching the **terminal objectives** or age-appropriate language.

With very young children in language intervention, a child-centered (as opposed to a trainer-centered) approach is very appropriate for facilitating content-form. Not only can child-centered approaches be implemented during planned intervention sessions, adaptations can also be implemented by caregivers during daily routines (Fey, 1986). Child-centered procedures are also called facilitative-play procedures, which are described in the paragraphs that follow.

Facilitative Play.   Facilitative play is one vehicle by which child-centered intervention can be applied. For the purposes of this discussion, facilitative play is defined as an activity in which (1) the child is free to select materials and the manner in which the materials are used, (2) the activity is used to create a highly accepting and responsive environment in which the child is motivated to communicate spontaneously with the clinician or caregiver, and (3) the activity is used as the context for applying child-centered language intervention procedures (Fey, 1986).

By using facilitative play, a skilled clinician can facilitate the emergence of a number of content-form interactions. These include, but are not limited to, increasing utterance length, expanding semantic categories, introducing morphological markers, developing more advanced sentence structures, and adjusting inaccurate syntactic arrangements of words in sentences.

Following the Child's Lead.   The fundamental facilitative play procedure is called following the child's lead, and it permeates nearly all procedures that characterize the child-centered approach. Following a child's lead involves three steps (Fey, 1986).

First, the clinician (or caregiver) sets up a situation that is likely to result in some communicative attempt on the part of the child, and then he or she waits for the child to say or do something that can be interpreted as an attempt at communication. For example, the clinician knows a child (Veronica) well enough to know that a ball is a favorite toy, so the clinician sets up the intervention room such that a ball is visible but not accessible to Veronica. Further, self-talk and parallel-talk may be incorporated in order to provide a linguistic model for the target word. By arranging things in this way, the clinician is reasonably assured that any overtures made in the direction of the ball can be interpreted as behavior intended to communicate a desire to have or play with that toy.

Second, having waited for the child to produce a behavior that can be reasonably interpreted as an attempt at communication, the clinician then proceeds to interpret the behavior as having meaning and some communicative intent. Continuing with the example of Veronica, once in the intervention setting, Veronica sees the ball, points to it, and says, "ba." The utterance *ba* may be interpreted in a number of ways, and it is up to the clinician to choose the likeliest possibility. For example, the utterance may be intended to point out that there is a ball "over there," or it may be interpreted as a request to obtain or play with the ball.

The child's behavior and the clinician's objectives may be used to interpret the intentions. For example, if the child points to the ball and then moves directly to the modeling clay, the clinician can be reasonably sure that the intent is merely to point out the presence of the ball in the room. However, if the child points to the ball and continues to gesture toward it, and perhaps even whine, the clinician can assume that the intent is to communicate a desire to either have or play with the ball.

Third, once the child has made the utterance and the clinician has interpreted it in some way, it is up to the clinician to give a communicative response that is intended to facilitate language development. Options for these kinds of responses include expansions, expatiations, recast sentences, and buildups and breakdowns.

Expansions. Expansions (Fey, 1986) are defined as contingent verbal responses that repeat a child's prior utterance while adding relevant grammatical, and sometimes semantic, details. When following the child's lead, using expansions is one option for responding to the child's behavior in such a way as to facilitate communication development.

In the example above, when Veronica says a word approximation meaning *ball* and continues to gesture toward the ball, the clinician can use expansions if an objective is to increase Veronica's utterance length to two words. Two-word utterances that can be modeled immediately subsequent to Veronica's single-word utterance include "Want ball," "Play ball," or "Ball down."

Once the ball is in the child's possession, expansions combined with self-talk or parallel-talk may be used to continue to model two-word utterances for Veronica. "Roll ball," "Throw ball," "Bounce ball," "Ball up," "Ball gone," and "More ball" are all examples of two-word combinations that may be presented as expansions to Veronica's single-word utterance. In each case, the utterance describes for Veronica something that she (or the clinician) is doing with the ball.

Expansions accomplish a number of objectives. Comprehension of the model is facilitated because the model is composed, in part, of something that the child has already said. Moreover, by expanding the child's utterance, the adult communicates that what the child says is important and worthy of attention. Further, expansions model appropriate and contingent conversational responses and are likely to facilitate the development of conversational cohesion.

Expatiations.   Expatiations (Fey, 1986) are similar to expansions and are defined as contingent responses that extend some aspect of the child's meaning by contributing new, but relevant, information. They do not necessarily describe something that the child is doing. Instead, they add new information or even suggest possibilities for things that can be done.

In the example used here, when Veronica's single-word utterance is expanded, in each case the expanded utterance describes something that Veronica or the clinician is doing. By contrast, an expatiation might describe the ball further by adding new information about the ball (e.g., "Red ball," "Big ball"), or it may suggest to Veronica something that she can do with the ball (e.g., any of the previously mentioned two-word sentence expansions, if spoken as a suggestion).

Expatiations are likely to facilitate language development in the following ways. Since the adult model is closely related to an utterance recently spoken by the child, it is likely that the more complicated adult model will be comprehended. If it is not comprehended immediately, then because of the relationship between the model and the child's utterance, the child is likely to search for a logical interpretation of the adult model. Further, expatiations foster an appreciation for the reciprocal nature of conversation in much the same way as expansions. That is, the child learns by firsthand experience that the utterance is worthy of adult attention and experiences conversation that is appropriate and cohesive.

Recast Sentences.   Recast sentences (Fey, 1986) are related to expansions and expatiations in that the child's own sentence is repeated in some modified form. Recast sentences, however, are somewhat more complicated in that the clinician changes the modality or voice of the sentence rather than simply adding grammatical or semantic markers. Statements may be changed to the question form, such that if the child says, "The baby is hungry," the clinician responds with, "Is she hungry?" Active voice may be changed to passive voice, such that the sentence, "The dog chases the cat," is changed by the clinician to say "The cat is chased by the dog."

All the objectives of expansions and expatiations can be accomplished by recast sentences. Further, recast sentences are useful for children who are working on more complex grammatical forms.

Buildups and Breakdowns.   Buildups and breakdowns (Fey, 1986) describe a three-part procedure that is applied to the child's own utterance and can be used to help a child understand the relationships between words in more complex sentences (Figure 4–4). The first step is for the clinician to expand the child's utterance, or build it up. For example, suppose that Veronica, in the

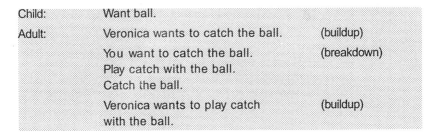

Child:	Want ball.	
Adult:	Veronica wants to catch the ball.	(buildup)
	You want to catch the ball.	(breakdown)
	Play catch with the ball.	
	Catch the ball.	
	Veronica wants to play catch with the ball.	(buildup)

Figure 4-4. Clinical example: Buildup and breakdown procedure.

example above, says, "Want ball." The clinician then builds up the utterance by saying, "Veronica wants to play catch with the ball."

The second step is for the clinician to take the expanded utterance and break it down into a series of repetitive and related utterances. Some possible breakdown sentences might be: "You want to catch the ball." "Play catch with the ball." "Catch the ball" (Figure 4–4).

The third step is for the clinician to build the utterance up again, by repeating the original expansion or some variation of it. The original expansion in this case is "Veronica wants to play catch with the ball" (Figure 4–4).

All the objectives accomplished by expansions and expatiations are also accomplished by the buildup-and-breakdown procedure. However, the method is not appropriate for children who have difficulty paying attention while the clinician goes through the three-step modeling process. Further, the procedure is probably most effective when it is combined with other facilitative play procedures such as parallel-talk, expansions, expatiations, and recast sentences.

School-Age Children.   Many school-age children and older preschoolers are able to benefit from intervention procedures that have more structure than the child-centered approaches. However, the basic principles of facilitative play are very appropriate for older language learners as well. That is, the clinical environment is one in which the child is motivated to communicate. It is an accepting environment where the child is able to experiment with language without fear of being criticized. Moreover, the child is allowed to select the materials whenever possible. Children work harder if they are allowed to participate in this way. Further, the clinician's response to the child's utterances is important since it demonstrates, in a nonthreatening way, some possibilities for alleviating the language errors that occur.

Interactive Language Development Teaching (ILDT).   ILDT is a procedure that combines structure with some flexibility, and it is ideal for groups of three to six school-age children (Lee, Koenigsknecht, & Mulhern, 1975). When using ILDT, each session lasts approximately 50 minutes and is divided into two parts.

The first part of the ILDT session lasts for about 30 to 35 minutes. During this time, the clinician tells a story that has been selected or developed specifically with consideration given to the intervention objectives of the children in the group. In determining the content of the story and in telling the story, some principles are followed. First, the theme and the characters of the story are familiar to the child. That means that the clinician may select from well-known stories, such as fairy tales and fables, or the clinician may write a story that uses real-life and familiar scenarios and characters, such as family and classroom routines. This principle is applied in order to minimize the attention that the child must pay to the new information, thus freeing him or her to focus attention on the target forms.

Second, in telling the story, the clinician restates important events frequently. This is in order to enable the children to hear the target structures repeatedly. Primary targets are modeled at least five times during the story, while secondary targets (those recently acquired or future primary targets) are presented at least three or four times.

Third, the use of simple props is encouraged. As their purpose is only to hold the child's attention during the telling of the story, props that lack detail are perfectly acceptable. Fourth, the children are encouraged to participate in telling the story. However, target responses are required only after sufficient models have been presented.

Fifth, because a number of children are in the group and they may not all have the same primary and secondary targets, the clinician plans the presentation of targets very carefully. Individualized stimuli are presented to each child and different questions are asked depending on which child is expected to respond.

Sixth, when a child makes an incorrect response to a question, the clinician has a number of response options that may be used to facilitate the child's producing the desirable grammatical form. These include giving a complete model that the child is required to imitate, giving a partial model that the child is required to repeat and complete, requesting that the child expand on the utterance, requesting a repetition, repeating the child's error in order to demonstrate its inappropriateness, and requesting a self-correction.

Once the story is complete, the children take a short break and then begin part two of ILDT, which is to participate in a group activity that continues the theme of the story and affords each child an opportunity to practice the targets. Part two activities require about 20 minutes of time, and they may be artistic, dramatic, or real-life in nature. During the activity, the clinician collects language samples to assess progress, models the targets in a meaningful context, and elicits the target responses from the children in spontaneous conversational speech.

Intervention Options for Children with Disrupted Language Content

The child with disrupted language content needs meaningful experiences that encourages him or her to have something of consequence to say. These experiences include experiences with objects (people, animals, things, or places), events (things that happen), relations between objects (the way in which people and objects are related to each other), and relations between events (the way in which events are related to one another in time and space and with regard to causality).

For children who have difficulty developing language content, practice experiences may be simple. Further, objects, events, and relations should be clearly labeled linguistically so that the child not only encounters a variety of concepts, but also experiences hearing the language used for the purpose of coding the experience. Self-talk, parallel-talk, reduced linguistic complexity, and facilitative play strategies, as described in the sections on facilitating content-form, may also be applied to facilitate the coding of language content.

Intervention Options for Unintelligible Children

When language form is disrupted to the extent that a child is difficult to understand, knowing whether comprehension is also impaired is critical to planning intervention. Therefore, some suggestions follow, both for unintelligible children with age-appropriate comprehension and for unintelligible children for whom language comprehension is also compromised.

When Comprehension Is Age-Appropriate.   When a child's speech is unintelligible and language comprehension is age-appropriate, it is probably disrupted form, and not content or use, that lies at the root of the communication disorder. Since speech is unintelligible, it is difficult to ascertain whether expressive language is at or below age level or to identify specific aberrant patterns of language expression. Moreover, since comprehension is within normal limits, there is no apparent need to address language from a receptive point of view. Therefore, it is critical to first improve intelligibility so that the child can be understood before determining whether any expressive language targets are to be addressed.

For unintelligible children, a phonological approach to intervention is often recommended. This involves the identification of phonological processes (patterned modifications of speech-sound production that are not consistent with the standard rules of the language). In general, phonological processes are simplified productions of standard phoneme sequences and words (Creaghead & Newman, 1989). Some examples are syllable reduction ([ba] for bottle), consonant sequence reduction ([bu] for blue), and stopping ([ti] for see) (Hodson, 1986).

Once the patterns are identified, then the patterns, and not the error phonemes, must be addressed in a very systematic manner. Addressing simplification patterns, or phonological processes, is a very efficient method for improving the intelligibility of an unintelligible child. These patterns are addressed through a cycles approach that combines auditory bombardment, visual and tactile stimulation, production practice, and semantic awareness. Complete descriptions of the approach are available (Hodson & Paden, 1991).

When Comprehension Is Compromised.   When compromised comprehension is concomitant to unintelligible speech, then, in addition to the phonological targets, discrete comprehension difficulties must be identified and targeted. This may be accomplished in much the same way as the cognitive milestones addressed in the previous section on the preverbal child.

Intervention Options for Children with a Pattern of Disrupted Language Use

A child whose language disturbance lies with the dimension of language use has age-appropriate ideas to communicate and communicates them clearly through the conventional linguistic system yet delivers the message in a way that is inappropriate. For example, children who have *attention deficit disorder (ADD)* often display symptoms of difficulties with the dimension of language use. Their apragmatic behaviors often include interrupting people, attempting to talk over the words of other people, making comments that are inappropriate or unrelated to the topic, and shifting topics without warning.

Some children with *learning disabilities, emotional disturbance,* and *mental retardation* also show symptoms of adversely effected language use. Any combination of the symptoms of disrupted language use (as described in Chapter 2) may appear in these aggregates of children.

Elective mutism describes a group of children whose language use is also inappropriate. Since the electively mute child chooses not to speak, speaker and listener roles are impaired, initiating and maintaining topics is not done, changing topics is unnecessary, turn taking is nonexistent, and paralinguistic aspects of verbal communication are absent. Paralinguistic aspects of nonverbal communication may or may not be appropriate, depending on the child.

Children who have been involved in extensive speech therapy are another group that may have difficulties with language use. Many of the symptoms appear to be the result of having spent a significant amount of time sitting across the table from an adult, and practicing the production of unrelated words or sentences and speech that is not meant to provide new information to a conversational partner.

Inappropriate communication behaviors that are sometimes noticed in long-term recipients of speech therapy seem to include the tendency to (1) produce or recite utterances rather than interact socially or exchange information, (2) shift topic without warning, (3) wait for instruction before taking a turn, (4) ignore nonverbal clues that communicate that clarification is needed, and (5) neglect to request clarification when needed. In short, speech is considered something to be practiced and not as a vehicle for meaningful communication.

Most of these problems can, and should be, avoided by using intervention techniques that are natural and communicative rather than those that are repetitive and devoid of context. Suggestions for natural, communicative strategies appear in the previous section, "Planning for Generalization."

Preschool-Age Children.   Regardless of the exact objectives that are to be addressed for the preschool-age child with disrupted language use, children benefit more from firsthand experience than from instruction. Therefore, if the clinical objective is for the child to successfully participate in rituals such as routine greetings and closings, then situations are set up that enable the child to first observe another person participating in the routine appropriately and then practice the routine with a real communication partner.

Some sample circumstances that may be used to facilitate the demonstration and practice of greeting and closing routine might include (1) arranging for another adult or child to enter the room periodically, (2) using puppets or dolls to demonstrate the routine and then participating in the routine with the child, or (3) using group intervention in which each child assists in demonstration and practice.

The use of puppets is practical for most settings where preschoolers receive clinical services. The demonstration steps may include (1) introducing the illustration, (2) using puppets or role players to illustrate the target, (3) briefly discussing exactly what happened immediately following the illustration, and (4) judging whether an illustrated behavior is appropriate or inappropriate.

The introduction to the illustration may include an explanation of the intervention objective, which should be modified to match the child's level of understanding. For example, if the objective is for the child to use greeting and closing rituals, then the introduction may include a story about people coming and going and the kinds of things they say when they first see each other and when they part. By the time the introduction is over, the child will be mentally prepared to pay attention to greetings and closings.

The illustration is carried out by puppets or role players. An example might be for the puppets to perform a series of several greetings and closings. Two friends meeting on the street, a visit to Grandma's, and seeing the teacher at the grocery store are some possibilities. The puppets carry out the routines, clearly demonstrating what one says and does when greeting someone and when terminating a conversation.

When the puppets have demonstrated greetings comprehensibly, the child may then participate in some discussion about what has happened. This may include a recount of the skits performed by the puppets. It may also include some speculation on what to do in similar circumstances not illustrated.

The illustration may take on a little more depth at this point, if desired. That is, the puppets may continue to perform but now, sometimes their behavior is appropriate and sometimes not. For example, during a set of follow-up skits, the puppets may forget to greet each other or they may greet each other in a rude way. This is the child's opportunity to judge whether the behavior of the puppets is appropriate or inappropriate. The discussion about the inappropriate skits may include some problem solving about how the unsuitable behavior makes the other person feel and what could be said or done that would be more apropos.

Following the illustration, the child has the opportunity to role-play in order to practice the language use objective. The practice steps may include (1) preparation for the practice skit, (2) role-play using puppets or other children, and (3) discussion of the performance with regard to the pragmatic target.

In preparing the child for the practice skit, it is important to make very clear exactly what roles are to be assumed by whom. The demonstration skits will probably have prepared the child adequately for the practice experience. Explanation of the details, however, may include telling the child the names and roles of the participants and the occasion and purpose of the meeting. Moreover, if it is the case that the puppet is going to behave inappropriately, it may be wise to inform the child of this in advance so as not to cause embarrassment or hurt feelings as a result of the performance.

The performance is an opportunity for the child to participate in a series of practice exercises with a puppet or role player. These may be similar to the illustration skits described previously.

Once the performance is complete, a discussion may follow. This includes comments about what has happened, and about what the characters did and said. It may also include a judgment of whether the puppets behaved appropriately, and if they did not, what they could do to improve their interactions.

Although it is not usually the case that a child is asked to use an inappropriate behavior during the practice exercise, be prepared for that possibility as well. If a child behaves inappropriately, the clinician should evaluate each situation individually. It may be wise to address the inappropriate behavior directly by asking the child to identify it and come up with some suggestions for alternative actions. However, with some children who are particularly sensitive, calling attention to an error in the presence of peers may be devastating and may discourage future willingness to participate in role-play activities.

School-Age Children.   By the age of 6, most children begin to benefit from instruction about language as long as it is appropriately combined with direct experience, while children age 8 and above have an even greater appreciation for metalinguistic training. For that reason, the suggestions for preschool intervention apply to this group as well. Further, with school-age children it is possible to incorporate more direct and abstract instruction and to increase the complexity of the tasks.

When Form, Content, and Use Are Separated

A child whose language is characterized by a separation of content, form, and use typically uses a language form that is not particularly meaningful in context. Examples are echolalia and perseveration. A child may repeatedly utter comments heard either in the home, at school, on the radio, or on the television.

In Chapter 2, an example was given of a child who repeatedly says, "Put the bear on Mary's bed, Suzy," regardless of whether the bear, Mary, or Mary's bed are even remotely accessible to Suzy. Other examples include the child who immediately repeats, verbatim, what has been said by another person (echolalia) or who repeats an utterance that was correct at one time but is no longer correct or accurate (perseveration).

Children who demonstrate behaviors characteristic of a separation of the language dimensions are often seriously mentally retarded, autistic, socially inappropriate, or emotionally affected. How well we are able to bring echolalic and perseverative behaviors under control is quite dependent on the degree of severity that characterizes the disorder. That is, a child who is mildly retarded (with an IQ of 55 to 69) may be capable of consciously controlling the occurrence of nonmeaningful utterances. By contrast, a child who is moderately or severely retarded (an IQ between 25 and 54) may have more difficulty identifying when a response is not meaningful in order to suppress it. For the profoundly retarded (an IQ below 25), the capacity for controlling meaningless utterances is usually minimal.

In children who are able to learn to control echolalia and perseveration, this is often done by calling the child's attention to the fact that the utterance is not related to the immediate context or ongoing events. Once this is pointed out, some suggestions for meaningful and contextually related utterances may be offered. Further, the client may be asked to produce some contextually relevant alternatives.

When Interactions Between Form, Content, and Use Are Disrupted

A child whose language behavior indicates a disordered interaction between the dimensions (i.e., content, form, and use) uses language that has an obvious contradiction between the content of the message and the way the message is delivered. The example given in Chapter 2 is the child who says, "Don't spank the baby," while hitting a rag doll.

Children whose dimensional interactions are disordered, as with those whose dimensions are separated, are often retarded or autistic. Further, the ability to bring the behavior under control is dependent on the degree of impairment. The suggested methods for accomplishing this are similar to those described in the preceding section on separation of content, form, and use.

When Attention Deficit Disorder Interferes

A child is diagnosed as having attention deficit disorder (ADD) when behavior indicates that he or she is highly distractible and inattentive. This condition typically impedes language acquisition, primarily in the dimension of language use. Further, if not addressed adequately in the preschool years, ADD has a negative impact on academic success. Therefore, the diagnosis of ADD significantly impacts the planning and implementation of the intervention program. It is important to address the attention deficits directly from the beginning of intervention, not only in order to increase the manageability of the child but also to prepare him or her to use social language appropriately and to succeed academically.

Since the child with ADD is characteristically distractible and inattentive, the two general goals that distinguish intervention for ADD are that the child learn to (1) manage distractions and (2) focus attention. In most cases, learning to manage distractions results in an increased ability to focus attention. Therefore, the two general objectives can usually be addressed simultaneously, as follows.

Managing Distractions.   In order for a child to learn to manage distractions, it may be necessary first to remove as many distractions as possible and then systematically to reintroduce them one at a time, as the child becomes capable of concentrating in their presence. At least three types of distractions may interfere with a child's ability to focus attention. They are visual distractions, auditory distractions, and psychological distractions. Any combination of the three may serve to prevent a child from completing work and behaving appropriately; consider all three when determining which distractions to bring under clinical control.

Managing Visual Distractions.   Visual distractions are the things and people that are present in the room and interfere with the child's ability to concentrate. Other children, the clinician, articles of clothing, jewelry, toys, intervention materials, papers, equipment, furniture, decorations, and clocks are a few examples. For the child with ADD who is visually distracted, initially these distractions are best minimized as much as possible. Thus, the child might be scheduled for individual sessions and seated at a table that faces a blank wall, with only the few materials necessary for the current assignment within view. Excessive verbal praise may be offered in an attempt to encourage continued work.

As the child becomes able to concentrate in this rather sterile environment, the clinician may add a few visual distractions, very systematically and one at a time. In order to achieve concentration, it may be necessary for the clinician to continually notice when the child becomes distracted and remind him or her to focus attention. However, it is ultimately the child's responsibility to identify distractions and return to task.

When the child identifies and resolves visual distractions independently, then it may be time to introduce additional distractor items. For example, a purposeful picture may be added to the wall. Then, as the child becomes able to autonomously focus attention even in the presence of the picture, an extraneous item may be added to the table or the table may be turned so that some of the room decorations are visible.

Eventually, it is hoped that the ADD child who is visually distracted is able to concentrate in a setting with an increasing number of miscellaneous distractions that include a variety of people and things. The preparation for that accomplishment involves achieving an internal locus of control for managing a few distractions at first and eventually a number of potentially interfering visual stimuli.

Managing Auditory Distractions. Auditory distractions are another type of distraction that may interfere with the ADD child's ability to concentrate. They include noises that occur in the room, such as sounds produced by air conditioning or heating systems, ambient noises in the corridor, clocks ticking, and conversations of other people who may be working in adjacent quarters. Regardless of whether a child has ADD, all these variables should be controlled to the best of the clinician's ability. In some settings, that may require negotiating for a private and reasonably quiet work area.

If auditory distractions are present in the room, they should be carefully controlled by the clinician in much the same way as the visual distractions. That is, you should begin with a reasonably quiet room. If the child tends to be distracted auditorily, systematically add one distraction at a time (e.g., soft background music, a clock ticking), never adding a new distraction until the child has achieved independent control of the auditory distractions at each level.

Managing Psychological Distraction. Psychological distractions are the most abstract and the most difficult to bring under control. If a child is distracted psychologically, intrapersonal communication (i.e., personal thought) interferes with the child's ability to concentrate. These thoughts may pertain to an anticipation of activities yet to come, preoccupation with the time, recollection of past events, or mental problem solving.

All people engage in these mental activities at least some of the time. However, when one's internal thoughts consistently interfere with the ability to focus attention and complete a task, then intervention is indicated.

As with the visual and auditory distractions, with psychological distractions it is necessary to begin with an external locus of control and gradually move toward an internal locus of control. Some steps toward accomplishing the independent control of psychological distractions may include the following: (1) Initially the clinician identifies the fact that the client is internally distracted and informs the client of the distraction, calling his or her attention back to the task. (2) After a number of distractions have been managed successfully in this way, the clinician begins to increase the subtlety of the signal so that the client is responsible to identify and control the distraction without direct instruction. (3) Once that has been accomplished, the clinician begins to demand that the client focus attention, without being told to do so, whenever an episode of distraction is called to the client's attention. (4) When the client is consistently taking the responsibility to return to a task after being informed of a mental distraction, the clinician may begin to request that when distraction is identified as present, the client specifically identify its source. (5) Eventually, the client recognizes when a mental distraction has interfered with the ability to focus attention, identifies the distraction, and returns to the task with no specific instructions from anyone.

Focusing Attention.   Simultaneous to teaching the child to manage distractions that interfere with attention, the clinician works with the child on improving the ability to focus attention. Being alert to factors that impact interest level, intensity of concentration, and duration of concentration is eminently important to achieving this.

Interest Level.   If a child has attention deficit disorder, his or her level of interest in the intervention activities is critical to focusing attention and to the success of the program. This is because attention to the task is necessary (1) for progress toward achieving language objectives, (2) for establishing a pattern of paying attention to the task while in the clinical environment, and (3) for eventually learning to consistently focus attention outside the clinical setting.

In planning intervention, select activities that are interesting to the child and use them for the greater part of the session. Interesting activities can be identified by questioning the child, the parent, the teacher, and significant others about the kinds of activities that typically hold the child's attention for more than a few moments.

Once a selection of interesting activities has been identified, they are then adapted to make them useful for facilitating the child's language learning needs. *For example, the activities described in Figures 4–2 and 4–3 (tea party and dress-up) are selected for the child only after determining that they are likely to hold attention for sufficient time to carry out the language-learning objectives. If there is no evidence that the activities in Figures 4–2 and 4–3 are likely to hold the child's attention, then they are not selected and, in fact, are replaced by activities that are more likely to interest the child. For example, if the child has an interest in a popular cartoon show, its characters may be used to achieve the objective of facilitating comprehension and production of third-person possessive pronouns instead of using the props suggested in the example.*

Initially, the goal is to achieve consistent attention for a period of time that is significantly longer than the baseline. If a session is 30 minutes long, a clinician may begin the program by planning to use a variety of high-interest activities for the entire session, with each activity being no more than 4 to 5 minutes in length. When consistent attention is achieved with extremely stimulating activities, then some more structured, more mundane activities should be introduced gradually. For example, once the child has established a pattern of focusing attention when engaged in the highly varied, stimulating procedures, then it is time to introduce one very short activity that is less interesting to the child, but not completely dull. The duration of the less-interesting activity may be from 1 to 5 minutes, depending on how long the child tolerates it without becoming significantly distracted. The timing for introducing the activity within the session is important. It may be best to initiate the less interesting activity about halfway through the session so that attention can be adequately focused before introducing it and also so the session can end after a significant period of highly stimulating work. With success the duration, number, and frequency of the less-stimulating activities can be increased gradually.

Intensity of Concentration.   In increasing a distractible child's ability to focus attention, a clinician must be mindful of the intensity of the child's concentration. For example, the quality of the concentration can vary throughout a session, even if the child does not appear to be actively distracted by internal and external stimuli. By paying close attention to signs that concentration is waning (e.g., wandering eyes or off-topic questions), a clinician may anticipate off-focus behavior before it occurs and then intercept it (by changing activities or by managing distractions) before it interferes with the goal of establishing a pattern of focused attention in the clinic.

Duration of Concentration.   Like intensity of concentration the clinician monitors the duration of each period of concentration. This is done so that (1) breaks in concentration can be predicted, and perhaps avoided, before they occur and (2) the clinician can monitor, and eventually extend, the typical length of concentration periods. Be aware that the length and intensity of concentration may vary for different levels of interest.

In the Case of Central Auditory Dysfunction

When a child is known to have central auditory dysfunction, two intervention objectives take priority. They are (1) to make auditory information accessible to the child and (2) to enable the child to gain the ability to manage distractions. The second objective was discussed in moderate detail in the previous section on attention deficit disorder.

The first objective, making auditory information accessible to the child, was not described previously because it specifically applies to children who have central auditory dysfunction. In order to accomplish this objective, one may systematically decrease the length and complexity of utterances spoken to the child, gradually increasing them as the child gains ability to handle incoming auditory stimuli. Moreover, systematically inserting meaningful pauses, emphasizing key words, and increasing visual and tactile cues all help to facilitate the processing of auditory information. Each of these modifications is utilized heavily at the initiation of the intervention program and then systematically reduced as the child gains the ability to make use of auditory information.

When a Child Is Electively Mute

Elective mutism was described in Chapter 3. In language intervention, it is important to break the aberrant communication pattern that has evolved without passing judgment on the caretakers or the child for having allowed the habit to become firmly established. Since the pattern emerges and is perpetuated in the context of the family or home, it is necessary to implement a family-oriented approach to intervention (see Chapter 5). In the family-oriented approach, the clinician guides the individual family members as they (1) identify their personal behaviors that serve to sustain the pattern, (2) make decisions about how they plan to change their own behaviors so as to encourage verbal communication, and (3) implement the changes.

In addition to involving the family, some modification can be made to increase the likelihood that the electively mute child will speak in the language intervention session. That is, children who do not wish to speak can be prompted to break the ice by a number of methods. A few minor adjustments have been found to facilitate a relaxed clinical atmosphere and are therefore appropriate for intervention in the event of elective mutism. These are the provision of culturally sensitive background music, use of the child's own familiar toys, and minimizing distractions in the clinical environment. However, providing a relaxed atmosphere offers no assurance that the child will talk. This is only a beginning. (Other suggestions were given in the section on nonverbal children earlier in this chapter.)

Removing all expectations of verbal communication is also essential to facilitating speech in elective mutism. Although removing expectations does not guarantee that the child will speak, neglecting to do so practically guarantees that he or she will not.

Additionally, we sometimes provide an electively mute child with a puppet or doll. Then, we speak directly to the puppet, waiting for a response from the child. By not speaking directly to the child and instead substituting the puppet, we create a situation in which the child is not the one who speaks since the words and sentences belong to the puppet. Even before an electively mute child speaks in an interpersonal exchange, the puppet technique can be used to gather information about the child's language abilities and to practice all types of linguistic patterns.

Beyond that, once the electively mute child begins to speak voluntarily, a language disorder is likely to become noticeable. Whether disturbed language is the cause or result of the elective mutism is difficult to determine, and probably irrelevant to the plan and outcome of treatment. It is incumbent on the clinician to accurately describe and treat the unique features of the language disorder as they emerge. Whenever there is a clinical history of elective mutism, it is crucial that the family participate in the language intervention program (see Chapter 5).

When Hearing Sensitivity Is Reduced

Speech-language intervention for the individual with reduced hearing sensitivity is often quite different from what is appropriate for individuals who have sensory access to spoken language. In addition to the degree of sensitivity reduction, timing and consistency of amplification and training as well as exposure to signed communication systems can strongly influence the outcome of the intervention program. An explanation of exactly how these factors are likely to impact intervention and some specific intervention suggestions are provided in the following sections.

Timing and Consistency of Amplification and Training. When an individual has reduced hearing sensitivity and he or she (or the family on the client's behalf) wishes to learn to understand and produce spoken language, then amplification and training are required—the earlier, the better. Three types of amplification devices are available: hearing aids, tactile aids, and cochlear implants. Regardless of the device used to enhance sound signals, if spoken language is to be learned, individuals with reduced hearing require access to amplification *and* training as early as possible. Spoken language is primarily an acoustic event and is best learned through accessing and comprehending its acoustic patterns.

The most common amplification device is the *hearing aid.* Types of hearing aids include body-type, all-in-the-ear, behind-the-ear (BTE), bone conduction, contra-lateral routing of signals (CROS), and extended-frequency hearing aids.

Regardless of type, most hearing aids are composed of three basic parts (Figure 4–5), the microphone, amplifier, and receiver. Sound enters the hearing aid through a microphone. The microphone changes the acoustic signal (i.e., sound) into an electrical signal. The intensity of the electrical signal is then increased through the amplifier. Finally, the amplified electrical signal passes through the receiver, where it is converted back into an acoustic signal that is much louder than the one picked up by the microphone. The magnified acoustic signal then leaves the hearing aid and enters the ear canal by way of an ear mold (Figure 4–5). It eventually travels through the air conduction pathway of the external ear toward the middle ear and cochlear (Figure 1–7) (Northern & Downs, 1991).

What we can expect a hearing aid to do is to magnify the sound so that the person with reduced hearing detects sounds that are otherwise inaudible. The difference between the minimum sound that a person is able to hear with

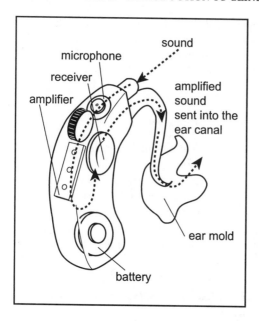

Figure 4-5. Basic parts of a behind-the-ear hearing aid: microphone, amplifier, receiver, ear mold. Adapted from "How to Buy a Hearing Aid" (ASHA).

and without hearing aids is called the functional gain. Although individual differences can be expected, Table 4–9 shows the approximate amount of functional gain that can be reasonably expected for four levels of reduced hearing (Northern & Downs, 1991).

Tactile sensory aids are another type of amplification device. Their function is to change auditory signals into vibratory patterns on the skin. By using the device, children with profoundly reduced hearing can be taught to recognize suprasegmental aspects of speech that are otherwise unavailable to them. These include distinguishing prosodic features of spoken language, identifying the number of syllables, and contrasting voiced/voiceless, nasal/oral, and stop/continuant phoneme pairs (Franklin, 1988).

Cochlear implants are the newest of the advances toward providing individuals with profoundly reduced hearing with clear representation of the

Table 4-9.

Approximate Functional Gain Reasonably Expected for Four Levels of Reduced Hearing

Degree of Hearing Loss (Unaided Thresholds)	Level of Sound Awareness with Amplification (Aided Thresholds)
100+ dB	45–55 dB
75–100 dB	25–50 dB
50–75 dB	15–30 dB
25–50 dB	0–15 dB

sounds of spoken language. The cochlear implant is a device that is surgically implanted in the temporal bone (Figure 1–7) behind the pinnae (Figure 1–7). The device's microphone receives sound and uses the sound to artificially stimulate the acoustic nerve. The acoustic nerve (Figure 1–7) carries the artificially induced acoustic signals to the brain where the signals are interpreted as sound (Loeb, 1985).

Certainly, the cochlear implant provides the most promise for the future with regard to providing people who have reduced hearing with a means for hearing and understanding spoken language. However, cochlear implants are not for everyone as they have not yet been refined to the point where they can provide the masses with natural hearing ability. Thus, the criteria for selecting cochlear implant candidates are rigorous.

Suggestions for Intervention.   Although making sure that amplification is available is an important step, it is not enough. The sound that the person hears through a hearing aid is a mechanical one, it may be very soft and the frequency configuration may be different from what is perceived through natural hearing. Therefore, if a person is to learn to identify and interpret the sound patterns of spoken language, it is critical that both amplification and training begin as soon as the hearing loss has been identified and that both amplification and training should be applied consistently throughout the language-learning years and beyond. Individuals whose amplification and training are delayed or inconsistent are at a distinct disadvantage for learning to use the information that is acoustically provided by the amplification device. In order to facilitate language acquisition through the auditory mode for individuals with reduced hearing sensitivity, the following principles and procedures are applied (Johnson & Paterson, 1991).

Adequate Aided Hearing.   The client must first have aided hearing that is adequate for spoken language acquisition. A number of steps can be taken to determine whether this is the case. Examination of the unaided audiogram is the first step. Clients with unaided thresholds as low as the following levels can generally be provided with sufficient gain to allow them to detect the essential speech cues: 250 **Hz** at 85 dB, 500 Hz at 100 dB, 1000 Hz at 115 dB, 2000 Hz at 115 dB, and 4000 Hz at 95 dB (Figure 4–6).

Anyone with a lesser unaided hearing sensitivity may not be a candidate for learning spoken language through the auditory mode. However, individuals with extremely low levels of hearing sensitivity may desire amplification so that some benefits can be gained from whatever levels of sensitivity are attained. Further, they may learn certain aspects of spoken language through tactile, kinesthetic, and visual stimulation.

Once a person has been fitted with an amplification device, the next step is to identify those with aided audition that is potentially usable for spoken language learning. The client's aided hearing potential for language comprehension and language learning may be indicated by comparing the aided

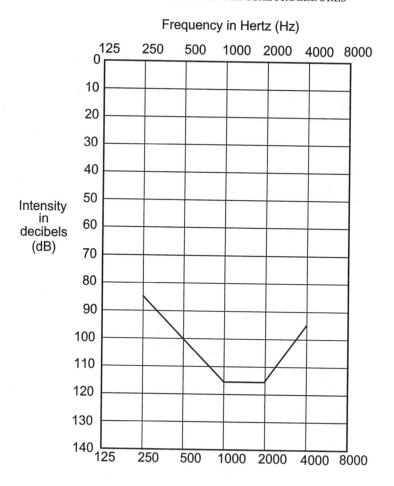

Figure 4-6. Evaluations of unaided thresholds: clients with unaided thresholds down to the solid line can generally be provided gain sufficient to allow them to detect essential acoustic cues of spoken language.

audiogram to Ling's banana-shaped curve, or "speech banana" (Ling, 1976). The speech banana was proposed as the lower limit for potentially usable aided hearing. These lower limits are, approximately, 50 dB or better at 250 Hz, 60 dB or better at 500 Hz, 65 dB or better at 1000 Hz, 60 dB or better at 2000 Hz, and 50 dB or better at 4000 Hz (Figure 4–7). Students with aided hearing levels at or above the banana-shaped curve are potentially good candidates for learning many of the auditory features of spoken language through the hearing mode.

A third step in determining whether a client can benefit from speech-language work presented in the auditory mode is the administration of the Five-Sounds Test (Ling, 1976). The test is comprised of five speech sounds ([u], [a], [i], [ʃ], and [s], which represent approximately the five routinely tested speech frequencies on an audiogram (250, 500, 1000, 2000, and 4000 Hz respectively). Clients as young as approximately 2½ can be taught to respond to this test.

On administering the test, the speech-language pathologist says each of the five sounds in random order while located in a position that does not allow the client to observe facial cues. The client may respond by using an age-

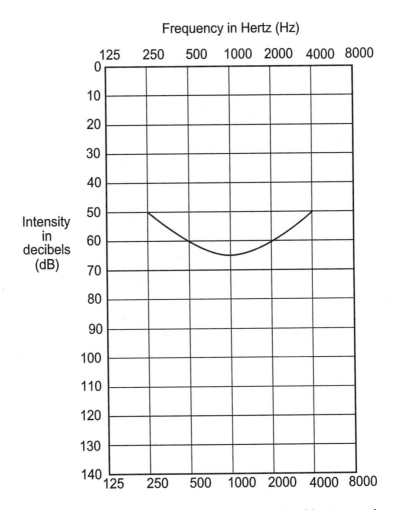

Figure 4-7. Ling's "speech banana," which was proposed by Ling as the lower limit for potentially usable aided hearing (Ling, 1976).

appropriate response such as repeating the sound heard, pointing to an icon representing the sound heard, raising the hand, clapping, or putting blocks in a box.

Three essential elements are gained through knowledgeable use of the Five-Sounds Test. They are (1) information about whether the hearing aid is working, (2) information about the client's frequency-response curve, and (3) approximately the most effective listening distance for the client on that particular day.

By taking the time to complete this procedure, we are likely to identify clients who can benefit from speech-language training by way of auditory stimulation. By so doing, those clients who have hearing sensitivity sufficient for learning the sound patterns of spoken language have the opportunity to do so and we do not frustrate those who are apt to derive more benefit from learning language through exclusively tactile, kinesthetic, and visual modalities.

Properly Working Amplification Device.   The client's amplification device must be working properly. The presence of the hearing aid in the appropriate place on the child's body does not necessarily indicate that the hearing aid power switch is on, that the aid is powered by its battery supply, or that it is working properly. Therefore, each time that the client arrives for assessment or intervention, it is important for the clinician to check the hearing aid and to teach the client and the client's parents to conduct the same check on a daily basis. A checklist for daily monitoring of hearing aids can be found in Appendix 4–6.

When a problem is identified, it is important for the clinician to be able to troubleshoot the hearing aid so that the exact nature of the problem can be identified and addressed as soon as possible. Appendix 4–7 provides methods for troubleshooting three common hearing aid complaints. The complaints are (1) that the hearing aid is not working properly, (2) that the hearing aid is not working at all, and (3) that the hearing aid is feeding back (e.g., squealing).

Confidence in Listening for Meaning.   The client must develop confidence in listening for meaning. This can only happen if listening for meaning and attending to sound are an integral part of the speech-language intervention program as well as of the child's home and academic environments. It may be that, as a profession, we are not yet in the habit of providing our clients who have reduced hearing sensitivity with ample opportunity to become confident with their ability to utilize the sound that is amplified through a hearing aid (Johnson & Paterson, 1987).

Appropriate Listening Distance.   The instructor's voice must be at an appropriate listening distance from the amplification device and ambient signal-to-noise ratio must be considered. The appropriate listening distance for a client on a particular day and in a particular physical location is determined by administering the Five-Sounds Test every time the client is seen for intervention. Auditory work is best presented at a distance for which success is achieved on the test.

Discrimination Practice.   Clients initially need some syllable-level and word-level discrimination practice to focus their attention and clear up auditory confusions. Listening practice with isolated speech sounds must be placed back into meaningful prosodic context as soon as possible. This is accomplished by embedding words in phrases and sentences for listening practice.

Active Participation.   The client must be an active participant in the listening process. Some techniques that can be applied to accomplish this end include asking the child to repeat what was heard, requiring early self-evaluation and self-monitoring, and encouraging production practice as soon as the client is ready.

Listening Practice without Visual Cues.   The client should have an opportunity to practice listening without benefit of visual cues. Mouth covering is not recommended because it interferes with the transmission of the signal and models a communication strategy that does not occur naturally in appropriate conversations. Instead, ask the client to listen, and not to watch, if the task emphasizes listening alone. Side-to-side seating, with the clinician slightly behind and on the side on which the client has the most hearing sensitivity, is preferred.

Involve All Sensory Modalities.   You should exploit to the fullest all sensory modalities when working with a client who has reduced hearing sensitivity. Although the emphasis is on maximizing audition for clients who have sufficient residual aided capacity, tactile, kinesthetic, and visual modes are very important and should not be ignored.

In fact, whenever a client with reduced hearing has sufficient residual hearing for learning language through auditory stimulation, then all sensory modalities should be used to their fullest potential in training. By way of contrast, when sufficient residual hearing capacity is not available to the client, then only the tactile, kinesthetic, and visual modes should be exploited to facilitate spoken communication.

Use of Sign Language Systems.   American Sign Language (ASL) is often used as a means of communication by many individuals with severely and profoundly reduced hearing sensitivity. ASL is a language that is quite different from spoken English in nearly all respects, including timing, syntax, morphology, and use of facial expression and body language. A unique and beautiful language, ASL is the native language of many members of the deaf community and an excellent way to communicate in approximate silence. Furthermore, it is a means by which many individuals with severe or profound hearing reduction spontaneously establish a dominant language, a criterion that appears to be critical to intellectual and cognitive development (Cummins, 1979).

A number of variations derived from ASL exist and are often used in an attempt to teach spoken English to the deaf through visual means. These alternate sign systems are called Manually Coded English (MCE) (Caccamise & Newell, 1983).

Pidgin Sign English (PSE) is a system of MCE that is widely used when deaf and hearing people interact, and it is well accepted by members of the deaf community. PSE combines the critical features of both English and ASL. ASL signs are basically connected in English word order, meanings of the ASL signs are maintained, and many of the spatial, directional, and temporal characteristics of ASL are preserved. PSE is a sign system that evolved naturally as a result of communication need (Caccamise & Newell, 1983).

Manually Coded English (MCE) includes a number of Manual English (ME) systems that were invented by hearing people for the purpose of teaching spoken English to the deaf. Seeing Essential English (SEE 1) and Signing Exact English (SEE 2) are examples of ME systems. These systems include signs borrowed from ASL and a number of invented signs and invented grammatical markers. Further, the ASL meaning of many borrowed signs is not preserved (Caccamise & Newell, 1983).

The Manual English (ME) systems are used primarily for teaching English morphology and syntax to deaf children. They are *not* particularly well received by members of the deaf community.

Regardless of the manual system that is used, signing does not necessarily assist deaf people in learning *spoken* English any more than knowledge of English assists people in learning Spanish or French. Even systems that preserve English grammar are not particularly effective in teaching *spoken* English to deaf people. This is because the visually represented grammar gives very little information on how the language actually sounds.

In fact, since various sign systems are often superimposed on spoken English for communication and training, the simultaneous use of speech and sign may at times interfere with an individual's opportunity to learn spoken language. Further, signing while speaking or speaking while signing may interfere with the clinician's ability to judge competence in the spoken language. A similar pattern has been noted in bilingual children who use two spoken languages, such that in bilingual language assessment it is recommended that only one language be used at a time because using two languages simultaneously impedes the clinician's ability to determine the client's communication abilities in each individual language (Kayser, 1993). The same is true of spoken and signed languages for the following reasons.

In **simultaneous communication,** prosodic changes occur. When used simultaneously, both speech and sign are accomplished more slowly, drawing out certain words, syllables, and signs in order to accommodate simultaneous production of two different languages. This effect is exaggerated for signing systems that attempt to represent all morphological and syntactic forms of

English manually, such as Seeing Essential English (SEE 1), Signing Exact English (SEE 2), Cued Speech, and finger spelling.

In simultaneous communication, lexical choices are affected. Communicators tend to select words and signs that have equivalent counterparts in both languages, and we avoid using words and signs that do not. This limits exposure to a variety of vocabulary options.

Linguistic interference also occurs in simultaneous communication, resulting in inaccurate conversational feedback. For example, I have a functional understanding and use of sign language as a result of having used it on a daily basis for 5 years and using it sporadically since that time. If a deaf client signs and speaks simultaneously, it is often the signed message rather than the spoken one that is understood. If, as a speech-language pathologist, I indicate that the message is clear, the individual with reduced hearing may misinterpret the feedback to mean that the spoken message is clear when in fact it is not. Further, if a clinician signs and speaks simultaneously during intervention activities, the person understands the signs and has no reason to pay attention to the available auditory characteristics of the spoken language. Therefore, the speech-language pathologist who uses simultaneous communication (speech and sign) predominantly deprives the person of the opportunity to listen to the spoken language and gain information about its auditory characteristics.

Despite these difficulties with simultaneous communication and manual systems, ASL and PSE are worthwhile as communication modes, and the ME systems are useful to demonstrate English morphemes and syntax. The early presentation of a manual system is one means for ensuring that individuals with severe or profound hearing loss have the primary language that is necessary for cognitive development. Sign language and simultaneous communication are also valuable and useful in a number of clinical situations. These include conversations not related to clinical assessment or intervention, providing instructions in the client's dominant language in order to assure that there is no misunderstanding regarding the clinical activity, clarifying information that has been misunderstood, and providing a visual demonstration of English morphology and syntax.

However, if sign language is used exclusively or if spoken language is not experienced without sign, the individual who desires to learn to communicate verbally is at a distinct disadvantage for learning to understand the acoustic patterns that constitute spoken language. Further, attempting to assess skill in either language during simultaneous communication is an exercise in futility. The only skill that is assessed accurately in the simultaneous communication mode is skill in using two languages simultaneously.

When Reading and Writing Difficulties Are Also Apparent

The profession of speech-language pathology is not formally designated for the teaching of reading and writing. However, a relationship exists between early language development and reading success. Therefore, the children that we see who have difficulty acquiring a first language in the preschool years are often at risk to experience difficulty in school when learning to read and write. Further, many of the school-age children who receive speech-language services are the same children who receive remedial instruction in the areas of reading and writing.

For that reason, we are concerned with some aspects of reading and writing development. Perhaps in some early language intervention programs it may be within our scope of practice to address risk for difficulty in learning to read and write.

One clinical activity that may serve to minimize risk of reading failure is to take measures to ensure that books and reading are regularly introduced to the preschool-age child in a sociable, enjoyable, interactive context. A particular type of book that may be especially helpful in this regard is a book of nursery rhymes, although many other types of books should be given serious consideration as well. Evidence has shown that better readers are likely to be quite familiar with nursery rhymes (Bryant, Bradley, McLean & Crossland, 1989). A nursery rhyme book can be incorporated naturally into the language-facilitation program, as many of them facilitate role-play activities such as "Ring Around the Roses," "Jack and Jill Went Up the Hill," and "Pat-A-Cake." Nursery rhymes also provide experience with rhyming and word play that are useful in facilitating language acquisition. Further, the language-play experience that is provided by nursery rhymes may be an important prerequisite to the metalinguistic development that is required for one to benefit from reading instruction.

Another speech-language experience, that perhaps lessens the risk of reading difficulties, is experience with narratives. Evidence has shown that poor readers also exhibit poor narrative skills (Norris & Bruning, 1988). Narratives and reading have a common factor, as both place the responsibility of creating the context on the one who is doing the narrating or reading. Experiential practice with all four types of narration may be beneficial. That is, in addition to facilitating language, the activity may also potentially reduce risk of failure in reading and academic achievement.

Once children with language difficulties reach school, there are a number of other things that speech-language pathologists can do to help mitigate the potential for serious reading and writing problems. First, if the child has been placed in special education for reading and writing difficulties, it behooves the speech-language pathologist to work cooperatively with the specialist who is directly addressing these academic concerns.

Second, if the child is diagnosed as having attention deficit disorder (ADD), we may incorporate into our intervention program several objectives to address this concern. (Several intervention options for ADD were presented earlier in this chapter.)

Finally, consider that the etiology of the language disorder may be the same as that which causes the reading and writing disturbance, as both spoken and written language require that one process and formulate symbolic information. Therefore, several language objectives can be included in the intervention program that may help the child with both spoken and written forms of language. These include, but are not limited to, objectives that address sound discrimination, auditory-visual associations, pattern recognition, and comprehending abstract information in the absence of context.

REGULAR EVALUATION OF PROGRESS

Essential to the effectiveness of the intervention program is the clinician's ability to continually evaluate (1) the changing needs of the client, (2) the benefit that the client gains from the program, and (3) the strengths and weaknesses of the program as administered. This requires some sensitivity to the client, clinical instinct, skilled observations of performance, continual problem solving, and a generous amount of adaptability on the part of the clinician. The regular collection of data is used to facilitate this process.

Regular Data Collection

Whenever a client participates in an intervention program, it is necessary to periodically evaluate progress toward both short-term and discharge objectives. Progress toward short-term objectives can be assessed informally as often as each time that the client is seen, because the frequency or duration of target behaviors can be measured at each intervention session.

Some clinicians measure performance throughout the session, accumulating masses of data. Others prefer not to use this method when working with children because (1) data collection throughout a session can interfere with one's ability focus on the objectives and procedures, (2) the child can be distracted by the data collection activity, and (3) the amount of data that is accumulated is often unwieldy.

Instead, it may be preferable to set a brief period aside at the end or at the beginning of each session, using that time for the sole purpose of data collection. That way, the clinician is free to focus attention and energy on the objectives and procedures for most of the session. Session-by-session data is collected in much the same way as the baseline data described earlier in the chapter. Once collected, the session-by-session data is compared to baseline (Table 4–4) and to the targeted degree of mastery as defined in the short-term objective (Table 4–5).

In a continuation of the example, John's baseline is 30 percent for the production of third-person possession. The short-term objective aims at an 80 percent degree of mastery, so it is expected that the session-by-session data will fall between baseline (30 percent) and target (80 percent), and that as time goes on, it moves in the direction of the target. For demonstration purposes, Figure 4–8 indicates session-by-session progress from baseline to completion.

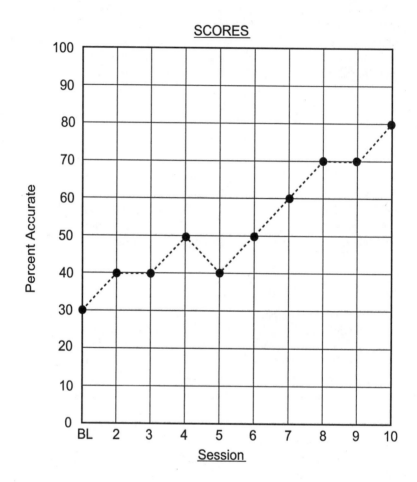

Figure 4-8. Clinical example: John's session-by-session performance on production of third-person possession as measured from baseline (BL) to completion.

Some clinicians prefer not to measure performance each and every time that the client is seen. Even so, a regular schedule of data collection, such as every other session, weekly, or biweekly, is advised.

The reasons for collecting regular data are many. For one, by frequently measuring performance the clinician is always aware of the client's status with regard to progress toward completion of short-term objectives. Moreover, any sudden changes in performance are readily apparent so the source may be identified and addressed as quickly as possible (Johnson, 1988).

Informal and Standardized Retesting

It is important to periodically ascertain the client's status in relation to the long-term objectives. Informal and standardized tests are used to accomplish this end.

An assessment is readministered under three circumstances. One is when the child is regularly scheduled for reassessment. Most states have regulations regarding how frequently a child is permitted to participate in a state-funded reassessment and this is not very often. Every two or three years seems to be somewhat typical. For children whose services are not supported by state funds, the guidelines do not apply. However, it is wise to establish at the beginning of the intervention program exactly how and when the child's progress toward long-term objectives are to be assessed.

Another circumstance that calls for reassessment is when the child has progressed such that the short-term objectives no longer apply and, therefore, additional testing may be needed to establish a set of new objectives. This can sometimes be accomplished through informal procedures. However, formal reassessment may be justifiable.

The other circumstance calling for reassessment is when the child has achieved a performance level that causes one to suspect that discharge may be appropriate. Formal testing may be done at this time to confirm whether the terminal objectives have in fact been met.

DISCHARGE AND FOLLOW-UP

Clients are discharged from an intervention program for a variety of reasons. In most cases, it is because the client has achieved all of the long-term objectives. This is of course desirable and is usually the case. However, a few clients are discharged for other reasons, such as not benefiting from intervention, not being likely to benefit from continued intervention, referral to another agency (e.g., due to a move, client's choice, or professional recommendation), and the client's choice to discontinue services for personal reasons.

Follow-up logically ensues after discharge. As with all other steps in the clinical process, follow-up is also documented, usually by a series of clinic file notes. Some possible follow-up options include scheduling a reassessment after a specified period of time and using a tickler file to make a phone call or send out a questionnaire after a predetermined date. The reasons for following-up on discharged clients is to identify individuals who may benefit from reinstating services, and to receive feedback from the individuals who have firsthand experience with the services provided at the center.

CONCLUDING REMARKS

Part 2 (Chapters 3 and 4) provides a fairly detailed introduction to traditional approaches for assessment and intervention. These and similar procedures are applied for the majority of young clients who receive language services. However, many clients have a number of special needs that require carefully planned modifications to the traditional methods. The next part (Chapters 5 and 6) offers an introduction to principles and procedures for addressing the special needs of the very young and of children who identify with a variety of cultural groups.

REFERENCES

American Speech-Language-Hearing Association (n.d.). How to buy a hearing aid [brochure]. Author.

Bryant, P., Bradley, L., McLean, M., & Crossland, J. (1989). Nursery rhymes, phonological skills and reading. *Journal of Child Language, 16,* 407–428.

Caccamise, F., & Newell, W. (1983). Terminology and brief descriptions of American Sign Language, Manually Coded English, and In-Group Signing. In W. Newell, S. Holcomb, B. R. Holcomb, D. Pocobello, K. Boardman, & L. Arthur (Eds.), *B-A-S-I-C S-I-G-N Communication.* Rochester, NY: National Technical Institute for the Deaf at the Rochester Institute of Technology.

Cole, M. L., & Cole, J. T. (1989). *Effective intervention with the language impaired child.* Rockville, MD: Aspen Publishers.

Creaghead, N. A., & Newman, P. W. (1989). Articulatory phonetics and phonology. In N. A. Creaghead, P. W. Newman & W. Secord (Eds.), *Assessment and remediation of articulatory and phonological disorders.* Columbus, OH: Merrill.

Cummins, J. (1979). Linguistic interdependence and the educational development of bilingual children. *Revue of Educational Research, 49* (2), 221–51.

Fey, M. E. (1986). *Language intervention with young children.* Austin, TX: Pro-Ed.

Franklin, D. (1988). Tactile aids: What are they? *Hearing Journal, 41* (May).

Hodson, B. W. (1986). *The assessment of phonological processes – Revised.* Danville, IL: Interstate Press.

Hodson, B. W., & Paden, E. (1991). *Targeting intelligible speech: A phonological approach to remediation.* San Diego, CA: College-Hill Press.

Johnson, B. A. (1988). Behavioral data and early evaluation of treatment outcome. *Human Communication, 6* (Sept.).

Johnson, B. A., & Paterson, M. M. (1987). Teaching spoken language to the deaf: Which modalities make sense? A poster session presented at the annual convention of the American Speech-Language-Hearing Association, New Orleans.

Johnson, B. A., & Paterson, M. M. (1991). Unique auditory language-learning needs of hearing-impaired children: Implications for intervention. A poster session presented at the annual convention of the American Speech-Language-Hearing Association, Atlanta, GA.

Kayser, H. (1993). Hispanic cultures. In D. Battle (Ed.), *Communication disorders in multicultural populations*. Boston: Andover Medical Publishers.

Lahey, M. (Ed.). (1988). *Language disorders and language development*. New York: Macmillan.

Lee, L., Koenigsknecht, R., & Mulhern, S. (1975). *Interactive language development teaching*. Evanston, IL: Northwestern University Press.

Ling, D. (1976). *Speech and the hearing-impaired child: Theory and practice*. Washington, DC: Alexander Graham Bell Association for the Deaf.

Loeb, G. (1985). Single and multichannel cochlear prostheses: Rationale, strategies, and potential. In R. Schindler & M. Merzenich (Eds.), *Cochlear implants*. New York: Raven Press.

Norris, J., & Bruning, R. (1988). Cohesion in the narratives of good and poor readers. *Journal of Speech and Hearing Disorders, 53*, 416–423.

Northern, H. L., & Downs, M. P. (1991). *Hearing in children*. Baltimore, MD: Williams & Wilkins.

STUDY GUIDE 4

1. Exactly what do you do to determine what needs to be accomplished by the intervention program?
2. Differentiate between long-term objectives and short-term objectives.
3. Exactly what do long-term objectives explicitly state? Exactly what do short-term objectives explicitly state?
4. What is a rationale? Why is a rationale statement included when writing intervention objectives?
5. Describe the relationship between short-term objectives and procedures. Describe the relationship between long-term objectives and procedures.
6. What is included in the written description of an intervention procedure?
7. Describe the format and purpose of an intervention plan.
8. What circumstances may warrant the revision of an existing intervention plan?
9. How does one determine prognosis? How does prognosis impact whether treatment is recommended?
10. What is included in the recommendations section of an intervention plan and why?
11. What does your signature on the intervention plan indicate?
12. How does one go about using results of intervention to establish new targets? Why might it be necessary to establish targets in this way?
13. Why are lesson plans necessary?
14. What is typically included in lesson plans?

15. How does one use antecedents and consequences to increase language behavior (A-R-C paradigm)?
16. Define and give examples of antecedents.
17. Define and give examples of consequences. Include information about the hierarchy of reinforcers.
18. What measures does a clinician take to control the physical environment?
19. What measures does a clinician take to control the linguistic environment?
20. Apply the A-R-C paradigm to the management of behavior problems.
21. Describe appropriate and inappropriate disciplinary actions.
22. How does one go about selecting the children for group intervention?
23. What measures does a clinician take to control the behavior of groups of children?
24. How does one plan for generalization? Why is it important to take these steps?
25. Describe some intervention plans for preverbal children.
26. Describe child-oriented intervention.
27. Describe facilitative play and how it may be used to accommodate language acquisition.
28. Describe the types of interactions that are suggested for speaking to preverbal children.
29. Differentiate between self-talk and parallel-talk.
30. Describe each of the following procedures and how they may be used to facilitate language acquisition.
    a. expansions
    b. expatiations
    c. recast sentences
    d. buildups and breakdowns
31. Describe interactive language development teaching (ILDT).
32. Describe intervention options for unintelligible children whose language comprehension is age-appropriate.
33. Describe intervention options for unintelligible children whose language comprehension is compromised.
34. What circumstances may precipitate a disorder in language use?
35. Describe some procedures that may be used to address difficulties with language use in preschoolers. How might these procedures be altered to address the needs of school-age children?
36. What can be done to address the needs of a child for whom the dimensions of language are separated or for whom the interactions between the dimensions are disordered?
37. Describe some procedures that can be used to address attention deficit disorder.
38. What are the fundamental intervention objectives for a child with central auditory dysfunction?
39. Describe some procedures that can be used to address elective mutism.

40. Explain the significance of timing and consistency of amplification and training with regard to individuals with reduced hearing sensitivity.
41. How does a hearing aid work and what can we expect a hearing aid to do for the person with reduced hearing sensitivity?
42. How much functional gain can we reasonably expect from a hearing aid? Since functional gain may be different for different amounts of hearing reduction, qualify your answer according to level of hearing sensitivity.
43. What are tactile aids and how are they used?
44. What are cochlear implants and how might they help a person with reduced hearing sensitivity? Are they always recommended? Why or why not?
45. Why is the provision of appropriate amplification alone not adequate if a person with reduced hearing wants to understand and produce the sound patterns of spoken language?
46. What procedures might you use to identify a person with aided audition that is adequate for spoken language learning?
47. What is accomplished by administering the Five-Sounds Test?
48. How often should a hearing aid be checked and by whom?
49. Describe the hearing aid check procedure.
50. Describe the basic procedures for troubleshooting a hearing aid that is either not working properly, not working at all, or giving feedback.
51. Describe a training procedure for assisting a person with reduced hearing if that person wishes to learn to comprehend and produce the sound patterns of spoken language.
52. How is sign language useful in speech-language intervention?
53. How might exclusive use of simultaneous communication interfere with one's opportunity to learn the actual sound patterns of spoken language?
54. Why is it important to continually collect data throughout an intervention program, and how is this done?
55. How often should informal and standardized testing be repeated and why?
56. What factors are considered when making a decision regarding the discharge of a client?
57. Describe an appropriate follow-up sequence.

Clinical Implications for Special Circumstances

Addressing the Language Needs of the Very Young

Collaborating With Families

LEARNING OBJECTIVES

At the conclusion of this chapter you will be prepared to:

- Discuss federal guidelines for the delivery of services to disabled preschoolers and their families and why these guidelines have increased the need for family-centered services in the field of speech-language pathology;

- Compare a family-centered model of clinical service delivery to a traditional model;

- Apply a number of suggestions for implementing a family-centered service delivery program;

- Plan and implement family-centered assessment sessions and intervention programs.

INTRODUCTION

Speech-language pathologists are finding that it is becoming increasingly necessary to address the communication needs of some individual clients by first addressing the needs that exist in the clients' family units. This is true because we serve an increasing number of individuals in the birth-to–age 3 population, an age group that responds better to idiosyncratically devised family programs than to relatively infrequent, one-on-one instruction from a stranger. It is when serving infants and toddlers that we are obliged to involve the family; however, family-centered procedures can, and perhaps should, be applied to selected clients at all ages.

PUBLIC LAW 99-457

One might be curious why the number of infants and toddlers served by speech-language pathologists has been on the increase. One reason is that the federal government is now required by law to financially support comprehensive early intervention for preschool children with disabilities, beginning at the time of birth (Houle & Hamilton, 1991).

In 1986, the Education of the Handicapped Act (now called the Individuals with Disabilities Education Act [IDEA], or PL 94-142) was amended by Public Law 99-457 (PL 99-457) (Houle & Hamilton, 1991). Compliance with Public Law 99-457 became mandatory in 1991. Prior to the passage of PL 99-457, its predecessor (PL 94-142) required that the federal government modestly support services for disabled preschool children aged 3 years and older. Further, PL 94-142 did not require that the government provide support services for disabled children below the age of 3. However, PL 99-457 has made significant changes in the federal support available to two age groups—3- to 5-year-olds, and newborn to 3-year-olds.

Three- to Five-Year-Olds

With the advent of PL 99-457, preschool children between the ages of 3 and 5 are now eligible to benefit from *all* services, rights, and protections that had previously been afforded to school-age children, with no cost to the parents (Section 619 of PL 99-457) (Houle & Hamilton, 1991). That is, any child over the age of 2 who is identified as having a disability is referred to the public schools or a state education agency so that services can be provided and federal funding obligations can be explored. Resulting services are documented and monitored by Individualized Education Programs (IEP). Although family-centered services are not required for children who have passed their 3rd birthdays, they are very appropriate for many 3- to 5-year-old children receiving Section 619 services.

The federal government supports the individual children who are eligible for services under Section 619 by providing money to the state of residence and by allowing the state education agency to oversee the services and the funds. In order for a state to qualify for such funding, all eligible children within the state must receive services.

Newborn to 3-Year-Olds

A disabled child below the age of 3 may be eligible for limited federal support under three conditions (Part H of PL 99-457) (Houle & Hamilton, 1991). (1) Any child who experiences developmental delays in one or more domains, as measured by appropriate diagnostic instruments, is eligible for federal support. The developmental realms that are considered include physical, cognitive, language and speech, psychosocial, and self-help and adaptive domains. (2) Any child diagnosed as having a physical or mental condition that has a high probability of resulting in developmental delay in any of the listed domains is eligible for federal support. Some conditions that may categorize a child as being at risk for delay include mental retardation, cleft palate, genetic syndromes, hearing impairment, as well as any other condition that is known to result in delay. (3) If a particular state has opted to provide services to children at risk for whom no delay or handicapping condition has been identified, any child for whom a delay is likely in the absence of intervention is also eligible for federal support.

No child in these three categories may be denied services because of inability to pay. However, for those who are able to pay, a sliding scale may be used to determine the exact proportion of the cost that is absorbed by the federal government to supplement the cost to the family. Services to individual infants and toddlers are supported by federal funding through money allocated to the state of residence. The agency through which the money is managed is designated by the governor of the state (Houle & Hamilton, 1991).

The Part H program is particularly important to the topic of this chapter because of its strong emphasis on serving families. It requires that the communication assessment include an evaluation of both the child and the family, with consideration given to the strengths and needs of all parties concerned (Houle & Hamilton, 1991). Further, intervention services are documented on an Individualized Family Service Plan (IFSP), which include objectives and procedures for the family as well as the child.

FUNDAMENTALS OF FAMILY-CENTERED CLINICAL PROCEDURES

With the implementation of PL 99-457 in 1991, the character of our profession has begun to change and may continue to do so remarkably as we begin to focus on the younger clients that we are required to serve as a result of

Part H of the amendment. The following comments describe some of the approaches that have been developed in order to better serve infants, toddlers, and their families. In general, when serving children below the age of 3, the family must be an integral part of the program. Nevertheless, the family-centered approach is used to benefit many clients at all levels.

Why Involve Families in Clinical Service Delivery?

Regardless of the age of the client, when we ask a family to participate in a clinical program, we are interested in linking the benefits of our professional expertise with the resources that are available to the particular family (Andrews & Andrews, 1990). As speech-language pathologists, we have the educational background, preparatory clinical experiences, and access to a wide variety of resources that enable us to develop objectives and procedures that specifically address the communication needs of our clients. On the other hand, each member of a client's family has a unique perspective on the client, the client's communication abilities, how he or she fits into the family unit, and the family's interactive patterns. Further, members of the family generally share love and respect with the client and are intimately connected to the client's everyday routines and experiences. *Our goal is to enhance our expertise by taking advantage of all that the family can contribute to the program and to enhance the family resources by sharing with them the benefits of our expertise.*

Family-Centered and Traditional Approaches Compared

In order to understand the family-centered approach to clinical-service delivery, it is helpful to identify similarities and differences between it and the more traditional approaches. Family-centered and traditional approaches are alike in that both (1) are initiated because an individual is experiencing, or is at risk for, difficulty with communication; (2) involve communication objectives determined as a result of a diagnostic evaluation and/or progress assessment; (3) make use of intervention procedures that are known to facilitate the achievement of communication objectives; (4) require that the family be consulted regarding background information, statement of the problem, expectations for intervention, and measurement of progress throughout an intervention program; and (5) may employ home assignments and home programs. On the other hand, differences exist in each of the following areas: hierarchy of authority, methods for developing objectives and procedures, clinical relationships, and scheduling of sessions.

Hierarchy of Authority. In the traditional approach, we generally accept that the clinician is the one who makes the major decisions regarding the service plan. This is because the clinician has educational background, clinical experiences, and access to resources, qualifying that individual to make such decisions competently. Certainly, in making clinical decisions, many clinicians go out of their way to seek input from the family so that family needs and concerns are considered regardless of whether the program is officially family-centered. Traditionally, seeking family input may be done after sessions, briefly at the end of sessions, at scheduled meetings, or over the telephone. However, consistent family input is not necessarily a part of traditional programs.

Conversely, using a family-centered approach, the family members attend and participate in every session, a strategy that enables family input to reach the clinician as each decision is made. Family input is always considered when making any decision that impacts the outcome of intervention.

Methods for Developing Objectives and Procedures.   The development and management of a personalized intervention program is a project that involves a number of types of clinical decisions, with the establishment of objectives and of procedures being two types that occur on an ongoing basis. Generally, when a traditional approach is taken, objectives and procedures are determined as a result of standardized and informal testing. Although family input is often sought, the clinician must specifically seek it outside the realm of the planned intervention sessions. Further, in the traditional model the goals and procedures are typically directed at changing the communication behavior of one person—the client.

On the contrary, when taking the family-centered approach to service delivery, family input is *always* sought at the time that the goals and procedures are determined. Goals and procedures are generated by the clinician, taking into consideration the resources, priorities, and opinions of the family members. Also, the goals and procedures of the family-centered program address the communication needs of the client *within the context of the family.* This means that some goals and procedures may require change in the behavior of the client and other family members, or they may require change in the family communication system as a whole.

Clinical Relationship.   In most traditional models, the primary clinical relationship is between the clinician and a client or group of clients. Although clinicians develop clinical relationships with family members as a result of brief conversations before and after traditional sessions and as a result of scheduled consultation or planning meetings, most contact with clients is outside of the context of the family.

By contrast, when implementing a family-centered program, the clinical relationship is between the clinician and every family member who chooses to participate in the program. Almost all contact with clients takes place *within* the context of family communication.

Moreover, in a family-centered program, a number of clinicians may work with one family. One model program suggests employing a clinical team comprised of a few clinicians who work directly with the family, and a few observers who do not have direct contact with the family but are only involved in program planning and providing feedback (Andrews & Andrews, 1990; Johnson, Maxfield, & Sheeler, 1992).

Scheduling of Sessions. In a traditional approach to clinical service delivery, sessions are scheduled frequently and with regularity. Traditionally clients know that they attend on specified days, such as every Tuesday and Thursday; every Monday, Wednesday and Friday; or on a daily basis. Further, service delivery programs are usually implemented during regular working hours (i.e., 9:00 A.M. to 5:00 P.M.) and they take place at a clinic or speech and hearing center.

There are a number of advantages to these traditional scheduling patterns. For example, regular appointments are more easily kept than irregular ones, and frequent appointments are necessary in order for the client to make sufficient progress, especially since traditional sessions comprise the majority of planned communication activities that address the intervention objectives. Furthermore, meetings scheduled during the day are convenient for many service providers, and with young children daytime meetings do not interfere with bedtime and mealtime rituals.

Scheduling family-centered services may be somewhat more flexible. Some clinicians prefer to continue with fixed scheduling so that appointments can be remembered and kept. Even so, the regularly scheduled meetings may be less frequent, with the amount of time between sessions depending on the needs and desires of the family combined with the professional opinion of the clinician. Once each week or every two weeks may be workable in some situations. In a family-oriented program, less frequency may be necessary because the actual work that is done toward achieving goals is carried out by family members on a daily basis in the context of the family.

Some clinicians and families may prefer to schedule sessions on an as-needed basis. This works well for families whose need for professional input varies. For example, a family may participate in a session on a Monday and then return on Thursday, perhaps because of difficulties experienced in carrying out the assignment or because the goal is accomplished very quickly.

Another family may participate in a session on the same Monday and continue to work at home for a week or two before returning. This may be the case if the assignment is fully understood and progress is continuing. In either situation, it is the family's responsibility to determine when it is time to return for another session and to contact the clinician for an appointment when the need arises. Of course a clinician may call families regularly (e.g., weekly) to maintain contact and reassure them that they should call for a return appointment when ready.

In scheduling a family-centered program, a clinician may consider combining family-centered with traditional sessions. Perhaps concurrent to a fixed schedule of frequent sessions having a traditional format, a family may have the option of arranging a family session every few weeks or on an as-needed basis. By so doing, a client may receive the benefits of both traditional and family-centered programming.

Another variation in scheduling that may be seen in family-centered programs is arranging for sessions to take place outside regular working hours. When this is initiated, it is usually due to difficulties with convening an entire family during the working day. The individual clinician or agency administrator determines whether participating in off-hour scheduling is possible. If off-hour scheduling is selected as an option for accommodating family needs, then methods for compensating work time and methods for ensuring safety and adequate clerical support after hours is necessarily explored.

Also, home visits are considered an option for family-centered services. Sessions do not need to be provided in the context of the clinic and, in fact, home sessions can be more beneficial in several ways. For example, by traveling to the home for some sessions, the clinician has an opportunity to directly observe, in a very natural setting, the family, its available resources, and its communication patterns. This enhances the clinician's ability to more fully understand the communication pattern, the context in which the communication pattern is developing, and the materials that are available in the home for carrying out the program activities.

Evaluating the Family-Centered Approach as an Option

Clearly, family-centered programs are the only alternative for some clients, such as the very young. In addition to being a very practical approach for preschoolers, the family-centered approach is mandated by law for children under 3 years of age who receive federal support.

However, for a number of clients over the age of 3, the family approach is only one of many alternatives, while for others, family-centered programs may be completely inappropriate. Before commencing the program, the clinician judges whether a family is likely to benefit from a family-centered service delivery model. This requires the evaluation of a number of variables, including the child's age and willingness to interact with strangers, language or dialect of the family, motivation and commitment of the family, potential for real communication within the clinical relationship, the family's perceived ability to understand and perform the activities, and the time available for the family to participate in the program.

Age of Client.   The law requires that any client below the age of 3 who receives services based on federal support must receive evaluation and intervention services in the context of the family. Therefore, only family-centered services are appropriate for most people in that age group. Regardless of the law, children below 3 generally benefit more from family-centered services than they do from traditional services.

For example, an infant who is identified as having a condition that is apt to result in a communication disorder is unlikely to benefit from sessions that take place a few days each week outside the context of the family. Instead, preparing the family members to facilitate communication during the daily routines is desirable. Although the need for addressing the problem within the family may decrease somewhat as a child approaches the third birthday, a family-centered model is probably the most effective choice for many preschool-age children.

Client's Willingness to Interact with Strangers. Regardless of age, some children hesitate to communicate with strangers. This is especially true of children who receive services because of elective mutism. It may also be true of children who present emotional or psychological disturbances. Often in a traditional program, if a client does not separate from the parents or if the client does not speak to the clinicians, attempts at intervention are impossible or unsuccessful. A family-centered program may be one strategy for initiating services with a client or family who have these behavior patterns.

Language or Dialect. Individual speech-language pathologists generally serve a number of clients whose dialect is different from their own. Although it is not appropriate for clinicians to attempt to change a client's dialectal pattern, it may also be impractical or unreasonable for the clinician to become facile in every dialect that is used in a particular region. Families, on the other hand, are adept at using the dialect that is common to their culture. Therefore, in order to provide services to a client in the dialect of the familiar culture, family-centered services may be employed more appropriately than traditional services. (See Chapter 6 for some suggestions.)

Motivation and Commitment. In order to benefit from a family-centered service program, the family must be motivated and committed to addressing the needs of the client within the context of the family. Further, each individual must be motivated and committed to making appropriate personal adaptations that enhance progress.

Motivation and commitment are difficult to judge. However, we rely on clues given by the family members to measure these attributes. For example, the response to your suggestion for family involvement may offer some indication as to the amount of participation that can be expected.

Once a family-centered program has begun, the demeanor of the family members at the initial and subsequent meetings may also prove revealing. Further, the amount of time that individual family members devote to the program activities may be used as a gauge to determine whether their motivation and commitment are adequate for success in a family program.

Real Communication. In family-centered programs, real communication is an absolute necessity. We expect the family to participate in generating the goals and procedures, and we depend on their honest input to ensure that the program adequately meets the needs of the client and family. We also depend on their consistent, straightforward information about whether assignments were completed, whether communications are understood, whether the goals and procedures are amenable to the family members' expectations, and whether the activities are able to be performed in the home. Therefore, we need evidence leading us to believe that candidates for family programs are willing to communicate openly and honestly with the clinician or clinical team.

Ability to Understand and Perform the Activities.   We are obligated to make certain that the activities are simple and doable. We are further obligated to explain the activities in language that is understood and used by the family, and to provide these simple explanations in writing. Regardless of the efforts that we make to facilitate family understanding, a small group of people may be unable to understand the activities or remember them long enough to carry them out successfully. Therefore, prior to engaging a family in a program, we may judge the likelihood of individuals comprehending and doing the activities. For some clients with these kinds of difficulties, modifications to a family program are in order.

Time to Devote to the Program.   Even with all the factors that point toward a potential benefit from a family-centered program, the family must be willing and able to set aside time that can be applied to the sessions and home activities. Families who lack time to attend sessions and carry out the activities of the program are likely to be disappointed with progress.

Suggestions for Implementing a Family-Centered Program

Successfully implementing a family-centered program requires that a clinician transfer a number of skills that have been successfully applied when using a traditional approach. It also requires that one extend the boundaries of clinical service delivery to include some nontraditional strategies, taking care to stay within the scope of practice that is appropriate for the profession of speech-language pathology. That is, the boundaries may be extended to include some techniques borrowed from counseling so as to facilitate group cooperation for the purpose of accomplishing clinical objectives. However, the boundaries are not extended to provide counseling services. The scope of this section, therefore, is to define and describe some of the traditional and nontraditional strategies that are common to family-centered services. The discussion begins with describing how we go about defining the family so that we can identify the individuals who appropriately participate in a family-centered program.

Define the Family. For the purpose of implementing a family-centered program, a family member is defined as any person who is significant to the client's communication environment and who is interested in participating in the program (Andrews & Andrews, 1990). For children, these may include parents, grandparents, siblings, aunts, uncles, cousins, stepparents, step-siblings, foster parents, neighbors, close friends, day care providers, and partners to single parents. The families of adult clients may include any or all of these, plus spouses, children, and home care providers. Everyone who spends significant time communicating with the client and who wishes to participate is invited to participate in the family program, regardless of the person's biological or familial relationship to the client.

Contact the Family to Arrange a Meeting. A hallmark of the family-centered approach is that the entire family participates in the sessions and that, with the guidance of the clinician, members of the family carry out the intervention program at home. Therefore, a family meeting is initiated at the suggestion of the clinician. In order to accomplish this, the clinician contacts the family and suggests that the whole family participate in the sessions. It is at this time that the clinician arranges for a family meeting and invites all individuals who communicate regularly with the client and wish to participate.

Furthermore, during the first contact, the clinician clearly explains to the family representative the exact purpose of involving the family in the program. The family needs to know that we hope to utilize their knowledge about their family member in order to better serve that person and that we plan to share our expertise and guide them as they carry out the major portion of the program at home.

Expressing to the family that we need their input in order to best serve their family member is important. It is also important to demonstrate our commitment to this concept by giving serious consideration to any suggestions that they raise and by somehow making use of every suggestion even if it must be seriously adapted in order to be clinically usable.

Facilitate Family Cooperation. The family-centered approach is an unfamiliar format to most people who seek professional assistance. A lifetime of experience leads most people to believe that when one consults a professional for help it is the professional who addresses the problem. For that reason, many initially hesitate to participate fully in the family-centered program. This pattern may cause a family to appear uncooperative when in fact they are simply responding to an unfamiliar schema by using familiar behaviors and patterns. Participation must be encouraged. The following strategies may be helpful in enhancing family participation.

We *tell them that we need their help,* giving them credit for being the experts about their family while acknowledging ourselves as experts on professional issues. It is important for the family to believe that they will contribute to the family-centered program as part of a team of experts. A family who has a member with a communication problem or with a high risk for a communication problem may already be feeling a sense of failure. The very fact that they have initiated the process of seeking clinical intervention is evidence that they feel somewhat helpless in addressing the problem independently. By emphasizing their ability to contribute to the process, we empower them to facilitate needed changes. By emphasizing that they are a part of a team of experts, we reassure them that they are not alone in attempting to solve the problem; and we give them hope that they will gain the information and resources needed to facilitate improvement in the communication skills of their family member.

We *create an atmosphere that welcomes participation* from every family member. Real and honest communication takes place only if the atmosphere is encouraging and nonthreatening. Since real communication is critical to the success of the program, the physical and emotional environments are friendly, our demeanor is calm and approachable, and our comments and questions are reassuring and positive.

As soon as possible, *we give the family members something to do* so they can feel they are exercising some control over the communication problem. This usually comes in the form of an assignment. A simple observation assignment can be given to a particularly receptive family representative as early as the initial contact so that the family can begin working on something concrete even before commencing the program. An example of an early observation assignment may be for each family member to write down the exact sequence of events for two attempts at communication between the time of the initial contact and the first family meeting (one successful attempt and one unsuccessful).

By the time the first family meeting is complete, every family member who plans to continue in a family-centered program will know of at least one activity or observation that they will accomplish prior to the next meeting. Regardless of the exact assignment that is given, it is important to make sure that it is one that provides an experience of success and distinctly addresses the individual needs of the client and family.

In addition to home assignments, family members can be given responsibilities *during* sessions right from the beginning of the first meeting. For example, when they arrive at the first family meeting, it is important to make known their exact in-session responsibilities. One responsibility that parents need to take in family-centered sessions is the responsibility to monitor the behavior of their own children. This, however, is not inherently clear to many parents unless it is explained to them because they have probably had experiences with classrooms and other instructive domains where a child's behavior is monitored by the professional while in the professional's environment. However, in the family-centered program, we want to empower the parents to take charge of their child. Therefore, we let them know the rules at the outset, and we also let them know that they are the ones to enforce the rules.

The rules should be few and simple, and each negative should be countered with a positive alternative. For example, for the sake of safety, we may have a rule that the children are not to play near the electric outlet. Instead of simply stating that the child is not to play in that corner of the room, we also tell the parents exactly which parts of the room are available for play and why.

By putting the family members in charge of the children and by keeping the rules simple, we give them a sense of control over their children's behavior. Hopefully, this will transfer into a sense of control over the communication problem, which is likely to foster a worthwhile feeling and thus facilitate cooperation.

Another responsibility that is communicated to the family at the outset is each family member's role as a participant in the program. This might best be communicated in a positive way, emphasizing the importance of their potential contributions to the outcome, as family participation is necessary both *during and between each session* of the family-centered program.

If a family is to cooperate, the family members must believe that their immediate concerns are being addressed. Therefore, we *ask them to describe their immediate concerns.* If we neglect to seek this input, the goals that we select may not be particularly meaningful to the family, thus creating a situation that works against our attempts at winning cooperation and making progress toward communication goals.

For example, suppose a family has a young preschooler who is old enough to speak in short sentences but has not yet uttered an intelligible word. Following the formal assessment, a clinical team may prepare to present a plan for facilitating approximations of single words. However, in this case, when asking the family for input, the team may learn that a major priority for the family is unrelated to the production of single words. For example, a family with a nonverbal preschooler may be reasonably interested in addressing some of the immediate communicative concerns, such as getting the child to indicate "yes" and "no" accurately or using gestures to accurately communicate certain basic needs and desires.

These kinds of objectives may not involve the utterance of a first word at all and some of them may be accomplished rather quickly. For example, having the child indicate "yes" and "no" may be learned by associating the child's positive and negative desires with physical manipulation of the head for nodding and side-to-side shaking. In the early stages of the program, *their* priorities take precedence so that a very real family need can be met and they can experience some personal satisfaction. By being willing to adapt our plan to accommodate their perceived needs, we demonstrate respect for the opinions of the family members, genuine interest in meeting their needs, and sincere concern for the client's success. Thereby, we pave the way for initiating goals that we believe are in the best interest of the client. That is, the family whose preschooler has not yet said a first word may be more accepting of our plan for accomplishing first-word production after we have shown them that we can address their perceived immediate needs (e.g., indicating "yes" or "no").

Professional judgment may prevent us from honoring some family requests as presented. For example, a person may want us to accomplish an objective that is outside the realm of our professional expertise, or someone may present an objective that is clearly in the long-range future for the client, given current levels and skills. In these cases, efforts are made to use a suitable part of the family's suggestion, demonstrate how an activity may work toward accomplishing the suggestion, or make an appropriate referral to a professional who is qualified to meet the family's immediate felt need.

If we want family members to cooperate with us, we must make an heroic *effort to understand the communication dynamics that typically occur in that particular family.* For example, every family works together differently and has a different communicative style. These factors may strongly impact the outcome of intervention, and if understood and directed properly they can often be used to the advantage of the client. By knowing (1) who is in charge, (2) how the people in the family relate to one another, (3) the typical vocabulary that is used and understood among the family members, (4) the problems that are faced by the family, (5) the experiences that the family members have undergone together, and (6) how the client fits into all of this, the clinician is able to address family needs in a meaningful way. This communicates to the family that they are understood; and people who believe that their position is understood are likely to cooperate.

Further, when observing the family and trying to understand that family's communication patterns, it is important to *look for something positive.* This may be somewhat difficult to do because we are often in the habit of looking for the patterns and behaviors that need to be changed. However, if we want the family members to feel that we understand them adequately and if we want them to believe that we are on their side, they must also believe that we see their family unit in a positive way. If whatever changes we recommend are preceded by a report of what the family members are doing well, they are often more apt to cooperate and less apt to see our suggestions as criticism.

We need to take care to *be reassuring,* and not cast judgment or criticize in any way. Families who are seeking professional help may already be experiencing a sense of failure or guilt and may unintentionally criticize or judge themselves and each other. If this is the case, they may see no reason to come to us for something that they are already doing themselves, without positive results. For that reason, regardless of what a person says or does in a family-centered session, it is imperative that the clinician refrain from passing judgment or making remarks that could be interpreted as critical.

In fact it is best to refrain from volunteering any evaluative comments or suggestions for change. Of course, eventually, suggestions need to be made since the purpose of the program is for the family and the client to benefit from our professional expertise. However, advice is more likely to be accepted if it is offered after a very positive communication atmosphere has been established by the clinician and in response to a specific request for input.

One thing that the clinician can do to take action toward developing a positive atmosphere is to make sure that at least one positive remark is communicated in writing each time the family meets. Planning to do this forces the clinician to look for something that the family does well, which helps one to view the family in a positive way, and projects a positive impression. Writing down one positive remark each time also gives the family some consistent, concrete evidence that they are succeeding. The positive comment can be given in writing on the assignment sheet that will be discussed shortly. (See Figure 5–1.) For example, a comment may be, "Mrs. (Client) listens very carefully to what the child says," or "Mr. (Client) speaks directly to the child when describing something that has happened." The positive comments are used to reinforce some behavior in the family that should continue and that is judged to be useful for achieving progress in the communication program.

Understand the Problem from Everyone's Perspective. Everyone in the family may see the problem from a different perspective. Everyone in the family has experienced the problem under different conditions, and each deals with the problem in a personal way. As the clinician, it is your responsibility to try and appreciate each person's experience, goals, and frustrations. By looking at the problem though each person's eyes, you will develop what is called a **polyocular view** of the problem (Andrews & Andrews, 1990).

In order to develop this polyocular view, you must have a plan for how you will come to understand all of the facets of the communication problem being experienced by each family member. One simple thing that can be done to accomplish this is to give each person the opportunity to respond to all substantive questions that are asked at any time during the program. For example, during an initial meeting, it is important to ask each person to describe what communication with the client is like personally. In a traditional model, we may pose a question like this to all members present at the evaluation interview, but generally when one individual responds, we move on to the next question without seeking a response from all other family members present. In a family-centered session, however, we seek to understand each person's perspective so we ask everyone to respond to each question.

Another strategy that can be used to assist in developing a polyocular view is to give the family members time to freely interact with each other. Although this strategy may feel awkward, it can provide a wealth of information about the interactive patterns that naturally occur in the family.

Handle Disagreements Carefully. Whenever a family congregates to discuss a problem that has been identified within the family, it is inevitable that disagreements will surface regarding how the problem should be handled. The degree of conflict depends on the history and communication patterns of those present. You, as the clinician, must learn to manage these disagreements successfully. The following suggestions may be helpful as you learn to handle conflict interactions.

Expect disagreements to arise. If you are overwhelmed by the fact that the family members argue during the session, you will become distracted from your purpose. Remember, you are there for the purpose of linking your professional expertise with the family's resources. All families have disagreements, and *how the family handles conflict is one of its resources.* Expect conflict to happen and when it does, view it as an opportunity to learn about how the family functions when disparity occurs.

Recognize your professional limitations: it is not your job to resolve the disagreements within the family. If their disagreements are so complicated that they interfere with progress, then refer the family for counseling so that conflict resolution can be facilitated by a qualified professional.

Never take sides. Whenever two family members disagree about how a problem should be handled, it seems natural for both parties to try and win support for their way of thinking. For example, in some families, one parent may believe that speech therapy should be composed of very structured drill work while the other parent believes in a less-structured approach. When these types of disagreements come up and when either or both people try to solicit your support, it is to everyone's best interest for you to diplomatically redirect the conversation, dismissing yourself of any commitment to either way of thinking.

Talk openly about disagreements in a positive way. When family members disagree, acknowledge the fact that opposing viewpoints have been identified. Then, try to use the disagreement to the advantage of the program goals. For example, cooperation may be facilitated if a clinician points out how fortunate the child is to have the advantage of experiencing both parents' perspectives. The child can learn to appreciate flexibility from one parent and structure from the other. Additionally, progress *and* cooperation may be facilitated if we create assignments that take advantage of both points of view. For example, if one parent desires a structured approach and the other is more comfortable with flexibility, the two family members can have separate assignments that are tailored to their individual strengths. The more structured activities can be carried out by one parent, while the other parent can do the activities that require spontaneity and flexibility.

Use Vocabulary That Is Used by the Family. We have already mentioned that in our conversations with the family we should be careful to observe their communication style so that we may understand it more completely. It is also very important to use these observations to become familiar with the type of language that is typically used by members of the family. Certain word choices may become evident upon observation. Knowledge of these lexical idiosyncrasies helps us to frame our suggestions in a way that makes sense to the family members. That is not to say that we should imitate them or use their dialect if it is not our own. Indeed, it may be ludicrous (and perhaps insulting) to do so. However, if the family says, "I want to be able to understand the way he pronounces his words," then your communication with them should use the word *understand* as opposed to more sophisticated words like *comprehension, comprehensibility,* and *intelligibility,* and the word *pronounce* as opposed to *produce, articulate,* or even references to phonology.

As a student in the process of acquiring a new set of professional terminology, it can be tempting to use the opportunity of a family meeting to practice the jargon that you are trying to master. Unfortunately, this habit interferes with communication when conversing with people outside the profession. (It is also unfortunate that the temptation does not end when we become certified and licensed.) Therefore, it is advisable that you establish the habit of simplifying your language and rephrasing professional jargon whenever you speak with families. In a family-centered program it is our responsibility to take these personal adaptations one step further, using the types of words and phrases that we have heard the family members using in conversations among each other. By doing so, we ensure that the message is understandable to the family members and we demonstrate that we relate to them and understand their problem in a very real way.

Assess Disorder in Context of Family Communication.   In addition to the formal testing procedures that assist in making a diagnosis and generating suggestions for intervention goals, we want to observe free and uninterrupted communication among the family members. We are particularly careful to look for communication patterns in the family that may have an impact on the identified communication disorder, how some of these patterns can be used to improve communication behavior, and how some of these patterns may need to be modified or redirected in order to facilitate desired change.

Standardized testing may be administered in the presence of the family, and in some cases family members may be given a specific job to do in order to assist in the testing procedure. If a family member assists in administering a standardized test, the exact nature of family assistance is documented in a prominent place on the test form and in the diagnostic report. The amount of assistance that a family member gives during formal testing can vary greatly and depends on need and on a professional judgment of that person's reliability as a tester. Regardless of the amount of involvement that a family member has, that person must receive specific instruction regarding the purposes and procedures of the test.

For example, even if a parent assists minimally, such as by encouraging the child to cooperate during the administration of the Assessment of Phonological Processes–Revised (APP-R), the parent needs to know that the test is being given so that we can record exactly how the child pronounces each of the words. The parent also needs to know that the specific stimulus words are the ones that the child should say and that we want to give the child the opportunity to pronounce the words spontaneously before providing any kind of model. Extensive demonstration may be used to support these instructions.

Parents who participate extensively in test administration also need to be apprised of the purpose of the test and the general procedural guidelines.

For example, if a parent complains that the child's speech is unintelligible but the child refuses to speak in the presence of the clinician, it may be necessary for the clinician to instruct the parent in detail and then watch from the observation room while the parent presents the items.

In this example, suppose the client refuses to speak in the presence of the clinicians and the parents report that the child's speech is totally unintelligible. For part of the testing protocol, a family member may show the APP-R stimuli to the client, encourage him or her to name the items, and elicit imitative responses where necessary, all while the clinicians record responses from the observation room. A tape recorder may be placed in the evaluation room so that responses can be verified at a later time. Although information gathered in this way is not useful for standardized scoring, it may be used to collect enough information to determine the phonological processes that are to be addressed and to collect a wealth of information about the family member's style of working with the client. As a result, the information may be very useful in helping to create idiosyncratic assignments that effectively use the family member's talents and abilities.

Agree on Changes in Behavior of Client and Family.   One of the purposes of initiating the clinical program is to facilitate changes in the communication behavior of the client. In the family-centered program, we may find that some of the client's communication behaviors are addressed most effectively by changing some aspect of family communication as well. Regardless of whose behavior is to be changed, the clinician and the family *must agree* on the changes.

Often, in order to ensure that the family is in agreement with the changes, before presenting any suggestions for intervention objectives we ask each family member to express an opinion of exactly what needs to change. We also ask them to suggest one thing that they would like to see accomplished by intervention. Many family members have difficulty with this task and need encouragement. They may hesitate because if they knew what needed to be done, they would not have sought professional help or because they have little confidence that their suggestions are worthwhile. Either way, they should be reassured that their opinions are wanted and needed.

Although some parents are able to make suggestions that are very specific and can be applied directly to the program (e.g., "I want the child to be able to indicate yes or no"), in most cases the suggestions are vague and need explanation before they can be used. For example, many people say, "All I want is to be able to understand my child," or "I just want my child to talk." Although vague, these suggestions can be used. For example, if the parent simply wants to be able to understand the child, then we know that our short-term objectives should clearly lead toward improved speech intelligibility.

Once we have sought specific input from the family we are ready to use all of the information that we gathered (i.e., through standardized and informal testing, as well as observations) for the purpose of developing a set of proposed objectives. These proposed objectives are presented to the family and the family has the opportunity to suggest changes, additions, and deletions. Everyone must participate in the process of developing the objectives to ensure that everyone is committed to addressing them in an agreed-on format.

Agree on Intervention Procedures. Once we have agreed on the changes that are to be made, we then agree on the procedures that will be used to accomplish the changes. In our experience, family members rarely have suggestions for clinical procedures, and in fact, if we ask them to suggest methods for accomplishing the needed changes, they have reason to question our professional competence. Therefore, a clinician might make some suggestions for approximately two procedures that can be used, allow them to choose between them, and encourage them to make adaptations to accommodate their lifestyle. These suggested procedures must be simple, easy to do, and clearly related to the objectives that have been established. Some families choose to apply all suggestions rather than only one, while other families prefer to only partially accept the suggestions, making adaptations to suit their own family resources. Since the family members implement the procedures, it is important that they understand the procedures, that they agree that the procedures can be accomplished by them in their home environment, and that they clearly see the relationship between the procedures and the agreed-on goal.

Guide Family Members in Implementing Intervention Procedures. The procedures that have been chosen to address the objectives are performed daily at home by specified family members. Since the clinician will not be present when the procedures are carried out, adequate family preparation is needed.

First, we demonstrate the procedure to the family members. Of course we prefer to engage the client in the demonstration activity; however, some clients may not interact with the clinician at first, so it is acceptable to engage a substitute for the purpose of demonstration at the initial family meeting. The demonstration should be sufficient in length to give the family members a clear sense of what to do.

We then ask the family members who will perform the procedure to demonstrate so that we can be sure that the procedure has been fully understood. Again, we expect the client to be involved in the demonstration but in the first session it may be necessary to use a substitute.

While the family demonstrates the procedure, the clinician looks for ways that the procedure or technique can be enhanced. If some modifications appear to be needed, the clinician fades into the demonstration, modeling the changes in a nonthreatening way. The clinician is very careful to avoid pointing out errors or undesirable behaviors. Families who demonstrate for clinicians are nervous enough without us confirming the fear that they may be criticized. It is usually unnecessary to point out people's weaknesses if we focus on developing their strengths (Andrews & Andrews, 1990).

For example, some families develop a habit of speaking in unusual voices to the client, such as in an inappropriately high pitch (almost a falsetto). They may do this because it attracts the child's attention and because the child imitates it more than any other speaking pattern. They may do it because they are at a loss as to how to facilitate communication and this pattern results in at least some attempts at imitation—even though inappropriate. Whether to address this apparently counterproductive communication pattern may be a point of deliberation for the clinical team. However, rather than telling the family what not to do, more may be accomplished by giving them some very simple and concrete activities that are likely to lead to immediate success. Then, as soon as the client begins to improve, the family members are often found to discontinue their inappropriate behavioral pattern. Perhaps this is because, when they discover some strategies that work, they no longer perceive a need to do the things that do not.

Once the procedures are agreed on and the clinician is certain that the family understands how to perform the procedures, the clinician provides the family with a list of goals and procedures in writing. (See Figure 5–1.) This helps them to remember exactly what to do, and why and how they should do it.

Agree on Home Assignment.   The family-centered program relies heavily on home assignments because although the clinical intervention is designed in the presence of the clinicians and family, most of the intervention that takes place is done by the family in the home by way of assignments. Therefore, the family and clinicians must come to agreement on the assignments during the family-centered session. The assignments include both activity and nonactivity types.

Activity Assignment.   The intervention procedures described in the previous section are a major part of the home assignments. They are developed, demonstrated, and refined in the session. Then the family takes the procedure home in the form of an activity assignment.

Nonactivity Assignment.   In addition to activities, we often want families to complete other assignments between sessions. For example, we may want them to observe the client or family unit for a particular behavior or pattern of behavior. There are a number of things that we can ask families to observe and document between sessions. Among these are interactive patterns, changes in performance, expressive lexicons, and nonverbal patterns.

If it is determined that a nonactivity (e.g., observation) assignment would benefit the client, then the assignment with its rationale is presented to the family and the family determines whether it can be done at home and whether they understand how it may result in desired progress.

Communicating Home Assignments. Activity and nonactivity assignments are given to the family in writing before the end of the session. The goals and activities should be simple and easy to understand. They should be written in the language that is typically used by the family, and it should be clear to the family members that the procedures will facilitate accomplishment of their goals. An example format for written assignments can be found in Figure 5–1.

FAMILY-CENTERED LANGUAGE ASSESSMENT

Each family-centered assessment session is different. However, the outline below describes a format that may guide you in planning for a family assessment meeting. The outline is meant to supplement the preceding section which includes details about the procedures that may be followed.

Date _____

Names of Individuals Present

_____

_____

Remarks

_____

_____

_____

The Goals

_____

_____

_____

_____

The Assignments

_____

_____

_____

_____

_____

Date of Next Meeting_____

Figure 5-1. Family-Centered Program: Assignment Sheet

Introduction

First, we introduce ourselves and allow the family members to introduce themselves. We establish each person's relationship to the child and purpose for attending the session. Then we establish the purpose of using a family-centered approach, delegate to the parents the responsibility of managing the children, and explain the order of events for the meeting: interview, assessment (standardized and informal), break, presentation of proposed objectives and procedures, demonstration, and assignments.

Explaining the order of events is consequential so that the group understands what is going to happen and why. For example, they need to know that we will take a break so that they do not become concerned that the break is taken because someone did something wrong. They also need to know that they will participate in the process of determining goals so that they are prepared to provide meaningful input. Further, they need to know that they will participate in a demonstration so they are not taken off guard when they are asked to show us how they will perform the activity at home. Moreover, they need to know that the clinician will blend into their demonstration so they can expect this to occur and then naturally look for the clinician to modify the procedure or technique.

Interview

We gather information about the client and the family, asking *each* person to respond. In addition to the standard case history intake, the kinds of questions that we ask include: "What do you hope to gain from this meeting?" "What is communication with the client like for you?" "What is the exact history of the communication disorder?" "Is there one thing that you wish the client could do that would meaningfully improve communication?" "Is there any behavior in the family unit that, if changed, would enhance the outcome of the communication program?" The answers to these questions will be considered when determining goals later on in the session.

Assessment

The assessment part of the meeting may include informal and formal assessment procedures. One informal procedure that may be used is the observation of the family. In order to accomplish this, we give the family members opportunity to interact with each other freely, observing for interactive patterns that may have an impact on the outcome of the program. This may be done spontaneously and is usually most effective if it is done once the family has become comfortable with the clinician.

Formal assessment may include the administration of standardized and non-standardized tests. If needed, family members may assist in test administration.

Break

The break is especially necessary if more than one clinician is involved. It gives the clinicians and observers the opportunity to discuss all that has been observed during the session, it gives the clinician who has been working directly with the family the opportunity to observe the family, and it gives the family the opportunity to relax for a few moments. In some situations a family may be given a short assignment for the break, such as filling out forms or making a list of toys at home that can be used for a home activity.

During the break, the clinician prepares a set of objectives that will be presented to the family for their consideration. In preparing this list, the clinician considers all of the input that the family has given about their expectations, all the communicative patterns observed and how they may impact the outcome of the program, and the results of the standardized and nonstandardized (informal) tests.

Presentation of Proposed Objectives and Procedures

During the break the clinician considers the input that has been given by the family and the results of the assessment. Consequently, a set of objectives has been prepared, addressing the client's needs and the family's concerns. The family now has the opportunity to suggest additions, deletions, and modifications during this problem-solving portion of the family meeting. Once the objectives have been agreed on, the clinician presents the procedures that will be used to accomplish the objectives. Again, the family has the opportunity to suggest adaptations to suit their lifestyle and communication pattern.

Demonstration

The agreed-on procedures are initially demonstrated by the clinician. Then, the family members who will perform the procedures demonstrate, with the understanding that the clinician blends in to encourage alternate strategies. The demonstration continues until the clinician is certain that the family members are comfortable with the procedures and willing and able to do them at home.

Assignment

The objectives and procedures are given to the family as part of the assignment. Another part of the assignment may be for the family to observe and document a particular behavior within the family unit. All assignments are given in writing to facilitate later recall.

FAMILY-CENTERED LANGUAGE INTERVENTION

A number of follow-up sessions take place after the initial family meeting for every family-centered program. Although each follow-up session is different depending on the exact needs of the family, the subsequent outline may be used as a guide. (Some similarity can be noted between the intervention session outline and the assessment-session outline that was just presented.)

Introduction

Occasionally, a family member joins the program after it has been going on for some time. In that case, the new person is introduced to the clinician and all aspects of the introduction may be reviewed (as described in the section on the assessment session).

Current Status Report

The family is given the opportunity to update the clinician on what has been happening in the home program since the last meeting. As clinicians, we are particularly interested in how the assignment went. In some cases, we find that the assignment was not done. If that has happened, it is usually because the assignment was not understood, was not liked, was not clearly connected to the goal, or was otherwise inappropriate. For that reason, we attempt to find out about this in a nonthreatening way so that we can increase the chances that future assignments will be completed.

This is also a good time to ask some questions that help you understand the family's expectations for the immediate future. This information provides insight for preparing proposed objectives and procedures later in the session.

Family Demonstration

The family demonstrates the procedure that has been done at home since the last session. The clinicians specifically observe for behaviors of the family members that need to continue and behaviors of the family members that would be more effective if they were modified. Clinicians also look for evidence of progress and behaviors of the client that need to be addressed.

Break

This break is similar to the one described in the section on the assessment session. It gives the clinicians and observers the opportunity to discuss all that was observed during the session, it gives the clinician who has been working with the family the opportunity to observe the family, and it gives the family the opportunity to relax briefly. During the break, the clinician prepares some proposed modifications to the program (e.g., goals and procedures). In preparing this list, the clinician considers all of the input that the family has given about their expectations, all of the communicative patterns that have been observed, and how each may impact the outcome of the program.

Presentation of Proposed Modifications to Program

During the break the clinician considers the input that was given by the family and the outcome of the family demonstration. As a result, some modifications to the objectives and procedures have been prepared. The family now suggests additions, deletions, and modifications to these suggestions.

Clinician Demonstration

This demonstration is similar to the one described in the section on the assessment session. That is, the modifications to the procedures or new procedures are demonstrated by the clinician. Then, the family members who will perform the procedures demonstrate with the understanding that the clinician fades in to encourage alternate strategies. The demonstration continues until the clinician is certain that the family members are comfortable with the modified procedures and that they are willing and able to do them at home.

Assignment

The modified objectives and procedures are given to the family as part of the assignment. Another part of the assignment may be for the family to observe and document a particular behavior within the family unit. All assignments are given in writing to facilitate recall.

Dismissal from a Family-Centered Program

As with all service delivery programs, when a clinician contemplates **dismissal,** a number of factors must be considered. In many cases, clients are discharged because they have reached expected performance levels; thus, intervention is no longer needed. We wish that all clients could be dismissed as a result of program success, but unfortunately, a number of other circumstances may contribute to the decision to discontinue family-centered, as well as traditional, services.

Lack of progress is one reason for discharging a client from a family-centered program. If discharge is considered due to lack of progress, the reason behind the lack of progress is identified and attempts are made to address any factor that may interfere with advancement toward the established goals.

In some situations, an interfering factor may be identified and addressed within the context of the family-centered program. For example, a family that consistently neglects to complete activities at home can expect that progress will be minimal. However, if the reason for overlooking the home program activities can be identified and accurately addressed, the client is likely to make progress toward the goals.

Situations may arise in which the interfering factor is identified but cannot be addressed within the context of the family-centered program. For example, a family's communicative patterns may reveal a number of dysfunctional relationships within the family structure, thus impeding any sort of positive change that can be facilitated by family communication. Serious interpersonal problems between family members, unwillingness of individuals to consider alternative communication strategies, and firmly established behavioral patterns that counteract attempts at facilitating positive change are all examples of patterns that may have a negative impact on progress. Families with these types of problems may be discharged from the family-centered program with a referral for counseling. In the meantime, the client may benefit from a traditional intervention approach.

The Last Session

Regardless of the reason for discharge, the final session of a family-centered program is marked in a positive way. Inviting additional guests to attend (e.g., classroom teacher, special education coordinator, neighbor, family members who have not been involved in the program), holding it at a different location, and providing refreshments are some strategies that may enhance the milestone value of the program's last session.

The last session is different from the assessment and intervention sessions described earlier in this chapter in that the purpose of the final session is to review the accomplishments made by the client and family during the program and to discuss any related future plans.

Every final session has its own personality. However, in a general way, it is constructive to give all individuals the opportunity to share their view of the accomplishments made though the program. An atmosphere of celebration is appropriate for all families who have completed a program, regardless of whether all objectives were met.

Follow-up Alternatives

Families who are discharged because of having met the goals of their intervention program should be followed informally for a period of time. For example, the clinician or a designee may contact them after a specified number of weeks or months to ask for a verbal status report. Another possibility may be for the family to return for reevaluation after a specified time, such as 6 months or 1 year.

Clinicians who have discharged a family that has not yet met the goals of the intervention program may have a number of follow-up alternatives. Some families may discontinue the family program and transfer immediately into a traditional program. The traditional program is one vehicle for continuing communication between the clinician and the family.

A referral is another method of follow-up that facilitates continued work toward the agreed-on objectives. The referral is made in order to address a situation that interfered with the program, so following through on the referral is one method that the family uses to continue to address the goals. Once referred, if the family agrees, the clinician may make regular contacts for a verbal status report or a reevaluation may be scheduled to take place at a specified time in the near future.

CONCLUDING REMARKS

This discussion on family-centered services will be followed by a discussion about serving the needs of individuals representing diverse cultural groups. This is an appropriate transition because, although the family is a tremendous resource for all clients, for clients whose background is unfamiliar, the family members are often able to provide the link between our professional and personal experiences and the valid communication needs of the child.

REFERENCES

Andrews, J. R., & Andrews, M. A. (1990). *Family based treatment in communicative disorders: A systemic approach.* Sandwich, IL: Janelle Publications.

Houle, G. R., & Hamilton, J. L. (1991). Public Law 99-457. *ASHA, 33,* 51-54.

Johnson, B. A., Maxfield, M. W., & Sheeler, B. W. (1992). Family program observation as an introduction to clinical procedures. A poster session presented at the annual convention of the American Speech-Language-Hearing Association, San Antonio, TX.

STUDY GUIDE 5

1. Why has the number of infants and toddlers served by speech-language pathologists been on the increase?
2. Prior to the implementation of PL 99-457, what was the obligation of the federal government to provide support services to disabled preschoolers?
3. Describe the services available to disabled preschoolers through Section 619 of PL 99-457.
4. Describe the services available to disabled preschoolers through Part H of PL 99-457.

5. Why is an understanding of Part H of PL 99-457 particularly important to the topic of family-centered clinical services?

6. What is our purpose when we involve families in the process of clinical service delivery?

7. Compare family-centered to traditional approaches for clinical service delivery. Discuss similarities and differences.

8. For the purpose of implementing a family-centered program, define the family.

9. What factors should be evaluated in determining whether a family program is appropriate, and why?

10. In contacting the family to arrange the first family meeting, exactly what should be communicated?

11. Why is it necessary to encourage most families to participate?

12. What is accomplished by emphasizing the family's ability to contribute to the intervention process?

13. What is accomplished by communicating that the family members are part of a team of experts when they participate in a family-centered program?

14. How might you create an atmosphere that welcomes family participation?

15. What is accomplished by giving the family members responsibilities and activities as soon as possible?

16. What are some immediate activities that family members can perform?

17. Who should control the children during the family meetings, and why?

18. Why do we ask the family members to define their immediate concerns before establishing program objectives and procedures?

19. What are some reasons for not addressing all immediate family concerns exactly as they are requested?

20. If it is decided not to address a family concern directly, what can be done to help the family understand that their concerns are a priority?

21. What is accomplished by making an effort to understand the communication dynamics that occur within the family?

22. Why is it sometimes difficult for us to identify the positive aspects of the family communication?

23. What is accomplished by relating positive aspects of family communication to the family members?

24. In a family program, what is accomplished by passing judgment and criticizing?

25. What should occur in the family program prior to offering any suggestions for changing an aspect of family communication?

26. What is accomplished by offering one positive comment in writing after each session?

27. Describe a polyocular view and explain why it is important.

28. How does one develop a polyocular view?

29. How can family disagreements be used to the advantage of the program?

30. What strategies might you use to manage family disagreements effectively?
31. In the family program, for what purposes do we listen for the type of language that is habitually used by the family?
32. What is meant by assessing the communication disorder in the context of the family?
33. How might family members be used to administer standardized tests?
34. Describe the process of determining objectives and procedures that meet with the agreement of the family.
35. Exactly what do we do to guide family members in implementing intervention procedures?
36. Describe the two types of home assignments that may be given.
37. What should be accomplished during the introduction of an assessment session?
38. What questions might be asked during the interview of an assessment session? How might the answers to these questions be used later in the session?
39. What is the purpose of the break that takes place during most family-program meetings?
40. During the assessment session, when is the demonstration over and why?
41. When a family has not completed an assignment, how should that be handled and why?
42. What are some reasons for dismissing a client from family-centered intervention?
43. What are some follow-up alternatives for families who are no longer involved in a family program?
44. How is the final session of a family program different from the other sessions that have taken place throughout the program?
45. Each of the following terms represent concepts that may need to be communicated to a family. None of the terms are inherently clear to lay people and should not be used without explanation. Consider each term and write exactly what you would say to a family member to express the concept that is represented by it.

a.	communication assessment	m.	presentation of stimulus items
b.	audiological evaluation	n.	language context
c.	test reliability	o.	language form
d.	test administration	p.	language use
e.	verbalizations	q.	content-form interactions
f.	language comprehension	r.	phonological processes
g.	language expression	s.	language sample
h.	pragmatics	t.	objectives
i.	syntax	u.	procedures
j.	semantics	v.	polyocular view
k.	morphemes	w.	below-age-level performance
l.	prosody	x.	at-age-level performance

y. PL 99-457
z. carry-over
aa. generalization
bb. articulation errors

cc. unintelligible speech
dd. pivot phrases
ee. telegraphic speech
ff. motherese

Introduction to Multicultural Issues

Identifying, Assessing, and Treating Children of Various Cultural Backgrounds

Barbara Ann Johnson and Teri Mata-Pistokache°

LEARNING OBJECTIVES

At the conclusion of this chapter, you should be prepared to:

- Discuss ASHA's position and plan for addressing the communication needs of people from various cultures;
- Discuss key terminology that is basic to the appreciation of multicultural concerns;
- Identify characteristics that impact language assessment and intervention for a small selection of minority cultures;
- Recognize that minorities are overrepresented in special education, understand why, and avoid referring minority children for special services unnecessarily;

°Teri Mata-Pistokache, M.S., CCC-SLP is Assistant Professor, Communications Disorders, University of Texas–Pan American, Edinburg, Texas

- Recognize levels of language proficiency and how they impact assessment and intervention for minority-language children;
- Identify available language assessment and intervention procedures that may be used for appropriately addressing the needs of minority children.

INTRODUCTION

The population of the United States is in the process of becoming increasingly diverse with respect to cultural and linguistic preferences. The 1990 U.S. census indicated that at least 25 percent of the nation was composed of people connected with racial and ethnic minority groups. Approximately 12 percent were African-American, 9 percent Hispanic, 3 percent Asian/Pacific-American, and 1 percent American Indian and Eskimo. The rate of population growth for these groups was reported as 110 percent for Asian/Pacific Americans, 55 percent for Hispanics, 38 percent for Native Americans and Eskimos, and 15 percent for African-Americans. By contrast, the rate of population growth for Americans of European (non-Hispanic) descent was reported at only about 3 percent (Taylor, 1993).

If these trends continue, by the year 2000, Hispanics will have increased by an additional 21 percent; Asian Americans, by an additional 22 percent; African-Americans, by about 12 percent; and European Americans (non-Hispanics), by a little more than 2 percent (Battle, 1993). It is estimated that by the year 2000, one-third of all school-age children will be identified with racial or ethnic minority groups (Spencer, 1986). Further, by the year 2010, it is estimated that one-third of the overall population will be composed of what is now considered to be the minority, and that by the middle of the twenty-first century, the so-called majority will be the minority (Taylor, 1993).

As a result of these demographic changes, speech-language pathologists are being called upon to serve increasing numbers of individuals from a wide variety of cultures, each having a unique set of normative behaviors, learning styles, social beliefs, and views of the world; each being diverse within itself; and each having unique and identifiable linguistic variations (Battle, 1993). For that reason, it is incumbent upon every speech-language pathologist and every student of speech-language pathology to become familiar with some basic principles for addressing the needs of individuals from a variety of cultural and linguistic backgrounds. Our further responsibility is to learn as much as possible about the cultural and linguistic characteristics that impact speech-language referral, assessment, and intervention of individuals who identify with various backgrounds.

This chapter is an effort to introduce these issues at the preprofessional level. For practical reasons, the information provided herein is meant as an introduction alone. Hopefully, the content encourages a fundamental appreciation of the importance of cultural and linguistic factors when addressing individual language needs. It also provides basic information about a few identified groups and encouragement to seek out more specific information regarding the languages and behaviors of cultural groups that you expect to encounter with relative frequency. Further, the chapter outlines some common inappropriate referral, assessment, and intervention procedures so that they can be avoided, and it offers suggestions for identifying, assessing, and treating the communication needs of minority-language children.

ASHA PREPARES ITSELF TO ADDRESS COMMUNICATION NEEDS OF MINORITY INDIVIDUALS

As the association that certifies professionals who serve individuals with communication disorders, ASHA recognizes the responsibility to prepare its membership to competently serve the growing number of individuals who identify with federally designated minorities. ASHA's position, commitment, and plan are described below.

ASHA's Position and Commitment

Speech-language pathology and audiology are among the few professions whose national organization (ASHA) has had a long-standing history of policies that oppose discrimination. Throughout the years, these policies have influenced where official meetings are held, restricted affiliations of elected officers, and defined ethical conduct associated with clinical practice. ASHA's policies opposing discrimination underlie the basic tenets of the association (Carey, 1992).

Further, ASHA has a history of having official policies that demonstrate commitment to promoting affirmative action. Appointments to committees and boards, selection of educational program faculty and topics, investments, and specific governmental lobbying efforts have all been influenced by ASHA's commitment to affirmative action (Carey, 1992).

Commitment to cultural diversity is evident in ASHA's governance structure, which includes committees on the status of racial minorities, cultural differences, linguistic differences and disorders, and political and social responsibility. ASHA is one of the few national professional and scientific organizations to carry a long-standing tradition (about 25 years) of maintaining a staffed unit within its national office dedicated solely to minority affairs (Carey, 1992).

Throughout the years, ASHA has promulgated a number of position statements, guidelines, and definitions regarding multicultural issues and linguistic differences. These documents have served to clarify issues that impact the professions and professionals, and they include such topics as social dialects, services to language-minority individuals, and language competence (Carey, 1992).

Resource development projects sponsored by ASHA have educated thousands of members across the country on **bilingual** issues and on communication disorders in multicultural populations. ASHA has conducted national conferences and institutes on underserved populations, Hispanic populations, minority recruitment, multicultural professional education, and historically Black institutions. The latest standards for ASHA certifications and accreditations require that individuals demonstrate multicultural literacy and that multicultural education begin at the preprofessional level (Carey, 1992).

ASHA's long-standing commitment to minority concerns has been demonstrated in many ways. Further, in 1992, "Multicultural Agenda 2000" was published in an effort to bring these operations together and move toward the future with a workable plan for addressing the needs of individuals who represent a diverse range of cultural backgrounds (Carey, 1992).

ASHA's Plan: Multicultural Agenda 2000

Multicultural Agenda 2000 seeks to improve the profession's commitment to minority cultures in six areas. They include (1) membership, (2) leadership involvement, (3) the ASHA national office structure and staff, (4) policies and programs affecting services, education, and research, (5) governmental and legislative efforts, and (6) public image.

Membership.   Regarding its membership, ASHA's plan is designed to increase the proportion of individuals who identify with federally designated racial/ethnic minority groups to 10 percent by the year 2000 (Carey, 1992). This is an increase of 6 percentage points over the 4 percent representation reported in 1987 (Cole, 1987).

Leadership.   Regarding leadership involvement, ASHA proposes to ensure that individuals who identify with federally designated racial or ethnic minority groups are afforded opportunity to participate in the leadership of the association. This includes a commitment to minority participation within the governance structure, within the special interest division structure, and in the design and implementation of all activities and programs sponsored by the association (Carey, 1992).

National Office Structure and Staff.   Multicultural Agenda 2000 makes a commitment to increase the proportion of individuals who are members of federally designated racial/ethnic minorities who are employed by ASHA in managerial positions. The objective is for the ratio of minorities in the national office staff to approximate minority representation within the association at large. A further objective is to assure the maintenance and prominence of minority programs in the national office organizational structure (Carey, 1992).

Policies and Programs Affecting Professional Services, Education, and Research.   Multicultural Agenda 2000 communicates to the ASHA membership that it is the responsibility of every ASHA member to upgrade personal knowledge and skill in order to appropriately serve and study multicultural populations (Carey, 1992). Resources and continuing education opportunities that encourage individuals to make this commitment have been sponsored by ASHA for a number of years. Further, certification and accreditation requirements take measures to ensure that, as you enter the profession, you have opportunity to understand this responsibility from the onset of your preprofessional education.

Governmental and Legislative Efforts.   ASHA is committed to promoting improved health care, educational opportunities, and overall quality of life for members of federally designated minority populations. Further, ASHA opposes acts that are contrary to such goals (Carey, 1992).

Public Image.   ASHA is committed to ensuring that in all its communication to the public, it presents an image that demonstrates recognition of the cultural diversity that characterizes the nation, ASHA's membership, and the people who are served by ASHA's certified professionals. Further, the commitment is not only to demonstrate recognition of diversity, but also to demonstrate ASHA's commitment to serving members of a wide variety of cultural groups (Carey, 1992).

CLARIFICATION OF TERMS

Terminology used to discuss multicultural issues can become confusing. We hope to unravel some of the confusion by providing definitions in this section. We begin with general terms that are used to describe populations, move on to terms describing attitudes about populations, and end with terms and concepts related to language and culture.

General Terms Describing Multicultural Populations

In order to understand the diversity that characterizes our nation, it is important to understand the differences between three concepts that are frequently confused with one another. The concepts are **race, ethnicity,** and culture.

Race.   The term race describes one's biological and anatomical attributes, such as skin color, facial features, and hair texture (Battle, 1993). Race is entirely a physical phenomenon determined by heredity. At this point in the history of physical anthropology, most consider that there are three distinct races of human beings — now termed Ethiopian (originating in the southern third of Arabia and sub-Saharan Africa), Palaearctic (originating in Europe, western Asia and Africa north of the Sahara), and Oriental (originating in Australia and eastern Asia) (Grolier's Academic American Encyclopedia, 1994).

Ethnicity. Ethnicity is described by one's race, origin, characteristics, and institutions (Battle, 1993). Ethnicity is determined by heritage and embraces the concept of belonging to a particular ethnic group. For example, ethnicity refers to the sharing of a unique social and cultural heritage passed on from one generation to the next. Ethnic heritage is frequently identified by distinct patterns of family life, language, recreation, religion, and other customs that cause certain individuals to be differentiated from others (Banks, 1987).

Ethnicity may sometimes be confused with race because ethnic groups often share the same racial or biological heritage. However, race represents a strictly biological concept, whereas the term ethnicity makes a statement about social and cultural history and about belonging to a group which may or may not be racially homogeneous. For example, Hispanics may be of the Palaearctic race if they are Mexican-American, but Hispanics may also include members of the Ethiopian race (e.g., some Puerto Rican individuals).

Culture. Culture is defined by the behaviors, beliefs, and values of a group of people who are brought together by commonalities. Explicit and implicit behaviors characterize each particular cultural group (Battle, 1993).

Explicit cultural behaviors are those characteristics by which the group is often recognized by outsiders. Explicit behaviors include distinguishing styles of dress, language and speaking patterns, eating habits, customs, and life-styles (Battle, 1993).

By contrast, implicit cultural behaviors are those that are not readily observable. They include such factors as age, gender, family, roles within the family, child-rearing practices, socioeconomic status, education, religion and spiritual beliefs, fears, attitudes, values, perceptions of what constitutes a handicapping condition, and exposure to and adoption of other cultural ways (Battle, 1993).

Culture is transmitted by ethnic groups through customary patterns, languages, and social institutions (Garcia, 1982). For example, Mexican-Americans as an ethnic group transmit Mexican-American culture by perpetuating a variety of cultural events. One example of a Mexican-American cultural event is the custom of celebrating *quinceañeras,* the commemoration of a young girl's passage to womanhood at the age of 15 years. For this important event, the young woman whose life is being celebrated chooses an elegant gown, traditional Mexican food is served, traditional Mexican music is played by a mariachi band, and religious customs are represented (e.g., the rosary, the Bible).

Further, the traditional language is incorporated in the many Spanish terms associated with the event even if English is the dominant language of the family. For example, the friends and relatives who sponsor the event are given the title of *padrinos* or *padrinas,* and these individuals receive special recognition at the banquet (e.g., *padrinos y padrinas del salon* are the individuals who finance the rental of the hall that is used for the *quinceañera's* festivities).

Terms Describing Attitudes toward Various Groups

Both positive and negative attitudes toward various cultural groups are evident in the world around us. The predominantly negative attitudes of **ethnocentrism** (which can be positive at times), **racism, prejudice, stereotype,** and discrimination are described first. The more supportive attitudes of **cultural pluralism** and **cultural relativism** are then described.

Ethnocentrism.   Ethnocentrism has two sides. As a dynamic social force, it can be either cohesive or corrosive.

Cultural Pride.   The cohesive side of ethnocentrism is the universal attitude of pride in one's ethnic or cultural group. **Cultural pride** can serve to draw people together by providing a group with solidarity. Pride in one's heritage is a cohesive force whenever it enhances self-esteem in the group and in the individual members of it (R. Garcia, 1982; S. Garcia, 1983).

Cultural Degradation.   Ethnocentrism is a corrosive social force when it causes bigotry, intolerance, alienation, or social dejection. **Cultural degradation** is a corrosive type of ethnocentrism, which occurs when groups are made to feel that their cultures are inadequate, backward, or inferior. Cultural degradation may result in attitudes of low self-esteem and self-rejection (R. Garcia, 1982; S. Garcia, 1983).

Cultural Chauvinism.   The other corrosive form of ethnocentrism is **cultural chauvinism.** This is the attitude that other groups are not only different but are also perceived as being wrong and inferior. Cultural chauvinism presumes that the people of one's own group are superior to members of other groups who are perceived as "barbaric," "uncivilized," or devoid of the "in" group's redeeming values and ways (Garcia, 1983).

Racism.   Racism is the attitude that one's racial group is inherently superior to another group (Garcia, 1982). Racism corresponds to both facets of the corrosive side of ethnocentrism—cultural degradation and cultural chauvinism.

Prejudice.   Prejudice is a negative *apriori* judgment about a group or about a group's individual members. The judgment is made without knowledge, analysis, or evaluation of the facts concerning the individuals who constitute the group (Garcia, 1982).

Stereotype.   A stereotype is an oversimplified, often negative concept about members of a particular group. The "tight Scotsman," the "rich Jew," the "sneaky Mexican," and the "Italian lover" are examples of ethnic stereotypes (Garcia, 1982).

Discrimination.   Discrimination consists of direct or indirect acts of exclusion, distinction, differentiation, or preference on account of group membership. Discrimination is based on racial or ethnic affiliation (Garcia, 1982) and other conditions that sometimes set individuals apart as different (e.g., handicapping condition, handedness, hair color, physique, or physical appearance). The attitudes of racism, prejudice, and stereotype are manifest in the act of discrimination.

Biases that result in discrimination are acquired through the teachings and beliefs that pervade homes, schools, and communities throughout humanity. Young people acquire these misconceptions and biases unless they are provided with information and experiences that teach about people of a variety of racial and ethnic backgrounds (Garcia, 1982).

Cultural Pluralism.   Cultural pluralism occurs when a number of diverse cultural groups coexist within the boundaries or framework of one nation, and these groups are mutually supportive of one another. A pluralistic society comprises people connected with diverse cultures, each having significantly different beliefs, behaviors, colors, and in many cases different languages (National Coalition for Cultural Pluralism, 1973).

Cultural Relativism.   A person who takes the position of cultural relativism views each ethnic and cultural group from its own vantage point. It takes the attitude that cultures are different but not necessarily inferior or superior. Cultural relativism requires that we perceive each culture (and its people) from its own unique perspective rather than solely from the perspective of one's own cultural sphere (Garcia, 1982).

In a climate of ethnocentrism, racism, prejudice, stereotypes, and discrimination, cultural relativism is not enough to counter the deep-seeded teachings of childhood. Its positive effects are quickly neutralized in the presence of extreme and firmly established forms of negativism (Garcia, 1982).

Beyond Cultural Relativism.   To proactively counter negative teachings, professionals need to go beyond taking a posture of cultural relativism. Therefore, we are all encouraged to carefully analyze our own covert and overt behaviors with regard to the negative attitudes and acts (ethnocentrism, racism, prejudice, stereotype, and discrimination). By taking this step we become able to identify our own attitudes or perceptions and increase our cultural sensitivity. It is important to increase personal awareness of negative attitudes and behaviors so that we can address them directly. For some people, recognizing negative attitudes may be a difficult task. For example, when dealing with clients whose cultures are unfamiliar, if opinions are particularly extensive and deep-rooted, significant effort is required to recognize them, make the necessary changes, and consciously oppose negative thinking patterns. Regardless, everyone who serves a clinical population must make the effort to identify and let go of any tendency toward intolerance of difference and the behaviors that are commonly associated with this thinking pattern.

Terms and Concepts Related to Language and Culture

Language and culture are interrelated and great diversity can be found across the nation, both between and within the various groups. However, it is sometimes wrongly assumed that all people share a similar culture and language. For that reason, people of minority language or minority dialect are sometimes evaluated for their proficiency in a language that is not related to the their cultural heritage or experience. Since this should not be the case, it is basic for speech-language pathologists and students of speech-language pathology to understand the dependent relationship between language and culture, the fundamental differences between language and dialect, the differences between language disorders and **language differences,** and the phenomena of **code switching** and **style switching.** The basic concepts are explained in this section.

Dependence of Language on Culture.   All humans are members of at least one cultural group, with definable implicit and explicit cultural behaviors. For each individual, communication patterns are determined by one's cultural orientation (Battle, 1993).

All societies have routines whereby children become socialized. This socialization process begins in the home via the interaction of the child and significant others. During this socialization period the child learns the cultural norms of the community which include the rules of appropriate behavior as well as the values and beliefs that underlie overt behaviors.

Linguistic and interactional demands that are placed on children vary across cultural groups. For example, it is through daily interactions with significant others that children acquire the linguistic systems and rules for participating in dialogues within that culture (Blount, 1982; Iglesias, 1985). Children begin to understand and then use the languages that surround them. It is through this process that language facilitates an unconscious transmission of values, beliefs, and culture across generations; thus acquisition of language also constitutes the acquisition of one's native culture (Ripich & Spinelli, 1985; Westby, 1988).

Language and culture grow up together over a period of history and within each person's lifespan, and the two function in harmony with one another. Much of culture is enacted and transmitted through language. The songs, hymns, and prayers of a culture; its folk tales and wise sayings; its appropriate forms of greeting and leaving; and its history, wisdom, and ideals are all wrapped up in its language. The memories and traditions of a culture are stored in its language.

Language and Dialect.

Language.   Language (as defined in Chapter 1) refers to the code whereby ideas about the world are expressed through a conventional system of arbitrary signals for communication (Lahey, 1988). Spanish, English, Navajo, and American Sign Language are examples of languages.

Dialect.   For the purpose of our discussion, the term *dialect* is used to describe a subset of the broader term, *language*. Dialect refers to phonemic, lexical, and semantic variations that occur within the language (Sapir, 1921) and are common to a particular group of people who are from the same region, of the same socioeconomic group, or share a similar ethnic heritage. For example, in 1800 Louisiana claimed three different varieties of French: "Louisiana Standard French," spoken by white descendants of the original French settlers; "Cajun French," spoken by Acadians expelled from Canada; and "Louisiana French Creole," a combination of French and West African languages spoken by the West Africans imported to work on plantations (Conklin & Lourie, 1983).

In this chapter, the broader term, *language*, is used when discussing both linguistic and dialectal variations unless the more specific term is required for the sake of accuracy. Although we recognize that dialectal differences are not exactly the same as language differences, the generalization of terms is necessary due to limitations in the scope of the chapter.

Code Switching and Style Switching.

Code Switching.   Code switching is the alternating use of two languages at the word, phrase, and sentence level, with a complete break between languages in phonology (Valdez-Fallis, 1978). An example of code switching between Spanish and English within the same sentence is *"Tienes una apple?"* ("Do you have an apple?").

Style Switching.   Style switching is the changing of linguistic form that occurs within a language. This includes changes within a dialect, such as switching from informal to formal language in order to accommodate situational demands (Labov, 1970). For example, when addressing one's peers, one might request a drink of water in a much different way than when addressing one's boss or university professor.

Style switching also includes changes from one dialect to another in order to accommodate a listener or conform to perceived social constraints. For example, most speakers of Black English have some facility in switching between Black English and Standard American English. In the case of this particular dialect, occurrences of style switching seem to depend on two factors: (1) skill with Standard American English and (2) perceived social consequences for using Black English or Standard American English in each particular situation (Seymour & Miller-Jones, 1981).

Language Differences and Language Disorders.

Language Differences.   For every cultural group, expectations about communication behavior and perceptions of what constitutes a communication disorder are unique. These expectations and perceptions are the product of the particular group's cultural values, perceptions, attitudes, and history (Battle, 1993).

Language differences occur whenever a variation of a symbol system is used by a group of individuals; this unique symbol system reflects shared regional, social, cultural, or ethnic factors. Language differences are typically characterized by variations in vocabulary, pronunciation, grammar, and pragmatics (Campbell, 1991).

An identified speaking pattern is considered to be a language difference and *not* a language disorder under each of the following circumstances: (1) the speaking pattern is universal to the social group or culture, (2) it is universal to the native region, (3) it is considered to be appropriate by the cultural group, or (4) it is explained by sociohistorical factors that describe the cultural group (Campbell, 1991).

Language differences do not require clinical intervention. In fact, language intervention is not appropriate when the pattern is characteristic of a linguistic difference, if in fact a concomitant language disorder is not identified.

Language Disorders.   As defined in Chapter 2, the term *language disorders* describes the language behavior of a heterogeneous group of children whose language is different from and not superior to the language of their same-age counterparts (Lahey, 1988). For the minority community, comparing a child's language to same-age counterparts means to compare one's language to the norms and expectations of the language community of which the child is a member (Peters-Johnson & Taylor, 1986).

In determining whether someone who identifies with a minority culture has a language disorder, the following criteria are considered. A language disorder is identified if (1) the speaking pattern is *not* universally used in the social or cultural group, (2) it is *not* universally used in the native region, (3) it is *not* considered to be appropriate in any situation for the native cultural group, and (4) the speaking pattern can be explained by cognitive limitations, sensory-input reduction, motor skills deficit, deficient social relationships, or it cannot be explained by sociohistorical factors that characterize the cultural group (Campbell, 1991).

Language Disorder Concomitant to Language Difference.   A language disorder can occur in a child who also demonstrates a pattern of language difference. A child whose language pattern does not correspond to the language patterns of the community is appropriately considered for intervention, whether a language difference is identified or not.

CHARACTERISTICS THAT IMPACT LANGUAGE ASSESSMENT AND INTERVENTION FOR SEVERAL MINORITY CULTURES

Basic information about select groups of cultural minorities is provided in order to introduce you to some patterns of behavior that may be encountered when meeting people outside your familiar cultural spheres. Only very fundamental information is included because the primary purpose of this chapter is to *introduce* you to the process of becoming a culturally literate professional. Further, it is both impractical and impossible to detail all the characteristics of all the cultural groups that may be encountered, as they are many in number and each identified group is strikingly diverse.

Hispanic Cultures

History.   Historically, Hispanic people (i.e., people of Spanish heritage) began to arrive on this continent more than 500 years ago, and perhaps more than 100 years before the arrival of travelers from the British Isles and western Europe. Much of what is now the southwestern United States was populated by Hispanics long before the territories became states. Much of Texas, New Mexico, Arizona, and southern California continue to be populated by people of Hispanic heritage whose families have lived in this country for many generations as well as those who have recently immigrated (Kayser, 1993).

In these parts of the nation, Spanish continues to be spoken. It is the dominant language of some and the secondary language of others who are bilingual; moreover, Spanish is the only language for some **monolingual** Hispanic-Americans.

The racial heritage of Hispanic people is varied. Some Hispanics are descendants of Native-Americans who settled in the Americas before the Spanish conquest. Other Hispanics are direct descendants of Spanish and European settlers. Still others have African-American ancestors, and a few are of Asian ancestry (Langdon, 1992).

Demographics.   Individuals from Spanish-language backgrounds already constitute the largest group of non–English background people in the United

States. After African-Americans, Hispanics constitute the largest minority group in the United States. If sustained immigration continues, Hispanics will become the dominant minority group by the year 2000 (Bouvier & Davis, 1982; United States, 1985).

The number of Hispanic Americans has increased dramatically during the past two decades, and accelerated growth is forecast for the next decade (Figueroa, Fradd, & Correa, 1989; United States, 1985). Thus, the number of individual Spanish speakers with limited English proficiency (LEP) and non-English proficiency will increase and the language skills of the individual people within the group will probably continue to vary tremendously (Oxford-Carpenter et al., 1984).

The largest concentrations of Hispanic people residing in the United States are found in the states that border Mexico—California has 34 percent and Texas has 21 percent of the total Hispanic population in the nation. Other states with high concentrations of Hispanics include New York, Florida, Arizona, New Jersey, New Mexico, and Colorado. The largest identified Hispanic group is Mexican (58 percent), followed by Central and South American (14 percent), Puerto Rican (13 percent), other Hispanics (9 percent), and Cuban (6 percent) (United States, 1990a).

Cultural and Social Aspects.   The heterogeneity within Hispanic cultures makes it impossible to easily characterize specific cultural features of Hispanic groups (Penalosa, in press; Erickson & Iglesias, 1986). However, a few common characteristics can be recognized. For example, older individuals may be given special respect because of their advanced age and experience; handshaking is accompanied by hugging and kissing upon greeting family and close friends; and family takes precedence over everything else, including job, school, and friendship (Langdon, 1992).

In social gatherings where adults and children are present, Hispanic adults have been noted to interact primarily with other adults. Adults do not ask children for their interpretation of events or emotional evaluations (Heath, 1986). Children are exposed to vocabulary related to names of relatives and relationships within the extended family (Guendelman, 1983), and Hispanic children are not usually asked to repeat facts or to predict what they will do.

Language.   Spanish continues to be a worldwide language. The United States is one of the largest Spanish-speaking countries in the world, behind Mexico, Spain, Colombia, Argentina, and Peru (United States, 1991). In 1976, the number of Spanish speakers in the United States was approximately 8.57 million, and it is projected to be 16.61 million by the year 2010 (Veltman, 1990).

There are significant differences among Hispanic children in terms of the quantity and quality of exposure to the English language. Some children are exposed to caretakers who model nativelike proficiency in both Spanish and English; others are exposed to nativelike modeling in one language and limited models in the other; and many are exposed to a mixed code of Spanish and English.

Distinct linguistic patterns emerge when an individual is consistently exposed to more than one language. The individual may (1) be of limited English proficiency, (2) demonstrate high levels of proficiency in one or the other language, (3) be of limited proficiency in both languages, or (4) exhibit high proficiency levels in both languages (Payan, 1984).

Spanish differs significantly from English in all dimensions. It is useful for clinicians to be aware of the major differences between the two systems so that differences due to second-language learning can be recognized as differences and not mistaken for disorders.

Phonology. Phonologically, Spanish has 18 consonants, including four semivowels, while English has 24 consonants with three semivowels. Spanish has five vowels, compared to 12-14 vowels in English. The following are examples of typical English productions specific to individuals whose first language is Spanish: [tʃ/ʃ] (chip/ship), [s/z] (price/prize), [t/θ] (tin/thin), [b/v] (imbite/invite, ban/van), [i/ɪ] (seek/sick), [ɛ/æ] (bet/bat), [æ/ɛ] (pat/pet), [ʌ/ɔ] (cut/caught), and [u/ʊ] (luke/look).

Syntax. Syntactically, there are several primary differences between the Spanish and English languages. Selected ones include differences in word order for changing grammatical meaning, differences in ways that number and grammatical gender are indicated, and differences in ordering adjectives and nouns in sentences.

In English, *word order* is important for communicating grammatical meaning. For example, if changing a statement to a question, one inverts the syntax of the noun and verb (e.g., "You [do] have an apple," versus, "Do you have an apple?"). The Spanish language, however, relies more on vocal inflection to communicate these types of grammatical changes (e.g., "¿*Tu tienes una manzana?*" literally means "You have an apple?" but if the intonation is raised at the end of the sentence, it becomes the question, "Do you have an apple?").

Spanish has a full set of *number and gender markers* to show adjectival and articular agreement with the noun. Therefore Spanish speakers use word endings to indicate both grammatical gender (masculine or feminine) and number (singular or plural) for all words that modify the noun; and the gender and number of the noun determine the word endings to be applied to all modifiers associated with it. In English, however, grammatical gender is not expressed and number is inflected for nouns and verbs only.

To demonstrate differences in the way number is grammatically expressed, in English one might say, "The frogs are jumping." The fact that there is more than one frog requires that the plural ending be added to the word "frog" and that the plural form of the verb "to be" be applied ("are"). The article "the," however, is the same for both singular and plural applications. By contrast, the same sentence in Spanish (*"Las ranas estan saltando"*) requires that the noun *(ranas)*, verb *(estan)*, and article modifier *(las)* all be inflected to indicate plurality. (If only one frog were jumping, one would say, *"La rana esta saltando"*).

Regarding grammatical gender, English nouns do not carry grammatical gender specifications. However, in Spanish, some words are grammatically feminine while other words are grammatically masculine. Therefore, in Spanish all modifiers that describe the noun reflect gender specification. The Spanish word for "frog" is *rana*. Since it is of feminine grammatical gender, the article is *la*, and any other modifiers that are added also carry a feminine grammatical marker. Thus, the phrase "the frog" is *"la rana,"* and "the frogs" is expressed as *"las ranas."* By contrast, the Spanish word for rabbit is *conejo*, which is grammatically masculine. The article is the masculine *el*, and all modifiers carry a masculine grammatical marker. Thus, the phrase, "the rabbit" is *"el conejo,"* and "the rabbits" is expressed as *"los conejos."*

To demonstrate the *ordering of nouns and adjectives* in the sentences, English adjectives generally precede nouns and bear no grammatical markers (e.g., "the white house," "the white cats"). In Spanish, adjectives are typically placed after the noun, and they must agree with the noun that they modify in both number and gender. For example, the Spanish word for "house" is *"casa,"* and the word for "white" is *"blanca"* or *"blanco,"* depending on gender (*"blancas"* and *"blancos"* for the plural forms). Therefore, the phrase, "the white house" is expressed, *"la casa blanca."* Similarly, "the white cats" is expressed, *"los gatos blancos."*

Attitudes toward Communication Disorders.   Unfortunately, there appears to be little reliable demographic data on the incidence of handicapping conditions in bilingual populations. This is partially because there are still large numbers of minority-language children whose conditions have either been misdiagnosed or undiagnosed (Ortiz & Maldonado-Colon, 1986).

Among many Hispanic and other minority groups, there is a tendency to attribute a child's "visible" handicap to an external nonmedical reason (Meyerson, 1983). This applies to communication disorders as well as other potentially handicapping conditions. For example, some Mexican-American mothers have been known to attribute their children's cleft palate to an eclipse during pregnancy (Meyerson, 1983, 1990). Others may attribute a congenital problem to a *"susto"* ("frightful situation") during pregnancy, to *"mal puesto"* ("witchcraft"), or to *"mal ojo"* ("evil eye"). Still other mothers report that their child's affliction is a direct punishment for wrongdoing. Among Cubans, a child's physical or mental problem is often attributed to *"empacho"* ("indigestion"), *"desmayo"* ("fainting spell"), *"decaimiento"* ("lack of energy"), or *"barrenillo"* ("obsessive thinking") during pregnancy (Queralt, 1984).

A belief in folk medicine *(curanderismo)* as part of a medical or rehabilitative process is common among some Hispanics. *Curanderismo* is practiced by *"curanderos"* ("healers") in Mexico or *"espiritistas"* ("spiritualists") in Puerto Rico. The *curanderos* use a combination of intense concern, rituals, herbs and herbal teas, oil massage, amulets, and prayers. Some groups seek medical care from physicians for physical problems, rehabilitation from rehabilitation specialists, and psychological support from *curanderos* (Meyerson, 1990).

African-American Cultures

History. Exactly how most African-Americans came to reside on the North American continent is a significant part of the African-American language and culture. Further, how the African-American culture and European-American culture met and evolved side-by-side is significant to the relationship that these two highly diverse groups presently share. Terrell and Terrell (1993) highlighted some of these significant events quite eloquently.

> African-Americans, also referred to as Black Americans, are currently the largest minority population in the United States. A highly diverse group of people, they can be very wealthy or very poor, or rural or urban dwellers. For all this diversity, the one factor that many African-Americans share is that they descended from Africans who experienced the forced emigration from their homeland to this country and the economic and political enslavement of an entire race of people, and who subsequently struggled to survive in and overcome a tradition of racism and discrimination. The various ways in which African-Americans have reacted and responded to this single, unifying factor have resulted in the elements of African-American culture as it currently exists. Included in this culture are attitudes, music, religion, and language styles. (p. 3)

Demographics. African-Americans constitute the largest minority group in the United States today. The African-American population includes not only African descendants but also immigrants from Caribbean nations.

More than half of the African-American population resides in southern states. About one-third resides in urban centers of the Midwest and Northeast, particularly in Chicago, Detroit, Baltimore, Washington, D.C., New York, and Philadelphia (Payne, 1986).

Cultural and Social Aspects. In many urban and working-class African-American families, mothers or grandmothers are recognized as the strong authority figure in the home. Males (e.g., brothers or uncles) may assume nonauthoritative roles (Payne, 1986).

In terms of language, a study of poor African-American families in Louisiana (Ward, 1982) identified some parent-child interaction patterns. Apparently, parents in the study interacted more with "lap babies" than with older toddlers who talked, children did not initiate conversation and were expected to make minimal responses when asked a question, and children were expected to listen and follow instructions as opposed to initiating conversations and selecting topics.

Five attributes are recognized as being characteristic of African-American families. These attributes are: (1) strong kinship bonds, (2) strong work orientation, (3) flexibility of family rules, (4) strong achievement, and (5) strong religious orientation (National Urban League, 1971).

Language.

Evolution.   Most of the Western Europeans who forced emigration upon Africans during the seventeenth century did not know the languages of the Africans, nor did the Africans know the languages of the Europeans. Further, it is likely that most of the Africans came from a variety of linguistic backgrounds, so they did not know each other's languages. With a need for communication between the groups and no common language, abbreviated patterns of communication developed. With continued use, rules, inflections, and other systematic linguistic patterns evolved (Terrell & Terrell, 1993).

The dialects that emerged are different from the dialects that evolved among European-American people in the same regions of North America because the African-American slaves were not permitted to become immersed in the language and culture of the European-Americans. Therefore, African-Americans had no way of knowing all the features of Standard American English, and they had no way of keeping up with mainline changes as the languages continued to evolve and mature. Therefore the two languages and cultures grew up side-by-side but independently (Terrell & Terrell, 1993).

Dialect.   A number of linguistic dialects are spoken among Black Americans in the United States. These include the Gullah dialect, which is spoken by persons living on islands adjacent to the coasts of South Carolina and Georgia. There are also various creoles such as Jamaican Creole English.

However, the most prominent linguistic system of African-Americans is known as Black English. Black English is the language that evolved among many African-Americans who underwent forced emigration in the nineteenth century, and it is one of many dialects of American English. Black English is a completely rule-governed linguistic system. The highest percentage of users of Black English are the African-American working class (Dillard, 1973). Many African-Americans do not use the dialect at all (Terrell & Terrell, 1993), and the extent to which a person identifies with African-American culture may influence the extent to which the person uses Black English and the density of the dialect (Terrell & Terrell, 1981). Some individuals vary their use of the dialect, switching codes to accommodate the communicative context and company (Terrell & Terrell, 1993).

Further, Black English is not used exclusively by African-Americans. Depending on the degree of socialization with Black English speakers, a number of Caucasians, Hispanics, and Asians use the dialect as well (Terrell &

Terrell, 1993). Many of the linguistic features of Black English and many of the diverse cultural characteristics that are associated with users of Black English are described in detail in a number of sources (Terrell & Terrell, 1993).

Phonology. There are many basic phonological rules of Black English that differentiate it from the Standard American English sound system. A few of these rules include (1) the silencing or substitution of medial and final consonants in words, (2) the silencing of unstressed initial phonemes and unstressed initial syllables, (3) the silencing of the final consonants in final consonant clusters, and (4) use of [skr] for [str] in the initial position of words.

Regarding the *silencing or substitution of medial or final consonants in words,* when using Standard American English one might say the words "nothing," "tooth," "they," and "protect." To represent the same concepts in Black English, one might say "[nʌtɪn]," "[tuf]," "[de]," and "[potɛkt]."

The *silencing of unstressed initial phonemes and unstressed initial syllables* can also be demonstrated. In standard English, sample words with unstressed initials are "about," "tomatoes," and "one" (as in "this one"). In Black English, these concepts might be represented by saying "[baʊt]," "[metoz]," and "[ʌn]."

With regard to *the silencing of the final consonant in a consonant cluster at the end of a word,* example words with final consonant clusters are "desk," "mind," and "missed" (pronounced [mɪst]). To represent these concepts when speaking Black English, one might say "[dɛs]," "[maɪn]," and "[mɪs]."

Some Standard American English words contain the [str] blend in the initial positions (e.g., street, string, straight). These words are often represented in Black English by substituting the [skr] blend. For example, "string" is pronounced "[skrɪŋ]" and "street" is pronounced "[skrit]."

Syntax. Black English morphology and syntactic rules are extensive and cannot be simplified to a few general rules. Examples are selected for discussion.

Inflection of verbs may be shown by examining changes in regular and irregular verbs and changes in noun-verb agreement (e.g., substituting "cash," "seen," and "done" for the Standard American English forms of "cashed," "saw," and "did"). Double modals are used in Black English (e.g., "used to couldn't" and "like ta"). The *-s* morpheme is often silenced for possessives (e.g., the Standard American English phrase "the boy's hat" may be represented by saying "the boy hat"). Comparatives and superlatives that are irregular in Standard American English are sometimes regularized in Black English (e.g., "stupidest" and "baddest"). Multiple negatives are used (e.g., "He didn't do nothing," and "Nobody didn't do it"). Additionally, irregular reflexive pronouns may be regularized (e.g., "hisself" and "theirself") (Terrell & Terrell, 1993).

Attitudes toward Communication Disorders.   Some African-American individuals may be embarrassed by certain disorders or have superstitions or religious beliefs about them. This applies to communication disorders as well as medical and physical disabilities. Folk medicines may be considered a "cure-all" for certain problems. Unfortunately little research is available to provide information on what members of African-American societies consider pathological and what to do about identified problems (Peters-Johnson & Taylor, 1986).

Native-American Cultures

History.   The Native-American cultures are the cultures native to the American continents. Native Americans populated the geographic region that is now known as the United States (and other parts of North America) for many centuries before any other people migrated to it.

Demographics.   The Native-American cultural group comprises nearly two million individuals who identify with approximately 500 specific tribal groups, each of which is diverse in both language and culture (Harris, 1993). Fifty percent of the population is under the age of 21 years (Dukepoo, 1980).

Each Native-American tribe has the status of a sovereign nation with a separate governing body. Each tribal government has a government-to-government relationship with Washington, D.C. This feature affects all aspects of Native-American life, and it is shared by no other minority group in the nation (Harris, 1993).

People who identify with Native-American culture reside in all 50 states, with most of the population being concentrated in California, Oklahoma, Arizona, New Mexico, North Carolina, and Alaska. There are 278 reservations and 209 Alaska-Native villages in the United States, many of which are isolated from major population centers. The tremendous size of some reservations and their remote distance from metropolitan areas profoundly affects socialization, language patterns, and accessibility to health and rehabilitative services (Harris, 1993).

More than half of the Native-American population reside in urban areas and not on the reservations or native villages. Urban dwellers are usually more educated, with lower unemployment rates, greater family income levels, and fewer dependent children than Native-Americans living on reservations. Regardless of location and acculturation into mainstream America, many Native-Americans maintain traditional life-styles and child-rearing practices (Harris, 1993; Miller, 1975; Red Horse, 1983).

Cultural and Social Aspects.   Native-American children frequently have numerous problems in academic performance due to cultural conflicts with the educational system and associated difficulties with the English language

(Cazden & John, 1971). The following is a list of characteristics common to Native-American children which often lead to teacher misconceptions and low teacher evaluations: (1) valuing cooperation over competition, (2) avoiding public recognition, (3) producing a lower level of language in English-dominated classrooms, (4) responding to authority figures by looking down or away, (5) valuing the present more than the future (which can result in difficulties with long-term planning), (6) offering less affirmative head-nodding, verbal interaction, and eye contact, and (7) tending to be visual learners, thus having difficulty responding to verbal instructions.

In Native-American families, extended family members are considered to be as important as immediate family members, sharing the same bond and level of intimacy. For example, with the Chippewa tribe the children of one brother are considered children of another brother. The Chippewa father teaches the children skills necessary for earning a living; the grandfather transmits philosophy, religion, knowledge of how to live a good life, and the way of the world; and the uncle is traditionally responsible for carrying out the task of disciplining the children (Basso, 1972).

Language.

Pidginization. **Pidginization** is a modification of a language that evolves for the purpose of communicating between people from dissimilar linguistic backgrounds. Short, simplified utterances that contain only substantive words are used (Terrell & Terrell, 1993). **Pidginized language** resembles telegraphic speech.

The rapid pidginization of Native-American languages has added to problems in English performance. Many tribal languages are rapidly losing lexicon and undergoing a process of syntactic simplification. For example, one Choctaw bilingual educator stated that the Choctaw spoken by tribal members in Oklahoma is considered "children's speech" by tribal members in Mississippi (Jacobson, 1979). Those students whose primary language is simplified Choctaw are sometimes severely handicapped in learning English as a second language.

Students who speak and write in pidgin Native-American English are often viewed as failing in academic settings. This is because many mainstream Americans view nonstandard English as a mark of poor education or an indicator of poor performance in school (Anderson & Anderson, 1983).

Language and Child-Rearing. Regardless of whether they have traditional or urban identity, the majority of Native-American families use child-rearing language practices that are incompatible with mainstream culture (Miller, 1975). For example, many Native-American mothers interact with their children silently and nonverbally. No matter how familiar they become with Euro-American culture, common language facilitation activities that include verbal interchange (e.g., story-time, peek-a-boo) are not typically practiced. Further,

Navajo mothers have been noted to interpret the language and behavior of active, verbal children as discourteous, restless, self-centered, and undisciplined (Guilmet, 1979).

Language Characteristics.   Over 200 different Native-American languages are spoken in the United States with dialectal variations within each. In order to demonstrate some characteristic differences between English and Native-American tongues, some characteristics of the Navajo language are selected for discussion.

Phonology.   The Navajo language differs from English in that final consonants are uncommon in Navajo and are not easily heard or produced when Navajo speakers begin to learn English (Harris, 1993). This presents problems with hearing and producing cognate pairs that differ by the final consonant only. Further, many morphological changes are made in English by adding consonantal suffixes (e.g., *-ed, -s,* or *-ing*). This is further complicated by the fact that there is no [ŋ] phoneme in Navajo. Therefore, the present progressive verb tense *(-ing)* is usually difficult to perceive and pronounce (Harris, 1993).

Syntax.   Navajo language has intricate verb structures that focus more on the aspect of motion and state than on the aspect of time. Number is not expressed in noun forms but in verb forms. Verb forms are singular, dual, and plural (one, two, and more than two). Third-person pronouns (e.g., *he, she, it, they*) do not exist. As a result, syntactic confusions are inevitable when Navajo speakers learn English as a second language (Harris, 1993).

Attitudes toward Communication Disorders.   Regarding health risks that impact communication development, Native-Americans have the highest prevalence of otitis media in the world (Stewart, 1986); and fetal alcohol syndrome (FAS) and fetal alcohol effect (FAE) present a major threat to the health and communication development of young Native-American children. Because of the high prevalence of these three disabilities, combined with environmental factors such as poverty and limited access to quality education, members of the Native-American cultural groups experience an increased risk for communication disorders. Further, necessary medical and rehabilitation services are often remote, impeding access to modern facilities and professionals who may address disabling conditions (Harris, 1993).

Historically, many tribes have considered the child with disabilities (including communication disorders) as a gift from the Creator. This was especially true of the mentally retarded. Today, however, attitudes toward handicapped individuals are less positive although there still seems to be an overall feeling of acceptance among most tribal members (Harris, 1993).

Asian-American Cultures

History.   Asian-Americans come from Asia or are descendants of immigrants from Asia. Asian immigrants have been coming to the United States for more than two centuries, dating back to 1785 (Cheng, 1993).

Asian-Americans may be the most extremely diverse of all of the cultural groups that have been discussed, as the Asians who have immigrated to the United States have come from a legion of historical, social, political, and linguistic backgrounds. The diversity ranges from affluent, well-educated, voluntary immigrants to those whose status is that of preliterate refugees. These groups differ greatly in their motivation for leaving their homelands, the effects of culture shock, and degree of acculturation upon arrival in the United States.

The number of identifiable Asian groups is more than 17, and it includes people from China, Japan, Korea, India, Vietnam, Cambodia, Laos, and various Pacific Islands including Guam, the Philippines, and Samoa. These individuals represent literally hundreds of languages and dialects (Cheng, 1993).

Demographics.   In the last two decades, the greatest number of migrants, immigrants, and refugees coming to the United States have come from Southeast Asia (Cheng, 1993). The Asian/Pacific Island population in the United States doubled between 1980 and 1990 (United States, 1990b). Asian people reside throughout the United States with the highest concentrations in California, Hawaii, New York, Illinois, and Texas (Ima & Rumbant, 1989).

Cultural and Social Aspects.   The Asian/Pacific populations hold a variety of religious, philosophical, and cultural practices. Major religions and philosophies include Buddhism, Confucianism, Taoism, Shintoism, Animism, Islam, and Christianity. Because of extreme cultural diversity, cultural generalizations are impossible to draw. For demonstration, we describe a few characteristics of some prominent Asian cultures.

Chinese.   In Chinese culture, respect for elders and the strength of the family unit are highly valued. One of the most important ideals of Chinese culture is the pursuit and maintenance of harmony. Value is placed on an outward calmness and on inner control of ill-favored emotions such as anger, jealousy, hostility, aggression, and self-pity. Openly confronting another person is viewed as undesirable. Education is considered to be extremely important. Chinese-Americans work hard to remove any linguistic and cultural barriers that may inhibit a good education (Cheng, 1993).

Korean.   Korean people have extended families that typically include three generations. The father is usually the head of the household and represents the family honor.

Teachers in Korea have a great deal of authority. Students are well disciplined and there are few delinquency problems in school.

Other Asians. In most Asian cultures, interactive patterns are very structured and predictable. An individual's status defines that person's role in a communication event.

The ability to work harmoniously within the group is highly valued over individual achievement. This includes being sensitive to the needs of others, showing emotional restraint, and working for the good of the group rather than for personal gain and recognition (Matsuda, 1989).

Language. Hundreds of distinct languages and their many dialects are spoken in East Asia, Southeast Asia, and the Pacific Islands. Since so many languages are represented, only a few are selected for discussion—Chinese, Korean, and Japanese.

Phonology. There are several major differences between the sound systems of *Chinese* and English. For example, Chinese words are composed of single syllables, making the rules for English syllabification and stress extremely difficult to master as a second language. As a result, speech may sound telegraphic and choppy. Further, few words have final consonants. Therefore, Chinese speakers often omit final consonants. Moreover, there are no consonant blends in most Chinese languages, making it difficult to master consonant clusters common to English.

The sound systems of *Korean* and English are quite different. In Korean, there are no consonant clusters in the initial and final positions of words, affricates do not occur in the final positions of words, and several distinctive feature classes do not occur, making sound substitutions necessary (e.g., [b/v], [p/v], [s/ʃ], [s/z], and interchangeable use of [l] and [r]).

Japanese has 5 vowels plus 18 consonants. Only the [n] consonant occurs in the final position. Double consonants such as [kk] and [pp] may occur. Difficulties noted in Japanese people learning English include adding vowels to word endings (e.g., [mɪlku]/milk) and the following consonant substitutions: [r/l], [s/z], [j/θ], and [b/v] (Cheng, 1993).

Syntax. *Chinese* grammar is noninflectional and does not use plural markers, tense markers, copulas, the verb *to have*, articles, or conjunctions. Pragmatically, Chinese people generally do not interrupt a speaker to ask questions. Therefore, in conversation, Chinese speakers may appear passive or nonparticipatory.

In *Korean,* there is no tonic word stress so that speakers may sound monotonous and have difficulty with interrogative intonation. Korean has no gender agreement, no articles, no verb inflections for tense and number, and no relative pronouns.

In *Japanese,* all verbs appear in the final position of the sentence. Personal pronouns are omitted since they are inferred by context. No distinction is made between singular and plural. For questions, interrogative markers are not needed at the initial part of the sentence because "yes/no" questions are marked at the end (Cheng, 1993).

Attitudes toward Communication Disorders. There are many different Asian/Pacific folk beliefs that relate to communication disorders and other potentially handicapping conditions. Levels of education, background, and personal experience shape individual reactions to folk beliefs.

Depending on geographic region and background, many Asian/Pacific people may view a handicapping condition as the result of wrongdoings of the individual's ancestors. Spiritual or cultural beliefs such as imbalance of inner forces, bad wind, spoiled foods, gods, demons, spirits, or "hot and cold forces" are thought to cause handicaps. Specifically, the Chamarro culture views a handicapped person as a gift from God and believes he or she belongs to everyone. The handicapped person is thus protected and sheltered by the Chamarro family (Cheng, 1989, 1993).

For Asians, illness may be treated with all available methods before consulting a physician. Treatments of disabilities or illness vary and may include options such as surgery, medication, therapy, acupuncture, massage, *cao* (coin rubbing), *bat fio* (pinching), *giac* (placing a very hot cup on the exposed area), steam inhalation, and herbs (Cheng, 1993). People may seek medical or rehabilitative assistance from a western-trained doctor (or specialist), a folk medicine man or woman, a faith healer, or a shaman.

Deaf Cultures

A cultural minority that is frequently ignored is that which characterizes the deaf community. This group of individuals has a unique language and culture that deserves to be recognized by our professions since a very high percentage of its members receive speech-language and audiology services. Since the group is not typically covered in writings that concern minority cultures as they relate to communication disorders, a fair amount of detail is included here.

The comments that follow result from five years of firsthand experience with people who identify with deaf culture. This experience was predominantly professional, educational, and social.

History. In general, deaf people have had to combat a long-standing history of being considered handicapped, and hence inferior, and are therefore intimately acquainted with stereotyping and discrimination. In spite of this historical pattern, attitudes toward the majority culture vary, depending on individual experiences and attitudes promulgated within the personal social spheres.

Demographics. People who identify with deaf culture include hearing and deaf people raised in families or communities having a high concentration of deaf people, deaf people who grow up attending schools for the deaf, and deaf people who become acculturated at a late age as a result of coming into con-tact with members of the deaf culture. Many deaf people seem to be **bi-cultural,** with deaf culture being either the dominant or secondary culture depending on exposure and opportunity. Some deaf people do not affiliate at all with deaf culture, either by choice or by lack of convenience.

Speech-language pathologists encounter people who identify with deaf cul-ture under a number of circumstances: (1) If employed by a school for the deaf, the students and many faculty members are likely to affiliate with deaf culture. (2) If providing services to a hearing or deaf child who has one or more deaf parents or deaf siblings, both the child and family members identify with the deaf culture to varying degrees. (3) Likewise, a number of deaf children and adults seek speech-language services in order to facilitate spoken com-munication.

Cultural and Social Aspects.

Third-Party Communication.   One aspect of deaf culture that is often mis-understood is the use of either a third party or a machine for the purpose of communication. Interpreters for deaf people, relay services, and telecom-munication devices for the deaf (TDDs) are commonplace among the deaf, and unfamiliar to those who have little exposure to deaf culture.

The use of *interpreters for the deaf* is particularly important to understand because interpreters are necessary to facilitate meaningful communication between deaf and hearing people if a common language is not shared. If using an interpreter, it is critical to understand that the interpreter is bound by a code of ethics which limits the exact nature of the services that the inter-preter is allowed to perform during the conversation. The sole function of the interpreter is to represent what you say to the client and what the client says to you, and to do *no more* than that. This means that if you make a mis-take in what you say, if you talk too fast for the interpreter to keep up, if your message is unclear, or if the client becomes confused, it is not the interpreter's role to inform you that a communication problem has occurred. It is your re-sponsibility to recognize signs of communication breakdown, just as if the in-terpreter were not present. In addition, it is not the interpreter's purpose to help the student with homework or to do tutoring.

Further, it is important to recognize that when using an interpreter some of what is said may be lost or not communicated as intended. Although the interpreter makes every effort to faithfully represent each person's words, it is not always possible for the interpreter to recognize or communicate the sub-tleties that convey the intent behind the spoken or signed words. In addition, communication takes place very quickly and translation is a complicated process; therefore direct translation is not always possible. Understandably, interpreters can fall behind or may find it necessary to summarize parts in order to keep up.

Telecommunication devices for the deaf are called TDDs and TTYs (short for teletypewriter) in the vernacular. They are electronic devices that are attached to a telephone, and they permit orthographic communication between two parties whose phones are *both* plugged into a TDD, independently. The keyboard of the device appears very much like a small typewriter with a liquid-crystal display showing the message as it is typed in. Printouts of the message are possible on some TDD models.

Users of TDDs develop fluency in an orthographic code that is basically incomprehensible to those not familiar with it. For example, when terminating a conversation, one types in *"SK"* to indicate that the conversation is over. If the other party agrees, then that person confirms by typing in *"SKSK."*

Communication relay systems are also important to understand, as they are consequential to the deaf community when communicating by phone to hearing people who do not have access to TDDs. Therefore, if you are contacting or being contacted by a deaf person (e.g., for making or cancelling appointments), you may use an unofficial or official relay system. In some cities, official relays are available and they can be called at various times of day or night to relay messages. In areas that do not have this support service, some deaf people set up their own unofficial relay systems with friends or relatives.

Access to News and Events. Because of difficulties with reading and writing and because of limited support services in most areas, many deaf people are unaware of significant news and events. For example, one deaf college student came from a city that had been affected by a newsworthy tragedy in which several lives were lost. Some months after the accident, upon returning from a visit home, he appeared to be very depressed. When questioned about this change in demeanor, he reported that when he was in his hometown on Spring break he learned that the father of his best friend had lost his life. When he mentioned his friend's name, it was recognized immediately as the surname of a person who had been killed in the tragedy that had been a top story in the national news several months prior. Because of lack of access to the news, the student had not even heard about the event until he went home and contacted his friend.

Newspapers that carry information about important events are written in complex language that may be difficult to follow unless reading skill is high. Although many news broadcasts are available with closed captioning, the comprehension of the captions is directly related to one's reading level, and closed captions are about as easy to follow as newspapers. Some areas of the country have simultaneous signed interpretation for news broadcasts, and this method is effective for deaf people who are fluent signers.

Family Structure. Deaf children grow up in families that represent a cross section of all of the diversity that characterizes the nation. However, a few circumstances sometimes occur as a direct result of having a deaf child in the family and these circumstances result in patterns common to deaf culture.

For some individuals, language competence for spoken communication may or may not develop. In these cases, if the parents do not sign and if the child's spoken skills are seriously compromised, communication within the family presents a serious problem.

It is very common for deaf children to grow up in schools for the deaf, which is a situation that changes family structure and influences the role the family plays in the child's upbringing. When a child lives away from home Monday through Friday for the entire school year, much of the parental-type nurturing is done by people who are not related to the child and do not have the same affection as does a parent. Further, the values that the child comes to embrace are sometimes remarkably different from the values of the family. Children are exposed to the values of their teachers and peers much more intensely than they are exposed to the values of their parents. Further, when a child is away for so much time, it takes a tremendous effort on the part of all family members to develop the closeness that sometimes comes naturally to families who are united throughout the year.

Also related to family life is the tendency for some parents to view their child as "disabled" and as a result to be protective or indulgent, mediating for a child for an unnecessarily long time after same-age peers are learning to survive independently. If this pattern continues for a number of years, it can lead to expectations about the world that are inaccurate, as well as disappointment and failure.

Relationship to Mainstream Culture. Regarding the relationship that deaf people share with the majority culture, many are members of it or intimately associated with it. However, the communication barrier often remains whenever deaf individuals interact with hearing people who are not familiar with deafness and deaf culture. Despite the awkwardness of the circumstance, in general it has been noted that most deaf people seem to appreciate efforts that hearing people make to learn standard systems of manual communication and are willing to patiently labor through sincere efforts to meet communication needs at least halfway.

Therefore, anyone who expects to interact with deaf people with regularity is advised to become familiar with American Sign Language (ASL) signs. Further, even if you are not planning to work with deaf individuals on a regular basis, be aware that you will find the need to communicate manually on some occasions. Therefore make the effort to learn at least the manual alphabet and basic signs necessary for communication survival.

Language. The native language of those who identify with deaf culture is American Sign Language, which was briefly described in Chapter 4. ASL is learned through context-embedded exposure to it during social interchange, just as is every other language (as described in Chapter 1). Consequently, being deaf does not automatically result in the opportunity to learn ASL. Many deaf people do not sign at all. Others have varying degrees of proficiency with ASL and English, depending on background and opportunity.

Many of the features of spoken language are not readily accessible to deaf people because of sensory input limitations. In order for a deaf person to acquire spoken language, intensive training is required. Few with severe or profound reduction in hearing acquire nativelike skill in spoken language, even with extensive training.

Spoken-Language Comprehension. Expectations regarding language comprehension are critical for communication with deaf people. Individual levels of skill vary proportionately to the degree of hearing reduction, exposure to spoken language, and history of effective training in spoken language. In most cases spoken-language comprehension is compromised.

Further, feedback indicating whether spoken communication is understood is often inaccurate for a number of reasons: (1) The person may believe that the communication is understood when in fact it is not. (2) The deaf person may use an ASL sign to indicate that if you continue to talk, comprehension may come. However, to someone not familiar with ASL, the gesture appears to be a green light to continue talking and the assumption is made that comprehension is occurring. (3) The deaf person may not want to indicate that the communication is not understood because of fear of being judged as lacking intelligence. This may be taken to the extreme of even overtly pretending to understand, when in fact the person does not.

Regardless of the reasons for these types of miscommunications, it is your responsibility to become sensitive to the very subtle cues that indicate that communication has begun to break down. For important communications, it is best to verify comprehension by asking the person to repeat the gist of the message (through whatever mode is useful), and also by presenting the same information through two or more modes.

Written Communication. Never assume that a deaf person understands written communication better than spoken communication. Usually, the person's knowledge of spoken English is similar to the same person's knowledge of English in its written form. Unless you are certain that the person's reading and writing skills are advanced, whenever verifying information in writing it is appropriate to keep the message simple and limit the writing to key words. Unless a person has had extensive opportunity to learn written language, long complicated notes are useless. They do not facilitate meaningful communication and they can serve to further complicate a misunderstanding.

Figurative Language. When you want your message to be understood, use literal, and *not* figurative, language. The comprehension of proverbs, metaphors, slang, and symbolic language comes with experience with the language; thus, the deaf individual whose facility with spoken language is compromised may become confused by abstract spoken expressions. Literal interpretation is always a possibility, so in some cases figurative language can cause a serious misunderstanding.

That is *not* to say that deaf people are incapable of comprehending and using figurative language. ASL is rife with figurative symbols, and they are used quite eloquently by individuals who are proficient in the language. For example, the ASL sign that one might use to instruct someone else to stop talking is a sign that, if taken literally, would mean to cut off the tongue with scissors.

In addition to figurative language, spoken humor may not be appreciated by a deaf person who is marginally familiar with spoken language. However, this is not a reflection of an overall inability to accept or deal with humor. Humor is a significant part of the deaf culture and ASL lends itself quite well to the use of humor.

Pragmatics.   *Eye contact* is very important to deaf communicators. However, it may not be the eye contact that is expected if one's primary experience is with hearing people. The eye contact that is important to deaf people, for the purpose of communication, may focus on the general personal space of the communication partner, with less visual attention being paid to the eyes and more attention being paid to the mouth and hands.

Similar to eye contact, *speaker-listener distance* may be influenced by acclimation to deaf culture. This is because when signing, people use all their personal space in order to perform the signs. In conversation, it is not expedient for distance between speakers to interfere with this personal signing space. Further, in order to appreciate the full effect of the communication event, one must stand back and take in the whole view.

Speech Intelligibility.   Partially intelligible and unintelligible speech are also common among the deaf. Therefore, what we do to try to understand an unclear message is important. Asking for a repetition is sometimes an appropriate action since most deaf adults are able to effectively repair unclear utterances. Requesting a written note is also appropriate; however, if skills in written language are affected, the note may be difficult to decipher. Another method of attempting to clarify a misunderstanding is to identify exactly what you do understand about the utterance and then ask key questions in order to fill in the gaps. This technique is useful when communicating with most people whose language is partially comprehensible, whether deaf or hearing.

Further, it is your responsibility to recognize when you have not understood the communication offered by a deaf person and to clearly communicate that fact, even specifically requesting clarification. The deaf person may not repair a misunderstanding unless you directly ask for a repair. Do not assume that a subtle signal or a puzzled look will result in an automatic attempt to clarify information.

Factors Influencing Language Dominance and Proficiency.   Language dominance and language proficiency in deaf people are influenced by a number of variables. Generally, the linguistic choices include spoken and manual communication systems and combinations thereof.

Competence in spoken language is possible. Extensive training is required, since deaf language learners have limited access to the audible characteristics of spoken language. Competence in manual communication is also possible. ASL, PSE, and other manual systems (described in Chapter 4) are available to many deaf language learners if they are exposed to the deaf cultural community and to instruction in the use of manual systems for communication.

In some cases, it appears that language competence does not develop adequately in either spoken or manual communication modes. When this happens, it is likely to be due to a lack of adequate exposure to spoken or manual systems. Under these circumstances, the consequences for cognitive development are grave.

Attitudes toward Communication Disorders.   Perhaps in an attempt to counter negative experiences that apparently result from stereotypes, many deaf people are resolved to demonstrate that deafness is *not* a handicap and that deaf people are capable of performing any task, given appropriate resources. Whether this is the attitude of most deaf individuals remains to be confirmed. However, the position has been stated publicly on many occasions.

OVERREPRESENTATION OF MINORITIES IN SPECIAL EDUCATION

As a result of current referral, identification, and assessment practices, many minority-culture children are overrepresented in special education, particularly in the language-related disciplines such as learning disabilities and communication disorders. These include children who identify with racial and ethnic minority groups, children who are linguistically different, and children of low socioeconomic background (Ambert & Melendez, 1985; Garcia, 1984; Mercer, 1972; Ortiz & Yates, 1983; Rueda, 1989; Shepard et al., 1981; Tucker, 1980). In a similar vein, children who speak languages other than English in the home are sometimes classified as having communication disorders, even if they are not truly handicapped (Shepard et al., 1981).

Apparently, many children with dialectal differences are often placed in articulation intervention, even if their speech-sound production patterns are consistent with the phonological rules of the community dialect. (For example, some Hispanic children may say "[ʃɛɚ]" for *chair* or "[bot]" for *vote;* and some African-American children may say "[bof]" for *both.*) Further, many children with linguistic differences are placed in language intervention, even through they use language that reflects opportunity and experience, or language that is appropriate for second-language learners.

Neglecting to consider levels of language competency (as described later in this chapter) is at the core of the problems related to referring children for special services unnecessarily. In addition, some likely reasons for overreferring children with language differences include stereotypes and misconceptions about racial and ethnic minorities, a scarcity of properly educated bilingual and minority-language professionals, and inappropriate clinical procedures. Each of these reasons is described in the sections that follow.

Stereotypes and Misconceptions

Stereotype is defined in a prior section as an oversimplified, often negative concept about members of a particular group (Garcia, 1982). Such concepts are potentially able to influence whether a child is referred for communication assessment and whether the assessment results in a recommendation for intervention.

Classroom Manifestations of Stereotyping.   Indications of stereotyping that are manifest in the classroom are important to understand because speech-language pathologists receive many of their referrals from classroom teachers who are often the first to notice that language skills do not adequately serve a particular child for academic success. Unfortunately, many educators carry stereotypical ideas about minority-language children that can result in both overreferral and underreferral (Hamayan & Damico, 1991). Further, these attitudes can result in low expectations for student performance and thus influence the way in which children are treated in the classroom (Brophy & Good, 1974; Eder, 1981; Good, 1986). Low teacher expectations are manifested by the identified instructional patterns that are listed in Figure 6–1.

In summary, our expectations affect the way we behave in situations and the way we behave affects how other people respond. Teachers expect specific behavior and achievement from particular students. Because of these expectations, some teachers behave differently toward different students. This teacher treatment communicates to each student what is expected. Imbalanced treatment influences self-concept, achievement, motivation, and level of aspiration. If stereotypical treatment is consistent over time, and if a student does not actively resist or change it in some way, it tends to shape achievement and behavior. With time, the student's achievement and behavior conforms more and more closely to that which is expected. Therefore, high-expectation students are led to achieve at high levels, while low-expectation students achieve at slower rates. In essence, a self-fulfilling prophecy occurs in that teachers have within their command to communicate expectations to children, shaping individual behavior toward expected patterns (Brophy & Good, 1974).

Effect of Stereotype and Misconception on Referral.   Studies carried out in the United States, Canada, and Britain show that many educators tend to have negative, stereotypical expectations of minority students. For exam-

(1) In general, teachers tend to wait less time for low-expectation students to answer questions.

(2) Teachers often give up on low-expectation students when they fail to answer questions correctly. Giving them the answer or calling on someone else are common but inappropriate teacher responses to student-response latency.

(3) Some teachers may inadvertently reward inappropriate behavior of low-expectation students. This is done by praising marginal or wrong answers and poor work. When students become aware of this pattern, it tends to discourage efforts.

(4) Low-expectation students are apparently criticized more than high-expectation students in parallel situations. Further, many teachers criticize misconduct while neglecting to give constructive feedback regarding poor academic work.

(5) Low-expectation students often do not receive praise in situations where other students are typically praised. Many teachers tend to fail to notice and praise hard work and improved performance that results from persistent effort.

(6) Teachers often fail to give low-expectation students meaningful feedback. Feedback that is given is frequently nonspecific or not particularly useful.

(7) Many teachers are inclined to call on low-expectation students less often.

(8) Some teachers tend to pay less attention to low-expectation students unless they are misbehaving. By doing this, they miss opportunities to reinforce good work. Further, many teachers fail to monitor what low-expectation students do and neglect to provide regular and timely feedback.

(9) Low-expectation students are sometimes segregated in seating patterns.

(10) Teachers generally expect and demand less of low-expectation students.(11) Some teachers allow other students to call out answers if the original respondent hesitates. This enables the more motivated students to take advantage of most of the public response opportunities. Further, it may demoralize less aggressive students who are trying to respond and/or reinforce slower students who are trying to avoid responding (Brophy & Good, 1974).

Figure 6-1. Manifestations of low teacher expectations, adapted from Brophy and Good (1974).

ple, kindergarten teachers in Toronto were asked to identify students whom they felt were likely to fail academically and those whom they felt would be highly successful. In the study, minority-language students were judged as about half as likely to succeed academically and about twice as likely to fail (Fram & Crawford, 1972).

A large number of studies have shown that many educators tend to use more positive interactions with students whom they perceive as high achievers as opposed to low achievers (Good & Brophy, 1971). In view of the fact that minority students are frequently and stereotypically perceived as low achievers, it is not surprising that they are also reported to experience less positive interactions with their teachers (Cummins, 1984).

As a result of preconceived ideas and resulting teacher interactive styles, the risk of inappropriate referral to speech-language and other special-education services is clearly inflated in the case of minority children from low socioeconomic status backgrounds. Children are referred even in the absence of cognitive, sensory input, motor skill, or social deficits that justify such a referral.

Effects of Stereotype and Misconception on Identification and Assessment.   Once referred, negative attitudes and low expectations can further affect performance and serve to perpetuate the stereotype. In assessment, all aspects of test selection, administration, scoring, and interpretation are potentially influenced by stereotyping. Results of traditional early identification measures often reinforce stereotypical expectations. This is *not* because the stereotypes are valid, but because few of the available standardized tools for identifying communication problems are appropriate for minority children (Fram & Crawford, 1972). The outcome is that either (1) erroneous screening and assessment results are regarded as valid, and thus intact children are identified as having potential problems (i.e., overreferral), or (2) problems identified through testing are viewed as a function of language and cultural barriers and as a result no intervention is recommended for children who would benefit from it (i.e., underreferral) (Cummins, 1984).

Common Misconceptions about Second-Language Learning.   Professionals and other school personnel (e.g., teachers, principals, diagnosticians) who work with minority-language children may not have an understanding of the process of second-language learning. This includes speech-language pathologists who are responsible for the diagnosis and treatment of language disorders in the population of minority-language children.

Research demonstrates that misconceptions are prevalent among speech-language pathologists in school settings. For example, in one study 20 masters-level speech-language pathologists were interviewed. All were employed by a school system in a community where 56 percent of the population was represented by Mexican-Americans and therefore each provided services to a high concentration of children who were learning English as a second language. In general, the following misconceptions were identified. Many clinicians *wrongly* assumed (1) that in order to be considered bilingual, the child would be required to speak Spanish and English with equal ability and with ability similar to that of monolingual English- or Spanish-speaking children; (2) that the optimum time for learning two languages is before the age of three years; (3) that the preferred method for learning a second language is for one person to speak language A while the other person speaks language B; and (4) that code switching is an indication of inadequate vocabulary and word-finding problems (Kayser, 1990).

These inaccurate beliefs reflect an incomplete knowledge of how children become bilingual, when children experience initial exposure to a second language, and how bilingual people use two languages socially when communicating with one another. Individuals who hold misconceptions are likely to misunderstand language-proficiency expectations among people who use two languages. **Misdiagnosis** and improper intervention are both likely results if misconceptions are not countered by adequate preparation for the task of serving bilingual and minority-language children (Kayser, 1990).

Lack of Properly Educated Bilingual and Minority-Language Professionals

A serious shortage exists in the number of professionals qualified to serve individuals who identify with ethnic and racial minority communities. Therefore many children who identify with ethnic or racial minority groups and receive speech-language services are assessed by people who are either unfamiliar with the minority language, unfamiliar with appropriate assessment procedures for that language and culture, or inadequately prepared to meet the needs of ethnic and racial minority children (Garcia, 1984).

In 1985, 91 percent of the certified speech-language pathologists who were surveyed reported that they had received no training pertinent to minority-language populations during their preprofessional and graduate level education (Campbell, 1985). In an informal review of 1986 applicants for the Certificate of Clinical Competence, only 8 percent of the newly graduated professionals had elected to take a course related to multicultural communication (Flint-Shaw et al., 1987).

Further, minorities represent only 4 percent of the certified speech-language pathologists and audiologists nationwide (Cole, 1987); and only 1% of ASHA's membership is proficient enough in any foreign language to provide clinical services to foreign-language speakers (American Speech-Language-Hearing Association, 1985). However, more than 25 percent of the population identifies with a racial/ethnic/cultural minority group (Taylor, 1993), and a healthy proportion of that 25 percent is likely to have a dominant language other than English.

It follows, then, that only about 4 percent of the professionals (at the maximum) are likely to be competent to serve at least 25 percent of the population needing speech-language services. Under these circumstances, there are two possibilities for service delivery to minority-language clients. (1) It is possible that minority professionals carry disproportionately large caseloads when compared to their colleagues. (2) In addition, it is probable that minority-language clients go without competent and appropriate services. That is, either speech-language pathologists who are not qualified in minority-language service delivery assess and treat the clients regardless of qualifications, or people who need intervention go without services at all.

Whether this pattern will change in the near future is uncertain, as minority students represent only about 9.6 percent of all students enrolled in speech-language pathology and audiology programs nationwide (Council of Graduate Programs, 1986), a proportion that still falls seriously short of the 25 percent representation of those needing services in the general population—and the 25 percent is continually increasing. Therefore, either a disproportionately large burden continues to rest on the shoulders of minority and bilingual speech-language pathologists, or many of the clients who identify with racial and ethnic minorities will continue to be served by people who are not prepared to meet their needs.

A third alternative exists: it is for members of ASHA and students of speech-language pathology, who are presently not culturally literate, to take advantage of continuing education opportunities and thereby *prepare to become involved* with the process of providing competent services to minority-language clients. (Some opportunities for professionals who lack specific competence in minority languages are described later in this chapter.)

Problems Caused by Inadequate Preparation.

Lack of Consideration Given to English Proficiency. Regarding bilingual individuals, there are three categories describing English proficiency as it relates to the identification of disorders—bilingual-English proficient, limited-English proficient, and those with limited proficiency in both languages. Understanding the differences between these categories is critical to diagnosis, valid intervention, and to the assignment of a qualified speech-language pathologist for intervention. Qualifications for working with each group are discussed in a later section ("Competency and Familiarity with Minority Language").

Lack of Consideration Given to the Levels of Language Competency. Four levels of language competency have been identified (Cummins, 1982). (See Figure 6–2, p. 311.) Their characteristics and how to apply them are described in detail in the section on considering language competency in second-language learners. The crux of the issue is that higher levels of language proficiency are considerably relevant for cognitive development and academic progress. It appears that these are the aspects that are often neglected in identification, assessment, and intervention. Further, it is the surface manifestations of linguistic proficiency that are frequently the focus of many clinical activities, yet surface skills do not necessarily prepare one for academic success. Failure to appreciate the differences between basic interpersonal communication and the higher-level cognitive-academic language results in a failure to assess and treat all levels of language proficiency—a practice that has unfortunate consequences for many minority-language students.

One unfavorable consequence is the identification of **pseudo-deficits.** That is, children whose exposure to the English language is compromised may not develop academic language proficiency equal to their peers (Fradd & Correa, 1989), and so when classroom performance is examined, they may take on the appearance of being language disordered, learning disabled, or intellectually deficient (Levin, 1985; Waggoner, 1984a, 1984b). As a result, pseudo-deficits (as opposed to true deficits) in language are identified. The pseudo-deficits are in fact *not* language disorders but evidence of gaps in the mastery of English (Ambert, 1986).

Another undesirable consequence of neglecting to consider levels of language competency is that children are often placed in the wrong treatment setting or classroom. That is, if the whole paradigm is not taken under advisement when determining language dominance, only the lower-level skills (i.e., familiar language with contextual cues) are commonly considered. If competence at the lower (i.e., basic interpersonal) level is confirmed, then the child may be placed in a learning situation (e.g., classroom or therapy environment) where higher skills (i.e., unfamiliar language and reduced contextual cues) are required for successful participation. As a result, the improperly placed child may appear to have academic difficulties that have no true relation to academic deficiency and the misplacement may have been avoided by properly considering all levels of language competency when making decisions about language dominance and classroom placement.

Inappropriate Clinical Procedures Commonly Used with Minority-Language Children

Inappropriate clinical procedures are identified as having been frequently employed when serving minority-language children. Some are described here so that you may recognize and avoid them.

Inappropriate Identification and Referral Procedures.

Referral Checklists. When referring children for special-education assessment (including speech-language referrals), educators may use checklists such as the one that appears in Table 6–1. The checklists are meant to draw teacher attention to behaviors commonly associated with learning problems and educational handicaps. If a child exhibits the behaviors on the checklist, some teachers refer children for special-education assessment. Unfortunately, close inspection of these types of checklists reveals a number of behavioral similarities between children who are rightfully referred for special-education assessment and minority-language children who do not need special services (Maldonado-Colon, 1985). It is common for behavior problem checklists that are designed to assist teachers in identifying educational problems (Table 6–

1) to include many characteristics of second-language learning and minority-language status. This results in confusion about what distinguishes language differences from language disorders and learning disabilities. This confusion results in overreferral for some minority-language children (Maldonado-Colon, 1985).

The confusion probably occurs because use of English for communication is typically reduced and perhaps compromised. As a result, culturally naive speech-language pathologists and educators may stereotypically (and inaccurately) view minority-language students as exhibiting speech and/or language disorders (Kretschmer, 1991). Learning style is another area that often diverges from teacher expectations and thus causes minority-language children to appear different (Trueba, 1987). (See column 5 of Table 6–1.) Inappropriate referrals and misdiagnoses are often the outcome when minority-language children are paired with educators who arbitrarily focus on language performance and learning style.

Academic Performance. Minority-language students may exhibit academic difficulties such as difficulty comprehending concepts that are presented in an unfamiliar language. These may lead to other academic problems in all areas including reading and writing. The result is that the child appears to be handicapped when in fact no true handicapping condition is present. These difficulties are often the result of lack of previous formal education, pedagogical orientation of the students' bilingual education program, or the extent and nature of the family's involvement and attitude toward education (Kretschmer, 1991).

Children are then referred for assessment on the basis of behaviors that do not fit the expectations of educators. As a result of erroneous referrals and inappropriately conducted assessment, it is often recommended that intervention ensue, not because special services are required, but because linguistic, cultural, economic, and other background characteristics are falsely interpreted as deviant. Speech-language pathologists and educators must be made aware that some behaviors, which although they do not conform to expectations of some cultural groups, are normal given an individual's cultural reference, social group, or prior experience. Such behaviors are better characterized as differences rather than deficits or handicaps (Ortiz & Maldonado-Colon, 1986).

As with the checklists, academic behaviors that are directly or indirectly related to linguistic proficiency constitute the most frequent reason for referral of minority-language children (Garcia, 1984; Maldonado-Colon, 1984; Ortiz & Yates, 1983). Research documents that many of the behaviors considered problematic by teachers are, in reality, characteristic of students who are in the process of normal second-language acquisition.

When children are referred for assessment based on environmental factors (e.g., teacher style, curriculum, or classroom organization) rather than on their own personal disability or need, this misclassification affects the over-

Table 6-1.   Learning Problem Checklist

The following checklist has been used to help educators identify children who may be experiencing learning problems. Note that many behaviors also typically characterize second-language learners (adapted from Ortiz and Maldonado-Colon [1986]).

Attention/ Order	Personal/ Emotional	Inter-personal/ Social	Adult Relations/ Authority	School Adaptation	Language
°short attention span	sad/ unhappy	few friends	talks back to adults	disrupts other students	speaks ex-cessively
°dis-tractible	°nervous/ anxious	verbally aggressive	intimidated by author-ity	speaks out of turn	°speaks in-frequently
talks excessively	°shy/timid	°°denies responsi-bility for actions	overly anxious to please	°°does not complete assign-ments	°uses gestures
°day-dreams	short tempered	instigates mis-behavior in others	°°passively uncoopera-tive	°°cannot work inde-pendently	°speaks in single words or phrases
unable to wait turn	°poor self-confidence	°°easily influenced	distrustful of adults	copies other's work	°refuses to answer questions
loud & noisy	extreme mood changes	bossy	refuses to accept limits	°°exerts little effort	°does not volunteer informa-tion
constant need for stimulation	cries easily	°°demands attention	°°defiant	°°lacks interest/ apathetic	°com-ments inappro-priately
hyperactive	unusual manner-isms or habits	inconsider-ate	ambivalent toward adults	frequently tardy or absent	°poor recall
°demands immediate gratifica-tion	°fearful	selfish	uses pro-fanity	°°gives up easily	°poor compre-hension
°disorga-nized	easily ex-citable	lies	°°clings to adults	°°cannot manage time	°poor vocabulary
°unable to stay on task	inappropri-ate emo-tional responses	steals	°overly dependent	°°lacks drive	°difficulty sequencing ideas
°appears confused	immature	jealous	°°seeks constant praise	°°disorga-nized	°difficulty sequencing events
	toileting problems	can't keep hands to self	rebellious	°°cannot plan	°unable to tell or re-tell stories
	°difficulty adjusting to new sit-uations	manipu-lates others	°°needs teacher direction and feed-back	°°unable to tolerate change	
	cruel	suspicious			
	uncoopera-tive	°cannot handle criticism			
	loses control	°°avoids competi-tion			
	overreacts	prefers to be alone			

(continues)

Table 6-1 (continued). Learning Problem Checklist

Attention/ Order	Personal/ Emotional	Inter- personal/ Social	Adult Relations/ Authority	School Adaptation	Language
		physically aggressive		°°sporadic academic perfor- mance	°confuses similar sounding words
				makes excuses	°poor pro- nunciation
				destructive	°poor syntax
				°°does not initiate	
				needs re- minding	

°Normal behaviors that often characterize culturally linguistically diverse children, resulting in inappropriate referrals.

°°Behavioral characteristics of culturally linguistically diverse children that are also frequently associated with learning disabilities.

all expectations and educational opportunities provided to these individuals. The end result is that students are made to feel marginal in their ability to succeed and they begin to act accordingly (Sinclair & Ghory, 1987). In turn, the pattern can result in reduced academic performance, social difficulties, and affective problems. The student *becomes* disabled, but the etiology is not related to some exceptionality inherent in the student. Instead, it is caused by the diagnosis or by some other factor external to the student (Cummins, 1986).

Inappropriate Assessment Procedures.   Some commonly used assessment patterns that are inappropriate for minority-language children have been identified. Misdiagnosis and overreferral are often the outcome of these practices. They are discussed here so that you may avoid using unsuitable techniques that may cause you to mistake minority-language children for children who indeed are in need of speech-language services.

Reliance on Traditional Test Batteries.   Although minority-language students can best be assessed by using a nontraditional informal approach to testing (discussed later in this chapter), many evaluators continue to rely solely on traditional test batteries (Westby, in press). While traditional assessment tools exist (e.g., standardized, commercially developed tests), their use with minority-language students has serious drawbacks. Lack of facility with standard English impedes performance for many children, making it difficult to obtain an accurate assessment of linguistic skills. Moreover, because standardized tests measure only select aspects of language, they do not reflect the students' overall proficiency and comprehension (Ochs & Schiefflin, 1979).

Contrived Assessments. Traditionally, language skills are assessed within isolated settings that specifically focus on distinct components of the linguistic system (Bates, 1976; Dore, 1975; Halliday & Hasan, 1976; Liles, 1987; Ochs & Schiefflin, 1979). Children are expected to demonstrate their abilities in artificial situations where language is isolated from meaningful context (e.g., picture pointing tasks, fill in the blanks). This method provides a way to scrutinize very specific language skills (Culatta, Page, & Ellis, 1983; Spinelli & Ripich, 1985). However, it is not always useful when assessing the language-learning needs of minority children and children with limited English proficiency, as contrived assessment situations reduce the probability of accessing and analyzing representative language (Spinelli & Ripich, 1985).

Inappropriate Intervention Procedures. Problems with the intervention that is applied in the case of minority-language children seem to result from the fact that most speech-language pathologists are not adequately prepared to address the needs of this population (due to inadequate knowledge about multicultural issues or lack of proficiency in the minority language). The lack of properly prepared professionals was discussed earlier in this chapter. In summary, the problem is that the number of bilingual and minority-language clinicians is disproportionately low (4 percent) when compared to the number of minority-language children who receive speech-language services (more than 25 percent).

The result is that (1) many inadequately prepared clinicians are not aware that some of the children on the caseload are not in need of services and (2) they then pursue intervention objectives that are not appropriate for meeting the language-learning needs of minority-language children. These include objectives that focus on linguistic differences, teaching English as a second language, and lower-level skills (e.g., drill activities with phonics as opposed to higher-level problem-solving activities). Further, intervention is often conducted in the native language of the clinician, regardless of whether it is the dominant language of the client.

PROVIDING EFFECTIVE CLINICAL SERVICES TO INDIVIDUALS WHO IDENTIFY WITH DIVERSE CULTURAL GROUPS

Whenever possible, it is expected that those who provide speech-language services to individuals of minority-culture background possess the qualifications and competencies that are necessary to effectively serve the language-learning needs of the individuals being served. For that reason, qualifications and competencies are described.

However, due to a shortage of personnel and a wide variety of cultures residing in certain geographic regions, circumstances exist that do not always allow for every minority-background child to be served by a professional who identifies with or completely understands the child's linguistic and cultural perspective. Therefore, some alternative suggestions are provided for those who encounter clients of minority backgrounds with whom they have inadequate direct prior experience.

Clinical Services Provided by Qualified Professionals

Qualifications of those who serve minority individuals are similar as for those who serve all clients, regardless of minority status. That is, qualified professionals are ASHA-certified (and state-licensed where required), have appropriate academic and clinical preparation for the population being served, possess a working knowledge of language acquisition milestones and processes, and are culturally literate. In addition, under ideal circumstances the clinician is a competent user of the minority language or dialect.

ASHA Certification.   Fundamental to all admonitions regarding service to any client, including minority-language individuals, is the principle that all clinical services are provided by competent professionals. First and foremost, the professional who treats the client is certified by ASHA or adequately supervised according to the association's guidelines.

Academic and Clinical Preparedness.   The ASHA-certified speech-language pathologists who provide clinical services are required to be prepared academically and clinically. Academic preparation includes course work and/or seminars and workshops that address the communication needs of minority-language clients. Clinical preparation includes supervised clinical practice or collaborative practice prior to taking on independent responsibility for addressing client needs.

The requirements of academic and clinical preparation are no different from the requirements that underlie all clinical service delivery. Certainly, no competent professional presumes to diagnose or treat a client without having adequate academic and clinical preparation for the specific presenting disorder (e.g., cleft palate, voice disorders, fluency disorders, or language disorders). By the same token, no competent professional presumes to diagnose or treat a minority-language client without adequate academic and clinical preparation. This is because, unless speech-language pathologists are prepared to understand linguistic differences through academic and clinical experience, assessment procedures often lead to inaccurate diagnoses, mislabeling (Cummins, 1984; Juarez, 1983), and inappropriate intervention.

Knowledge of Language-Acquisition Milestones and Processes. Central to appropriate language assessment for minority-language children is knowledge of language acquisition milestones along with awareness of proficiency levels and cultural differences. General patterns of language acquisition are probably similar across languages and cultures (Brown, 1973; Seymour & Miller-Jones, 1981; Seymour & Seymour, 1977; Slobin, 1985). However, differences may exist in the emergence of specific linguistic features that are unique to a particular group.

For example, first words emerge at about 10 to 12 months of age, and this is true cross-culturally. However, the specific words that are expected may be different for children in different cultures depending on the objects, events, and relations that they experience with frequency and perceive to be important. This occurs because children learn words that are related to topics adults feel children should know.

Cultural Literacy. As communication specialists, it is important for each not only to identify the characteristics of our own native cultures and communication patterns, but to make the effort to become functionally literate with regard to cultures other than the ones with which we personally identify. To become culturally literate, one must come to understand that culture involves much more than characteristics of language and dialect. Culturally literate professionals understand that one's culture permeates every dimension of communication. We must appreciate that each individual who seeks to benefit from our services views the world in a way that can only be completely understood through the eyes of the culture with which that person identifies (Battle, 1993).

Competency and Familiarity with Minority Language. In addition, adequate familiarity with the minority language is required if one is to competently provide speech-language services to minority-language people. The number of bilingual speech-language pathologists who are available to serve the growing number of individuals with a primary language other than English is quite small and constitutes only about 1 percent of the certified members of ASHA (ASHA, 1985). However, a much greater proportion of the population served by ASHA-certified professionals prefers to use a language other than Standard American English.

Individuals who wish to consider themselves bilingual for the purpose of providing services to minority-language clients should compare their skill to ASHA's definition (Cole et al., 1988) before attempting to become involved in the process of providing clinical services to bilingual people and to those with limited English proficiency. (ASHA's definition for bilingual speech-language pathologists and audiologists is in Appendix 6–1.)

ASHA's Committee on the Status of Racial Minorities (ASHA, 1985) has recommended competencies for assessment and remediation of communication disorders of minority-language speakers. They are as follows:

Serving Bilingual English-Proficient Clients.   Clients in this group are bilingual. They have nativelike control of English and may or may not have comparable control of the minority language. Speech-language pathologists who provide services to bilingual English-proficient clients must be able to distinguish between dialectal differences and communication disorders and they must understand the minority language as a rule-governed system. Knowledge of the phonological, grammatical, semantic, and pragmatic features of the minority language is essential. Further, it is necessary to have knowledge of nondiscriminatory intervention procedures ("Social Dialects," 1983). (Suggestions are introduced later in this chapter.) For bilingual English-proficient clients, it is not essential that the speech-language pathologist be proficient in the minority language.

Serving Limited English-Proficient (LEP) Clients.   These are clients who are proficient in their native language which is *not* English and have limited command of English. For this group, assessment is conducted in the native language. In order to be competent to assess limited English-proficient clients, clinicians *must* have native or near-native fluency in both the minority language and in English. Qualified clinicians are able to describe the process of speech and language acquisition for bilingual and monolingual individuals and how those processes are manifested in the oral and written modes. Further, clinicians are able to administer and interpret both standardized and informal assessment procedures and are able to distinguish between communication differences and disorders. Clinicians are also able to utilize intervention techniques to treat minority-language individuals with communication disorders and recognize cultural factors that may affect the speech-language services that are provided to minority-language individuals.

Some parts of the United States have high concentrations of a variety of diverse cultural groups, and therefore, a wide assortment of languages are represented. It is not possible for clinicians to be fluent in every language. Therefore, some suggestions for clinicians are offered in the next section of this chapter ("Alternatives for Professionals Who Are Not Bilingual or Not Adequately Prepared for Minority-Language Children").

Serving Clients Who Are Limited in Both the Minority Language and English.   These individuals possess limited communicative competence in both the minority language and English. For clients in this category, communication should be assessed (objectively and subjectively) in both languages to determine language dominance. (Procedures are explained in the section on assessment that appears later in this chapter.) The results of the bilingual assessment then determine the languages to be used in intervention.

All of the competencies required for assessing limited English proficient clients are also recommended for assessing individuals in this group. (See the previous section.) If intervention is to be provided in the minority language, one adheres to the competencies recommended for providing intervention to limited English-proficient students. If intervention is to be provided in English, proficiency in the minority language may not be necessary.

Alternatives for Professionals Who Are Not Bilingual or Not Adequately Prepared for Minority-Language Children

Regardless of your cultural orientation or background, if you continue to pursue a career in the profession of speech-language pathology, it is inevitable that you will have occasion to provide clinical services to a variety of individuals who are members of cultures other than the one with which you identify. In some cases, you may reside in an area with a large concentration of people who are members of cultures other than your own. In that case, if at all possible, it is your responsibility to become familiar with the cultures and linguistic features that characterize the people of that region since you are likely to be called on fairly often to serve members of that group.

On the other hand, individuals from a variety of unanticipated cultural groups may seek your services and you may have no way of predicting in advance the specific cultural groups so that you may study the characteristics. Further, in some regions so many cultural groups are represented that it would be impossible to become completely familiar with each. Regardless of whether you serve a large or small number of individuals of any particular cultural group, each individual deserves to be served competently and each person deserves to be treated with respect. The following general guidelines and collaboration strategies may be used to facilitate the process, but they are *not* meant to substitute for educating one's self about a number of discrete cultural groups whenever possible.

General Guidelines.

1. In communicating with individuals from cultural groups other than your own, you should learn the name of that culture as assigned by its members—and use it (Battle, 1993). Outdated and/or ethnocentric terms are not appropriate as they have been discarded by the group for a reason. Therefore they are likely to offend.

2. Avoid the use of generic terminology as substitutes for more descriptive racial or ethnic terms (Battle, 1993). For example, it is easier to use a generic term, such as "cultural minority," than it is to learn the name of a cultural group as assigned by its members, but a negative attitude is clearly communicated by such practice.

Further, the generic term that you choose may not be particularly accurate. For example, referring to a child as "multicultural" may not be particularly accurate if the child is predominantly familiar with only one culture.

3. Be aware of words, images, and situations that suggest that all or most members of a racial or ethnic group are the same without taking into account variations within the group (Battle, 1993). Make no assumptions about the

individual person's beliefs, behavioral patterns, and personal status based solely on your knowledge of race, language, or apparent cultural affiliation. Physical appearances and first impressions may be misleading. Further, each cultural group is diverse within itself. Therefore, specific personal characteristics, if they are significant to language assessment or intervention, are best determined on an individual basis.

4. Be aware that some terms have negative racial, ethnic, or socioeconomic connotations. A number of terms imply that European-Americans are the standard by which all other groups should be evaluated (Battle, 1993). Some examples include "culturally disadvantaged" and "minority." Other evaluative terms include reference to "good" and "bad" language or imply that the characteristics of a dialect or language difference are "errors" or "error patterns."

Some individuals may need to learn to overhaul thinking patterns and carefully monitor communication registers so that negative, racist, and ethnocentric thinking patterns can be changed and so that clients can be effectively served. If you are a person who is apt to say that someone is a member of a particular culture *but* has some other positive quality, if you are likely to poke fun at a distinctive group when you are in the company of those who do not identify with that group, or if you occasionally preface comments with "I'm not prejudiced, but," then you probably are at risk to make ethnocentric comments that offend people. Such thinking patterns are difficult but not impossible to overcome.

5. Avoid using expressions that reinforce racial and ethnic stereotypes. These include expressions that employ color-symbolic language (e.g., "black humor," "yellow") and slanglike reference to racial or ethnic groups (e.g., Indian giver) (Battle, 1993).

6. Be aware of the nonverbal sources of miscommunication between people from different cultural groups. These may include acceptability of touching, appropriate speaker-listener distance, suitable topics for conversation, and styles of greeting (Battle, 1993).

7. Be aware of verbal sources of miscommunication between people from different cultural groups. Suitable word selections, topic management styles, and extent of small talk are some examples of verbal behaviors that can result in misunderstanding when people communicate cross culturally (Battle, 1993).

Collaboration Strategies.   It is recognized that not all speech-language pathologists possess the recommended competencies to serve minority-language children. Therefore, some alternative strategies are suggested so that those with limited skill are able to make the most of the available resources, enabling them to enhance their service to minority-language clients. Speech-language pathologists who are not bilingual are encouraged to take each of the following steps whenever appropriate (ASHA, 1985).

1. Establish contacts with ASHA-certified individuals who are bilingual/bicultural. In some settings, the bilingual contacts may be hired as consultants in order to accommodate the needs of minority-language children.

2. Establish a clinical cooperative. By doing so, a district or group of agencies may employ an itinerant speech-language pathologist whose primary role is to serve the needs of minority-language children.

3. Establish networks with professionals who work in a variety of settings. By so doing, the available means are multiplied through interagency sharing of equipment and human resources. Networks are also valuable for the purpose of recruiting individuals who are competent to serve minority-language populations.

4. Establish the agency as a clinical-fellowship site or graduate-practicum site for individuals from programs with adequate training in minority-language service delivery. Graduate students and recent graduates from such programs are a valuable resource when assessing and treating individuals with minority-language dominance.

5. Establish **interdisciplinary teams.** If bilingual speech-language pathologists who are knowledgeable about serving minority-language populations are not available for collaboration, then explore the possibility that such individuals may be available in other professions, such as psychology and special education. If such individuals are available and willing to participate, an interdisciplinary team may be established in order to guide decisions made with regard to minority-language children.

6. Use interpreters and translators. The use of interpreters and translators is appropriate under three circumstances: (a) when the speech-language pathologist does not meet the recommended competencies for serving minority-language children, (b) when an individual who needs services speaks a language that is uncommon to the geographic region, and (c) when there are no trained professionals with proficiency in the minority language who are available to provide services.

Considering Levels of Language Proficiency in Second-Language Learners

The issue of language proficiency is central to the process of identifying and treating minority-language children. It seems that when people learn a second language, competency is achieved at basic levels of communication earlier and perhaps more completely than at more advanced levels. Recognizing these levels is at the core of language assessment and intervention since misunderstandings surrounding these levels often lead to misdiagnosis and ineffective intervention practices.

In the mid-1970s, the distinction between levels of language proficiency was formally identified (Skutnabb-Kangas & Toukomaa, 1976). Apparently, Finnish immigrant children who were either born in Sweden or who immigrated at a relatively young age (e.g., preschool) appeared to converse appropriately and comfortably in everyday, face-to-face situations regardless of whether using Swedish or Finnish. For the same group literacy skills were considerably below age expectations in both languages. As a result of studying this observation, a distinction is recognized between four levels of language proficiency (Cummins, 1984). These levels are best understood by examining the quadrants that appear in Figure 6–2. An expanded explanation of the figure follows.

Language Competency as It Relates to Language Context.   The horizontal continuum (Figure 6–2) relates to the range of contextual support for expressing and comprehending the meaning of language. The extremes of this continuum are described in terms of *context-embedded* versus *context-reduced* communication (Cummins, 1982).

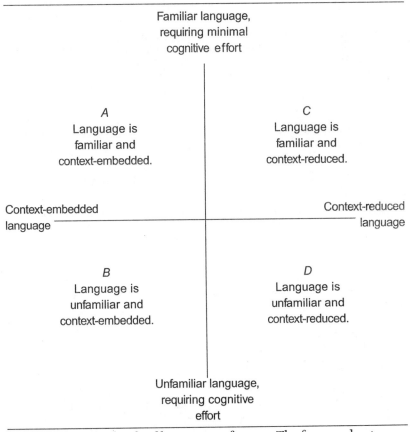

Figure 6-2.   Four levels of language proficiency: The four quadrants are used to describe four levels of language proficiency (adapted from Cummins, [1984]).

In context-embedded communication (left side of the horizontal continuum), language is supported by a wide range of meaningful cues (Cummins, 1982). For example, when baking cookies and talking about the ongoing activity, the words correspond to the events as they occur. That is, events (e.g., stirring, mixing, pouring), objects (e.g., flour, sugar, salt, dough, spoon), and relations (e.g., in, around) are pointed out at about the time that they appear. Since the contextual cues are available to facilitate comprehension and production, context is said to support language. Therefore language, under these circumstances, is considered to be context-embedded. Sample activities presented in Chapter 4 (Figures 4–2 and 4–3) are examples of activities that lend themselves to context-embedded communication.

On the other hand, for context-reduced communication (right side of horizontal continuum), contextual cues are absent and the child is forced to rely on linguistic cues alone (Cummins, 1982). For example, explaining how to make cookies in the absence of supporting materials or demonstration is a task in which the context is seriously reduced. In this case, interpretation and formulation of messages depends heavily on knowledge of the language itself.

The amount of context that is available to facilitate language comprehension and production ranges from situations in which nearly all language is supported by context (e.g., demonstration) to situations in which negligible language is supported by context (e.g., lecture). This range is represented by the horizontal continuum of Figure 6–2.

Language Competency as It Relates to Familiarity with the Language.
The vertical continuum (Figure 6–2) relates to degree of mastery for the type of language that is used in the situation. The upper end of the vertical continuum consists of communicative tasks and activities in which language is largely familiar, and therefore little cognitive energy is required for successful participation (Cummins, 1982). An example of familiar language is memorized rituals such as conventional greetings and closings (e.g., "Hello." "How are you?" "Fine, thank you, and you?") and small talk.

At the lower end of the continuum are tasks and activities in which the communicative tools are not yet familiar, thus major cognitive effort is required (Cummins, 1982). An example of language that is *not* familiar is language whose content is not known, such as an explanation concerning a new concept. Memorized rituals do not meet the requirements of this type of conversational schema.

Four Levels of Language Competency. The two continua intersect, forming a set of four quadrants (Figure 6–2). These quadrants are used to define four levels of language proficiency that are situation dependent (Cummins, 1982). They are described as follows.

Basic Interpersonal Communication Skills (BICS). The upper left quadrant (A) of Figure 6–2 describes a situation in which the context provides ample cues (context-embedded) and the language that is required is familiar. The type of communication required by this situation is called basic interpersonal communication skills (BICS). Competency at the BICS level is superficial.

An example of a BICS situation might be a conversation about an impending storm while standing outside looking at the sky. Perhaps one might point to the thunderclouds and say that it is going to rain so it is not a good day for a picnic (Fradd, 1987). The language is context-embedded because all the objects, events, and relations are clearly visible while being represented linguistically. The language is not cognitively demanding because words, morphological markers, and syntactic relations are all familiar.

Many second-language learners achieve competence at the BICS level after approximately two years of exposure (Cummins, 1982), and this is long before competence at the three higher levels can be expected. This was the case with the Finnish immigrants described previously.

Unfamiliar Language in Context-Embedded Situation.   The lower left quadrant (B) of Figure 6–2 describes a situation where, although adequate contextual cues are available, the language that is required is not familiar (Cummins, 1982). The demand in this situation is to use contextual cues to decipher and produce unfamiliar linguistic concepts.

Tasks in this quadrant require some familiarity with symbols in order to respond correctly. Interaction with another person is not necessary to complete the task and students may be expected to function alone. Activities in Quadrant B are more interpersonal than in Quadrant A, and they usually involve some type of reading and writing in addition to conversation.

Tasks in Quadrant B are those with which the child has had a great deal of prior experience. For example, a child is learning to play a board game specific to a familiar sport and the game requires the child to combine or associate known vocabulary that is related to a well-known sport and apply it to the board game (Fradd, 1987).

Interactive Language Development Teaching (ILDT) (Lee, Koenigs-knecht, & Mulhern, 1973), an intervention technique described in Chapter 4, is another example of a Quadrant B language activity. Recall that for ILDT, a familiar theme is used to facilitate the teaching of unfamiliar linguistic concepts.

Familiar Language in Context-Reduced Situation.   The upper right quadrant (C) of Figure 6–2 describes a situation in which, although the required language is familiar, the language used in the situation is not supported by contextual cues (context-reduced) (Cummins, 1982). This situation places demands that are not required in the conditions of Quadrants A and B. That is, language must be comprehended and produced in the absence of adequate contextual evidence.

The language in Quadrant C is still interpersonal but task demands are cognitively demanding. Other people are usually involved in providing contextual support. An example situation might be using props to solve mathematical word problems while studying with a friend (Fradd, 1987).

Cognitive Academic Language Proficiency (CALPS). The lower right quadrant (D) of Figure 6–2 is the most difficult in that contextual cues are not available and the required language is not yet mastered. Since this circumstance describes the language requirements of many academic classrooms, the communication required is described in terms of cognitive academic language proficiency skills (CALPS), which requires approximately 5 to 7 years to achieve (Cummins, 1982).

CALPS tasks are usually performed alone. As tasks become more context-reduced, they also become more individualized and less interpersonal or interactive. An example is listening to a lecture and then completing a writing exercise based on the lecture. Another example is solving word problems individually (Fradd, 1987).

Comprehensive Language Assessment: Suggested Procedures for Minority-Language Children

For minority-language children, a comprehensive language assessment ideally begins with preassessment and then a determination of language dominance, two procedures that are not typically done with those not having minority status. Further, the ideal assessment protocol for minority-language children requires that the clinician be abreast of a number of alternatives to the available standardized tools. The discussion that follows addresses each of these issues.

Pre-Assessment. The assessment of any student with limited English Proficiency (LEP) or culturally linguistically diverse (CLD) background is preceded by collecting information related to the reason for the referral. The process is called *preassessment* or *prereferral,* and through it the communication disorder is carefully considered in terms of whether referral for assessment is an appropriate step and in terms of whether the child's needs can be aptly met without intervention (Barona & Santos de Barona, 1987). The following five criteria are considered in the pre-assessment process.

Experiential Background of Teacher and Child. When considering whether to refer a child for testing, it is important to determine whether the experiential background of the teacher or student contributes to the perceived problem. For example, an educator who does not have training or experience with diverse cultural backgrounds should consider whether the child's learning problems are teacher induced. Further, the child's academic background (e.g., school attendance, change in school), family background (e.g., mobility, lifestyle), and medical background (e.g., sensory problems, history of illnesses) should be scrutinized to identify any historical variables that may contribute to the communication difficulties.

Culture of Teacher and Child.   The cultural backgrounds of both the teacher and the student must be considered. If the teacher is not familiar with the child's culture or if the child's culture is different from that of the school, then it is possible that cultural variables contribute to the apparent communication problems.

Language Proficiency of Teacher and Child.   In making a referral based on academic performance, one considers whether the teacher and the child share a common language. Further, the child's proficiency in the minority language and English are taken into account.

Teaching Style of Teacher and Learning Style of Child.   Consideration is given to whether the teaching style of the teacher matches the learning style of the student. Learning styles are often influenced by cultural orientation, so teachers may need to adapt their style to match the learning needs of minority-language children.

Perceptions and Expectations of Teacher and Child.   How teachers and students view one another can also influence academic performance. Teachers who carry negative attitudes toward cultural diversity may impede academic success. Further, due to their background, some students view school as unnecessary or irrelevant.

When to Refer for Assessment.   The assessment proceeds only after all possible explanations for the difficulties have been explored and after all questions concerning the adequacy of such efforts have been satisfied. While the assessment process itself involves many areas that require sensitivity and skill, it is equally important that the steps leading up to the referral reflect an awareness of the role that language and cultural diversity may play in the communication problems experienced. In particular, an assessment is conducted only after evidence has been gathered proving that the learning environment is not deficient. This evidence includes confirmation that the educational programs in use are appropriate for the ethnic, linguistic, and socioeconomic groups being served and that these programs have been implemented effectively.

Classification of Disorder for Follow-Up.   As a result of assessment, the child's learning problem is described according to one of three categories that describe the child's problem in terms of how it is to be addressed (Adelman, 1971). The three categories are Learning Problem Type I, Type II, and Type III.

Type I. A Type I Learning Problem is identified if the assessment reveals that the child's problems result primarily from deficiencies in the learning environment. This is not considered to be a disorder, and the problem is addressed by modifying the learning environment so that it accommodates the learning needs of the child. Language intervention is not recommended and, in fact, the process ends with preassessment procedures as described previously (Adelman, 1971). An example of a Type I classification is a minority-language child who is referred for speech-language assessment but is found to have language that is within normal limits when taking cultural and environmental factors into consideration.

Type II. A Type II Learning Problem is considered to be a minor disorder. For this classification, the problem is found to result from a combination of deficiencies, some of which can be attributed to the child and some to the environment. Type II problems are often addressed adequately by making modifications in the learning environment. Although language intervention is not necessarily recommended, the speech-language pathologist may work cooperatively with the academic teacher in order to recommend appropriate modifications to the academic environment (Adelman, 1971). An example of Type II classification is a minority-language child who experiences academic difficulties related to second-language learning, requiring that adaptations be made to the classroom in order to accommodate the child's academic and language-learning needs.

Type III. Type III Learning Problems are identified when the problem is found to result primarily from deficits in the child's performance and potential for language acquisition. Type III problems are clearly considered to be disorders and special placement is required in order to address the needs of the child. Speech-language intervention is recommended if language-learning needs are identified (Adelman, 1971). An example of a Type III classification is a child who language performance is found to be compromised due to cognitive, sensory, motor skill, or social deficits, even when taking cultural and environmental factors into consideration. All of the etiological factors described in Chapter 2 have potential for causing such a deficit.

Determining Language Dominance of Child. As suggested in the section on language differences and disorders, the standard that is used to determine whether a child's speaking pattern is due to a difference or a disorder is the language pattern of the child's own community. Determining the exact nature of the community language may be somewhat complicated, as people who identify with ethnic and racial minorities often experience exposure to the minority language with a range of dialect densities, various codes, Standard American English and variations of it, and code switching (Seymour & Miller-Jones, 1981). Furthermore, some language patterns carry a social stigma or penalty (Irwin, 1977), a circumstance that leads to perceived obligation to conform to Standard American English regardless of which linguistic style is preferred (Shuy, 1971).

Therefore, once the child has been referred, the first step in a comprehensive individualized assessment is to determine language status or language competency for both the language of the home and the language of the classroom (Kayser, 1989; Wilkinson & Ortiz, 1986). This measure is important for children who may have been exposed to two or more spoken languages or dialects, and it is also important for deaf individuals who use spoken and signed languages with varying degrees of proficiency.

The purpose of the language competency assessment is to identify the child's stronger language (language dominance) and to identify level of competency for each language. (Competency levels are discussed in a previous section of this chapter.) This information about language dominance is used to determine the languages to be used in the assessment and the testing instruments to be administered. Information about language dominance is also considered in interpreting test results and in developing recommendations for intervention if appropriate. By carefully identifying the child's stronger language prior to beginning the assessment, we decrease potential for misidentification, assuming that assessment is conducted in the appropriate languages by a competent individual who is properly prepared for the task (Wilkinson & Ortiz, 1986).

All of the procedures described in the following paragraphs are meant to be used in a systematic and quantifiable fashion. Further, none are intended to be used alone. Instead, they are applied in combination in order to comprehensively determine the child's language preference, dominance, and competence in a variety of domains and with a variety of communication partners (Kayser, 1989).

Standardized Instruments. Existing standardized procedures alone are not recommended for determining language dominance (Wilkinson & Ortiz, 1986), as they tend to reduce the examination of the complex phenomena of bilingualism, linguistic preference, and language dominance to a simple survey of lexical and phonological properties of each language. Instead it is recommended that information about the child's language preferences be obtained from language sampling under a variety of circumstances, from observing the child's use of language in group situations and in the classroom, and from questionnaires about the child's language use practices and preferences (Kayser, 1989).

Language Sampling. General procedures for conducting and analyzing a language sample are presented in Chapter 3. However, in the case of children who identify with a minority culture, it is recommended that the sample be elicited in a minimum of three contexts (e.g., home, school, and clinic) and with a minimum of three different conversational partners (e.g., siblings, peers, and clinician) (Kayser, 1986).

Culturally salient materials are selected to elicit the sample and measures are taken to ensure that the child is comfortable enough to produce language that is representative (Seymour & Miller-Jones, 1981). Further, the child's language is compared to the language of other children from the same cultural and ethnic community (Kayser, 1989).

For example, culturally salient materials are materials that are likely to be found in the child's cultural sphere, that represent the culture's people with reasonable accuracy, and that can be applied to familiar traditions and folkways. The child should have access to choose from a variety of toys, books, and materials with which the child can readily identify. Therefore, a selection of picture books showing people from a variety of races and cultures are made available, the dolls and action figures include people with a range of appearances, and objects for discussion include those things that are likely to be found in the child's home and community environments. Further, the child should not be quizzed with regard to any items that are not chosen or items with which the child is not likely to be reasonably familiar.

Language preference is tentatively identified by systematically observing the code selected by the child under a variety of circumstances and by systematically observing the child's responses to both linguistic patterns as they are presented by several communication partners.

Observing and Charting Language Behavior in Classroom. Two methods for observing and charting behavior are recommended when attempting to identify the linguistic behaviors used by children in group interaction. As with language sampling, it is important to pay particular attention to the language of choice and the responses to each linguistic pattern as it is presented. The two methods for accomplishing these are the scan technique and the focal technique, which are described as follows (Kayser, 1989).

When using the *scan technique,* an observer attends to the behaviors of a particular child for a specified period of time that is relatively brief (e.g., 10 minutes), records exactly what the child does and says, with whom the child interacts, and any other notable data regarding that particular child. Then the observer moves on to pay attention to the behavior of a different child in the group, repeating the procedure until all children of interest are observed and adequate data is collected on each (Kayser, 1989).

When using the *focal technique,* the observer concentrates on watching the behaviors of one child in the group over an extended period of time (e.g., 1 hour). The focal technique may be applied over a period of several days in order to gain accurate and complete information about the child's linguistic patterns in the classroom (Kayser, 1989).

Questionnaires. Questionnaires are applied in order to gain information from a number of individuals who interact with the child on a regular basis. Parents and teachers are some examples of people who may be asked to complete a questionnaire or participate in a questionnaire interview. The goal of the questionnaire procedure is to obtain an accurate description of language proficiency and language preference for several domains from the perspectives of a number of people who are well acquainted with the child (Kayser, 1989).

The Assessment Battery.

Testing in Both Languages.   Federal and state policies mandate that the evaluation be conducted in the child's primary language unless it is not feasible to do so (PL 94-142). Whenever assessing children who are possibly bilingual or bidialectal, it is always appropriate to test in *both* languages (Kayser, 1989; Seymour & Miller-Jones, 1981). That is because language disorders affect common underlying language processes (Cummins, 1982, 1984); it is *not possible* for a bilingual child to have a disorder in one language and not the other. Therefore, if a child is to be considered for intervention, assessment criteria must include evidence that the disorder exists in the native language system as well as in standard English (Juarez, 1983). A minority-language child is judged as having a language disorder only if (1) the language behaviors are *not* characteristic of people from the same cultural group who speak the same language or dialect and who have had similar opportunities to hear and use the language, and (2) this is found to be the case for the minority language as well as for English (Mattes & Omark, 1984).

Evaluator with Nativelike Fluency in Both Languages.   Valid non-discriminatory assessment is carried out by an evaluator who has nativelike fluency in *both* languages and is familiar with regional variations of the minority language (Ortiz et al., 1985). In addition, the evaluator has all of the qualifications that are described in an earlier section of this chapter and in Appendix 6–1.

Natural Communication as Opposed to Standardized Tests.   Standardized English tests are not recommended when assessing the communication behaviors of children who identify with minority cultures (Seymour & Miller-Jones, 1981; Taylor & Payne, 1983). This is because test construction, test administration, content, tasks, numbers of minority students used in determining normative data, and inevitable potential for misinterpretation of results are bound to lead to conclusions that do not reflect what the individual child knows about the language (Ambert & Dew, 1982; Kayser, 1989). Instead, assessment of minority-language students is geared toward natural communication, utilizing measures that address all levels of language mastery (Wilkinson & Ortiz, 1986).

A few standardized tests are available for testing children of minority culture. The standardized approach to testing is a western European social-communicative event (Heath, 1984) and therefore may be unfamiliar to many children who identify with cultures other than those derived from or strongly influenced by western Europe. Further, the test items of most standardized tests do not represent the linguistic experiences of many children (Kayser, 1989). For these reasons standardized tests, as they exist, are not recommended for assessment and diagnostic purposes (Seymour & Miller-Jones, 1981). Therefore a number of alternatives are recommended in order to improve the language-assessment practices that are used when testing minority children. Alternatives to standardized instruments are suggested (Kayser, 1989).

Alternatives to Standardized Testing. One alternative to standardized testing is to *systematically modify a standardized procedure.* A test procedure may be modified in order to help elicit the information necessary to accurately determine communication skill within the familiar cultural/ethnic community, while utilizing an existing standardized instrument (Kayser, 1989). Whenever any modification is applied to a standardized procedure, it may influence test validity and reliability, so all modifications must be recorded on the test form and in the assessment report.

Since the validity and reliability of the results may be affected by the modifications and since normative data of most standardized tests does not apply to many members of minority cultures, the scoring and interpreting of test results are done with a great deal of caution and with more regard paid to language-acquisition milestones than to the client's standing in relation to published norms. The following modification procedures are sometimes applied to standardized tests in order to gain more accurate assessment information (Erickson & Iglesias, 1986; Kayser, 1989; Weddington, 1987).

1. Reword the test instructions.

2. Provide additional time for the child to respond.

3. Continue testing beyond the recommended ceiling.

4. Record all responses, particularly when the child changes or explains an answer, makes additional comments, or performs a demonstration.

5. Compare the child's answers to the child's dialect or to features known to characterize first- or second-language learning. Rescore articulation samples and expressive language samples, giving credit for language variations or language differences.

6. Develop several additional practice items for each subtest so that the process of "taking the test" is clearly established prior to formally beginning the actual test procedure.

7. On picture recognition tests, request that the child name the picture in addition to pointing. By doing this, you may ascertain whether the standardized response is appropriate to the child's cultural community.

8. When a child's response appears to be incorrect according to the test manual, request that the child explain why the seemingly incorrect

answer was selected. It may be that the child's response is completely logical when cultural experiences and expectations are considered.

9. If a child has had limited experience with books, line drawings, or standardized testing procedures, and if picture identification is required by the test, you may request that the child identify the actual object, body part, action, or photograph if needed. By doing this, you may learn whether a particular response is related to level of experience with the testing process as opposed to language competence.

10. Complete the testing in several sessions if necessary.

11. Omit items that you expect the child to miss because of age, language, or culture.

12. Change the pronunciation of vocabulary words if a particular pronunciation is common to the child's cultural experiences.

13. Use different pictures if the ones provided by the test are potentially subject to cultural bias.

14. Accept culturally appropriate responses as correct, even if they are not listed as correct in the test manual.

15. Have a parent or other trusted adult administer the test items if it encourages responding or if it provides a way to administer the test in the child's familiar dialect.

16. If necessary, repeat the test stimuli more times than specified in the test manual.

Adapting a test is a second alternative, which is different from modifying a test in that when a test is adapted (or revised), the task, and perhaps the content of the instrument, undergo substantial changes. Tests are adapted for the purpose of including stimuli that are culturally meaningful to the client in order to comply with the assessment objective of obtaining true information about the child's language, so that it can be described accurately (Gavillan-Torres, 1984; Weddington, 1987).

However, when a standardized instrument is adapted, a new instrument evolves. Although the revised test may be more likely to provide nonbiased and accurate assessment results, it is neither norm-referenced nor standardized; hence, it does not profess to have the same validity and reliability as does the standardized instrument. Therefore, the standardized normative data that are included in the original test manual are *not* applicable for use with the adapted instrument. Instead, part of the process of adapting the test may include the development of normative data that apply to the local culture (Erickson & Iglesias, 1986).

Test adaptation is a complicated process that involves a cooperative effort among a number of professionals. The endeavor involves making culturally relevant changes in both the content of the test and the tasks that the test requires the child to perform (Kayser, 1989).

In order to accomplish this, the test and its contents are viewed by a number of bilingual or bidialectal specialists. These include at least two bilingual or bidialectal academic teachers from different levels of academic teaching (e.g., primary and secondary), at least one speech-language pathologist, a psychologist, a special education teacher, and a bilingual or bidialectal member of the community (Kayser, 1989). Suggestions are available for making effective adaptations to existing standardized instruments (Kayser, 1989).

Language sampling is a third alternative. General procedures for language sampling are described in Chapter 3. Further, more specific guidelines and comments on using a language sample for the purpose of partially determining a child's language proficiency are included in a previous section of this chapter.

In addition, language sampling is an important part of the assessment battery for children who identify with minority cultures. Because of its flexibility, language-sampling procedures can be used to eliminate many of the cultural-bias problems associated with standardized test administration and therefore yield a wealth of information about the child's actual communicative competence (Seymour & Miller-Jones, 1981).

A fourth alternative is the use of *criterion-referenced procedures*. Criterion-referenced testing follows the analysis of a representative language sample and it is different from both language sampling and standardized testing. Criterion-referenced testing is different from language sampling in that the latter is quite flexible, while the former is structured and seeks to probe performance in very specific areas that are explicitly described with regard to performance criteria in advance of the testing (Gorth & Hambleton, 1972).

Criterion-referenced testing is different from standardized testing in that psychometric norms are not used. Instead the clinician who applies criterion-referenced procedures uses knowledge about the sequential order of language acquisition and cognitive development as a reference when evaluating the child's performance on the criterion-referenced tasks. The purpose of criterion-referenced testing is to follow up on the results of the language sample and thus pursue in greater detail the areas of concern identified by sampling (Seymour & Miller-Jones, 1981).

An example of criterion-referenced testing is the systematic evaluation of a child's achievement of an identified developmental or language milestone. For instance, if a child is 20 months of age yet lacks vocabulary and does not yet join words to form short sentences, one might systematically investigate whether the cognitive concept of object permanence has been acquired. Knowing that object permanence usually becomes complete between 10 and 18 months of age, it is expected that the average 20-month-old child grasps the concept. To systematically test this concept, one might provide situations that involve the disappearance of a desired object or event, carefully observing the child to determine (1) whether the child looks for or requests the absent object or event and (2) the frequency and duration of the child's attempts to retrieve the object or event.

Documentation of Linguistic Differences and Socioeconomic Status.   Further, as part of the assessment, a number of questions are asked in order to understand the cultural and environmental factors that may influence the child's language development. The extent to which both languages are used within the family and external to the family, and family attitudes toward both languages and cultures are important to identify. In addition, the literacy activities of the family and community are useful to recognize in order to gain a complete understanding of the linguistic opportunities that are accessible to the child (Kayser, 1989).

Language Intervention: General Suggestions for Minority Children

If intervention with minority-language children is to be effective, it must be **culturally valid.** That is, it must be offered in the context of the values, attitudes, and wishes of the familiar culture. This includes giving consideration to attitudes toward communicative disorders and what to do about them, as well as incorporating the cultural and linguistic experiences that are indigenous to the child's world (Westby & Rouse, 1985). Further, in a general sense, effective intervention strategies take into account factors that include the child's facility with language at all levels (see BICS and CALPS earlier in this chapter), individual academic skill, reception- and response-modality preference, and preferred cognitive style. A few key intervention considerations are outlined as follows.

Native-Language Instruction.   Competent client participation requires that the client grasp exactly what the task requires and accurately comprehend feedback regarding performance and instructions on how to achieve success. When the primary mode of instruction is Standard English, minority-language clients are at a decided disadvantage. In a sense, they are denied access to instruction unless some provision is made to assure that they understand what is required (Tikunoff, 1987).

For that reason, we are advised not to restrict use of first or dominant language by second-language learners (California, 1984). Concepts, knowledge, and skills are most effectively taught through the language that is most familiar to the child. Further, the mother tongue is not only the best instrument for learning (especially in the early stages), it is an essential part of the child's sense of identity (Anderson & Boyer, 1970).

Utilize Home-Cultural Information during Instruction.   Children learn the rules of discourse naturally in their homes. This allows them to participate socially with other members of the family and community. When a child is a member of a minority culture, the familiar rules of discourse may not transfer easily for use in school and other unfamiliar circumstances. This is because the rules of classroom discourse usually reflect those of the majority culture, which may be different from the discourse rules that are familiar to minority-language children. When coupled with insufficient English-language skills, minority-language children are deterred from participating competently in instruction until they understand and master the majority-culture rules of discourse.

For this reason, effectiveness of instruction may be enhanced by structuring cooperative working situations where minority-language students are allowed to talk as they work, helping each other with task completion. Also, a clinician may respond to or use referents from the student's home culture to enhance instruction. For example, with a Spanish-speaking Hispanic child it is appropriate to use the term *"mi hijito"* ("my little son"), in order to convey fondness and belongingness. One may also take into account, and make use of, preferred learning and social-interactive styles (Peters-Johnson & Taylor, 1986). It is recommended that clinicians make use of materials that are designed specifically for linguistically and culturally diverse children. This includes commercial materials as well as books, toys, and household items that truly represent the activities and people of the home culture. Moreover, motivators and reinforcers that are compatible with the child's culture and experience are preferred.

As a general rule, when a clinician accommodates the rules of discourse to suit the minority culture, learning is more likely to occur (Tikunoff, 1987). These include adapting rules of discourse, selecting materials, and checking personal attitudes.

In addition, minority-language students may be confronted with classroom demands that convey values and expectations that conflict with those of the home culture. In this case, clinicians are obligated to ensure that minority-language students understand the cultural values and expectations that are required to succeed in traditional academic settings. Even so, minority-language students must *never* be led to perceive a priority of rightness when the classroom values and norms conflict with their own (Tikunoff, 1987).

Comprehensible Input. In order for students to acquire language, they must be able to understand what is being communicated to them. Comprehensible input refers to meaningful language that is useful in achieving proficiency, so comprehensible input is basic to effective instruction (Krashen, 1981). Effective intervention is organized to provide students with comprehensible input, that is, meaningful language that they can comprehend and apply.

There are at least three things that a clinician must do in order to generate effective intervention programs that provide comprehensible input to minority-language children. The clinician must (1) assess the student's level of linguistic function, (2) determine the task demands of the intervention activity that is under consideration, and (3) reconcile the discrepancy between the child's level of linguistic function and task demands (Tikunoff, 1987).

Beyond that, it is important to be able to accommodate the child's level of linguistic function so that the demands of the intervention task can be met successfully. Some suggestions for accomplishing this are as follows.

Nonlinguistic Means for Encouraging Comprehension.   First the clinician may encourage comprehension through the use of nonlinguistic cues. Gestures, pictures, audiovisual materials, and facial expressions are all helpful in providing a nonlinguistic environment that is conducive to understanding spoken or written language (Krashen, 1982).

High-Context and Low-Context Activities.   The clinician may prepare a combination of high-context and low-context activities to be used in intervention (Westby & Rouse, 1985). High-context activities include tasks such as making cookies from a recipe, talking about the calendar or weather, and recapping the events of the day. By contrast, low-context activities include conversations about things that are not present in the immediate context. For reinforcement, a family member may help with low-context activities at home (Westby & Rouse, 1985). For example, some family members can read a library book with the child, and clinicians can teach family members how to ask appropriate questions and how to talk about the story with the student as they read together.

Social and Academic Goals.

Consideration to Academic Level and Social Skills.   Consideration should be given to developing goals in both academic and social language skills (refer to CALPS and BICS earlier in this chapter). Minority-language individuals master aspects of social and academic language at different rates and with different degrees of proficiency. Grade level, previous education experience, gender, ethnicity, first-language skills, age of arrival to the country, and previous opportunities for learning English all contribute to the success of the intervention program and should be considered when developing goals and procedures (Fradd & Weismantel, 1989).

Gradually Reducing Context and Increasing Cognitive Demands.   A major aim of language development for second-language learners is to develop students' ability to manipulate and interpret cognitively demanding context-reduced text. A key to why minority students often fail to develop high levels of second-language academic skills is because their initial instruction has emphasized context-reduced communication (i.e., instruction in English that is unrelated to prior out-of-school experience). This can be prevented by increasing contextual cues when presenting the second language to the child, thus increasing comprehensibility of the less familiar language. Then, by gradually reducing the availability of contextual cues, the child is prepared to comprehend and use the second language in cognitively demanding, context-reduced situations (see the discussion on BICS and CALPS earlier in this chapter).

CONCLUDING REMARKS

The comments on multicultural issues conclude this introduction to language disorders in children. Each topic covered in this volume deserves to be followed by more detailed study as you proceed with your preprofessional and graduate education. Throughout your education and career, you will continue to add to this groundwork as new information becomes available to you and as you come into contact with the many individuals whose rate or pattern of language acquisition requires clinical attention.

REFERENCES

Adelman, H. (1971). Learning problems. In D. Hammill & N. Bartel (eds.), *Educational perspectives in learning disabilities.* New York: John Wiley & Sons.

Ambert A. N., & Melendez, S. E. (1985). *Bilingual education: A source book.* New York: Garland Publishing Co.

Ambert, A. N. (1986). Identifying language disorders in Spanish speakers. In A. Willig & H. Greenberg (Eds.), *Bilingualism and learning disabilities: Policy and practice for teachers and administrators.* New York: American Library.

Ambert, A., & Dew, N. (1982). *Special education for exceptional bilingual students: A handbook for educators.* University of Wisconsin-Milwaukee: Midwest National Origin Desegregation Assistance Centers.

American Speech-Language-Hearing Association. (1985). *Directory of Bilingual Speech-Language Pathologists and Audiologists, 1985–1986.* Rockville, MD: Author.

Anderson, G. R., & Anderson, S. K. (1983). The exceptional Native American. In D. R. Omark & J. G. Erickson (eds.), *The bilingual exceptional child.* San Diego, CA: College-Hill Press.

Andersson, T., & Boyer, M. (1970). *Bilingual schooling in the United States.* Austin, TX: Southwest Educational Development Laboratory.

ASHA. (1985a, June). Clinical management of communicatively handicapped minority language populations. *ASHA,* 29–32.

ASHA. Committee on the Status of Racial Minorities. (1985b). Clinical management of the communicatively handicapped minority language populations. *ASHA,* 27(6), 29–32.

Banks, J. (1987). *Teaching strategies for ethnic students.* Newton, MA: Allyn & Bacon.

Barona, A., & Santos de Barona, M. (1987). A model for the assessment of limited English proficient students referred for special education services. In

S. Fradd & W. Tukinoff (eds.), *Bilingual education and special education.* Boston: College-Hill.

Basso, K. I. (1972). To give up on words: Silence in western Apache culture. In P. Gigiolo (Ed.), *Language and social context.* New York: Penguin Books.

Bates, E. (1976). *Language in context.* New York: Academic Press.

Battle, D. E. (Ed.). (1993). Introduction — which is written by Battle. *Communication disorders in multicultural populations.* Boston: Andover Medical Publishers.

Blount, B. G. (1982). Culture and language of socialization: Parental speech. In D. A. Wagner & H. W. Stevenson (eds.), *Cultural perspectives on child development.* San Francisco: Freeman.

Bouvier, L. F., & Davis, C. B. (1982). *The future racial composition of the United States.* Washington, DC: Demographic Information Services Center of the Population Reference Bureau.

Brophy, J. E., & Good, T. L. (1974). *Teacher-student relationships: Causes and consequences.* New York: Holt, Rinehart, & Winston.

Brown, R. (1973). *A first language.* Cambridge: Harvard University Press.

California State Department of Education. (1984). *Studies on immersion education: A collection for United States educators.* Sacramento: Author.

Campbell, L. R. (1985). A study of comparability of master's level training and certification requirements and needs of speech-language pathologists. Unpublished doctoral dissertation, Howard University.

Campbell, L. R. (1991). Second language dialect instruction. A miniseminar presented at the Mid-South Conference in Speech-Language Pathology, Memphis, TN.

Carey, A. L. (1992). Get involved multiculturally. *ASHA,* May, p. 34.

Cazden, C. B., & John, V. P. (1971). Learning in American Indian children. In M. Wax, S. Diamond, & F. Goeting (eds.), *Anthropological perspectives on education.* New York: Basic Books.

Cheng, L. L. (1989). Service delivery to Asian/Pacific limited English proficient children: Management of the communicatively handicapped minority-language populations. *Topics in Language Disorders,* 9(3), 4–14.

Cheng, L. L. (1993). Asian-American cultures. In D. E. Battle (ed.), *Communication disorders in multicultural populations.* Boston: Andover Medical Publishers.

Cole, L. (1987). Minority brain drain in human communication sciences and disorders. Rockville, MD: American Speech-Language-Hearing Association. [Unpublished manuscript]

Cole, L., Delgado, L. L., DeVane, G. F., Holliman, D. G., Kayser, H., Nelson, J. E., Simpkins, W. T., White, D. W., & Douglass, R. L. (1989). Bilingual speech-language pathologists and audiologists [official statement of ASHA]. *ASHA,* 17–88.

Conklin, N. F., & Lourie, M. A. (1983). *A host of tongues: Language communities in the United States.* New York: Free Press.

Council of Graduate Programs in Communication Sciences and Disorders.

(1986). *1985–1986 National Survey Report.* Tuscaloosa, AL: Author.

Culatta, B., Page, J. L. & Ellis, J. (1983). Story retelling as a communicative performance screening tool. *Language, Speech & Hearing Services in the Schools, 14*(2), 66–74.

Cummins, J. (1982). The role of primary language development in promoting educational success for language minority students. In J. Cummins (ed.), *Schooling and language minority students: A theoretical framework.* Los Angeles: California State Department of Education Evaluation Dissemination and Assessment Center.

Cummins, J. (1984). *Bilingualism and special education: Issues in assessment and pedagogy.* San Diego, CA: College-Hill.

Cummins, J. (1986). Empowering minority students: A framework for intervention. *Harvard Educational Review, 56*(1), 18–35.

Dillard, J. L. (1973). *Black English: Its history and usage in the United States.* New York: Vintage Books.

Dore, J. (1975). Holophrases, speech acts, and language universals. *Journal of Child Language, 2,* 21–40.

Dukepoo, F. (1980). *The elderly American Indian.* San Diego, CA: San Diego State University Center on Aging.

Eder, D. (1981). "Ability grouping as a self fulfilling prophecy: A microanalysis of teacher-student interaction." *Sociology and Education, 54,* 151–61.

Erickson, J. G., & Iglesias, A. (1986). Assessment of communication disorders in non English proficient children. In O. Taylor (ed.), *Nature of communication disorders in culturally and linguistically diverse populations.* San Diego, CA: College-Hill.

Figueroa, R., Fradd, S. H., & Correa, V. I. (1989). Bilingual special education and this issue. *Exceptional Children, 56,* 174–78.

Flint-Shaw, L. M., Kayser, H., DeVane, G. F., Holliman, D. G., Brown, H., Hardwick, H. A., Nelson, J. E., Reveron, W., Turner, E. G., Cole, L., Douglass, R. L., & Leslie, C. P. (1987). *Multicultural professional education in communication disorders: Curriculum approaches.* Rockville, MD: American Speech-Language-Hearing Association.

Fradd, S. & Correa, V. (1989). Meeting the multicultural needs of Hispanic students in special education. *Exceptional Children, 45*(2), 105–10.

Fradd, S. (1987). Accommodating the needs of limited English proficient students in regular classrooms. In S. H. Fradd & W. J. Tukinoff (Eds.), *Bilingual education and special education: A guide for administrators.* Boston: Little-Brown.

Fradd, S. & Weismantel, M. J. (1989). *Meeting the needs of culturally and linguistically different students: A handbook for indicators.* Boston: College-Hill Press.

Fram, I., & Crawford, P. (1972). An examination of the relationship between sex, birthdate, and English as a second language and teachers' predictions of academic success. Research report 0N00494. New York Board of Education.

Garcia, R. L. (1982). *Teaching in a pluralistic society: Concepts, models, strategies.* New York: Harper & Row.

Garcia, S. B. (1983). Effects of student characteristics, school programs, and organization on decision making for the placement of Hispanic students in classes for the learning disabled. Unpublished doctoral dissertation, University of Texas at Austin.

Garcia, S. B. (1984). Effects of student characteristics, school programs and organization on decision making for the placement of Hispanic students in classes for the learning disabled. Unpublished doctoral dissertation, University of Texas at Austin.

Gavillan-Torres, E. (1984). Issues of assessment of limited English-proficient students and of truly disabled in the United States. In N. Miller (ed.), *Bilingualism and language disability.* San Diego, CA: College-Hill Press.

Good, T. L. (1986). What is learned in elementary schools. In T. M. Tomlinson & H. J. Walberg (eds.), *Academic work and educational excellence: Raising student productivity.* Berkeley, CA: McCutchan.

Good, T. L., & Brophy, J. E. (1971). Analyzing classroom interaction: A more powerful alternative. *Educational Technology, 11,* 36–40.

Good, T. L., & Brophy, J. E. (1973). *Looking in classrooms.* San Francisco: Harper & Row Publishers.

Gorth, W., & Hambleton, R. (1972). Measurement considerations for criterion-referenced testing and special education. *Journal of Special Education, 6,* 303–14.

Guendelman, S. (1983). Developing responsiveness to the health needs of Hispanic children and families. *Social Work in Health Care, 8,* 1–15.

Guilmet, G. (1979). Maternal perceptions of urban Navajo and Caucasian children classroom behavior. *Human Organization, 30*(1), 87–91.

Halliday, M. A. K., & Hasan, R. (1976). *Cohesion in English.* London: Longman.

Hamayan, E. V., & Damico, J. S. (1991). *Limiting bias in the assessment of bilingual students.* Austin, TX: Pro-Ed.

Harris, G. A. (1993). American Indian cultures: A lesson in diversity. In D. E. Battle (ed.), *Communication disorders in multicultural populations.* Boston: Andover Medical Publishers.

Heath, S. B. (1984). Cross cultural acquisition of language. Paper presented at the annual meeting of the American Speech-Language-Hearing Association, San Francisco.

Heath, S. B. (1986). Social cultural contexts of language development. In S. B. Heath (Ed.), *Social and cultural factors in schooling language-minority students.* Sacramento: Bilingual Education Office of California State Department of Education.

Iglesias, A. (1985). Communication in the home and classroom: Match or mismatch? *Topics in Language Disorders, 5,* 4.

Ima, K., & Rumbant, R. G. (1989). Southeast Asian refugees in American schools: A comparison of fluent-English proficient and limited English proficient students. *Topics in Language Disorders, 9*(3), 54–75.

Irwin, R. (1977). Judgments of vocal quality, speech fluency, and confidence of southern black and white speakers. *Language and Speech, 20,* 261–66.

Jacobson, B. (1979). [personal communication cited by Omark & Erickson 1983]. In D. R. Omark & J. G. Erickson (eds.), *The bilingual exceptional child.* San Diego, CA: College-Hill Press.

Juarez, M. (1983). Assessment and treatment of minority-language-handicapped children: The role of the monolingual speech-language pathologist. *Topics in Language Disorders, 3*(3), 57–66.

Kayser, H. (1986). An ethnography of three Mexican-American children labeled language disordered. *Monograph of Bueno Center for Multicultural Education, 7*(2), 23–42.

Kayser, H. (1989). Speech and language assessment of Spanish-English speaking children. *Language, Speech, and Hearing Services in Schools, 20,* 226–44.

Kayser, H. (1990). Social communicative behaviors or language disordered Mexican-American students. *Child Language Teaching and Therapy, 6*(3), 255–69.

Kayser, H. (1993). Hispanic cultures. In D. Battle (ed.), *Communication disorders in multicultural populations.* Boston: Andover Medical Publishers.

Krashen, S. D. (1981). Bilingual education and second language acquisition theory. In California State Department of Education (ed.), Schooling and language minority students: A theoretical framework. Los Angeles: California State Department of Education, Evaluation, Dissemination, and Assessment Center.

Krashen, S. D. (1982). *Principles and practices in second-language acquisition.* Oxford, UK: Pergamon Press.

Kretschmer, R. E. (1991). Exceptionality and the limited English proficient student: Historical and practical contexts. In E. V. Hamayan & J. S. Damico (eds.), *Limiting bias in the assessment of bilingual students. Austin, TX: Pro-Ed.*

Labov, W. (1970). The logic of non-standard English. In F. Williams (ed.), *Language and poverty.* Chicago: Markham.

Lahey, M. (Ed.). (1988). *Language disorders and language development.* New York: Macmillan Publishing Company.

Langdon, H. W. (1992). The Hispanic population: Facts and figures. In H. W. Langdon & L. L. Cheng (eds.), *Hispanic children and adults with communication disorders: Assessment and intervention.* Gaithersburg, MD: Aspen Publishing Co.

Lee, L., Koenigsknecht, R., & Mulhern, S. (1975). *Interactive language development teaching.* Evanston, IL: Northwestern University Press.

Levin, H. M. (1985). *The educationally disadvantaged: A national crisis.* Working paper no. 6. Philadelphia: Public/Private Ventures.

Liles, B. Z. (1987). Episode organization and cohesive conjunctives in narratives of children with and without language disorder. *Journal of Speech and Hearing Research, 30,* 185–96.

Maldonado-Colon, E. (1984). Profiles of Hispanic students placed in speech, hearing, and language programs in selected school districts in Texas. Unpublished doctoral dissertation, University of Massachusetts, Amherst.

Maldonado-Colon, E. (1985). *The role of language assessment data in diagnosis and intervention for linguistically/culturally different students.* Reston, VA: Eric Clearinghouse on Handicapped and Gifted Children.

Matsuda, M. (1989). Working with Asian parents: Some communication strategies. *Topics in Language Disorders, 9*(3), 45–53.

Mattes, L. J., & Omark, D. R. (1984). *Speech and language assessment for the bilingual handicapped.* San Diego, CA: College-Hill Press.

Mercer, J. R. (1972). *Labeling the mentally retarded.* Berkeley: University of California Press.

Meyerson, M. D. (1983). Genetic counseling for families of Chicano children with birth defects. In D. R. Omark & J. G. Erickson (eds.), *The bilingual exceptional child.* San Diego, CA: College-Hill Press.

Meyerson, M. D. (1990). Cultural considerations in the treatment of Latinos with craniofacial malformations. *Cleft Palate Journal, 27,* 279–88.

Miller, D. (1975). *Native American families in the city.* San Francisco: Institute for Scientific Analysis.

Miller, D. (1975a). Native American families in the city. In G. Powell, J. Yamamoto, A. Romero, & A. Morales (eds.), *The psychosocial development of minority group children.* New York: Brunner/Mazel.

National Coalition for Cultural Pluralism. (1973). Appendix A: Statement by the Steering Committee of the National Coalition for Cultural Pluralism. In M. Stent, W. Hazard, & N. Rivlin (eds.), *Cultural pluralism in education: A mandate for change.* Englewood Cliffs, NJ: Prentice-Hall.

National Urban League. (1971). *The state of Black America: The strengths of Black families.* New York: Author.

Ochs, E. & Schiefflin, B. (1979). *Developmental pragmatics. New York:* Academic Press.

Ortiz, A. & Yates, J. R. (1983). Incidence of exceptionality among Hispanics: Implications for manpower planning. *Journal of the National Association of Bilingual Educators, 7,* 41–54.

Ortiz, A., & Maldonado-Colon, E. (1986). Reducing inappropriate referrals of language minority students in special education. In A. Willig & H. Greenberg (Eds.), *Bilingualism and learning disabilities: Policies and practices for teachers and administrators.* New York: American Library Publishing Company.

Ortiz, A., Garcia, S. B., Holtzman, W. H., Jr., Polyzoi, E., Snell, W. E., Jr., Wilkinson, C. V., & Willig, A. C. (1985). *Characteristics of limited English proficient Hispanic students served in programs for the learning disabled: Implications for policy, practice and research.* Austin: University of Texas at Austin, Handicapped Minority Research Institute on Language Proficiency.

Oxford-Carpenter, R., Pol, L., Lopez, D., Stupp, P., Gendell, M., & Peng, S. (1984). *Demographic projections of non-English language background and limited English proficient persons in the United States to the year 2000 by state, age and language group.* Rosslyn, VA: National Clearinghouse for Bilingual Education.

Payan, R. (1984). Language assessment for bilingual exceptional children. In L. M. Baca & H. T. Cervantes (eds.), *The bilingual interface.* St. Louis, MO: Time Miror/Mosley.

Payne, K. T. (1986). Cultural and linguistic groups in the United States. In O. Taylor (ed.), *Nature of communication disorders in culturally and linguistically diverse populations.* San Diego, CA: College-Hill.

Penalosa, F. (in press). Chicano English. In L. Cole & V. Deal (eds.), *Communication disorders in multicultural populations.* Rockville, MD: American Speech-Language-Hearing Association.

Peters-Johnson, C. A., & Taylor, O. L. (1986). Speech, Language, and Hearing Disorder in Black Populations. In O. L. Taylor (ed.), *Nature of Communication Disorders in Culturally and Linguistically Diverse Populations.* San Diego, CA: College-Hill.

Queralt, M. (1984). Understanding Cuban immigrants: A cultural perspective. *Social Work, 29,* 115–21.

Red Horse, J. (1983). Indian family values and experiences. In G. J. Powell (ed.), *The psychosocial development of minority group children.* New York: Brunner/Mazel.

Ripich, D. N. & Spinelli, F. M. (1985). *School discourse problems.* San Diego, CA: College-Hill.

Rueda, R. (1989). Defining mild disabilities with language-minority students. *Exceptional Children, 56,* 121–28.

Ruiz, N. (1989). An optimal learning environment for Rosemary. *Exceptional Children, 56,* 130–44.

Sapir, E. (1921). *Language: An introduction to the study of speech.* New York: Harcourt Brace.

Seymour, H. N., & Miller-Jones, D. (1981). Language and cognitive assessment of black children. In N. J. Lass (ed.), *Speech and language advances in basic research and practice,* Vol. 6. New York: Academic Press.

Seymour, H. N., & Seymour, C. M. (1977). A therapeutic model for communicative disorders among children who speak Black English vernacular. *Journal of Speech and Hearing Disorders, 42,* 247–56.

Shepard, L., & Smith, M. L.; with Davis, A., Glass, G. V., Riley, A., & Vojer, C. (1981). *Evaluation of the identification of perceptual-communicative disorders in Colorado.* Boulder: University of Colorado, Laboratory of Educational Research.

Shuy, R. (1971). Sociolinguistic strategies for studying urban speech. *Bulletin of the School of Education* (Indiana University), *47,* 1–25.

Sinclair, R. L., & Ghory, W. J. (1987). Becoming marginal. In H. T. Trueba (Ed.), *Success or failure? Learning and the language minority student.* New

York: Newbury House.

Skutnabb-Kangas, T., & Toukomaa, P. (1976). *Teaching migrant children's mother tongue and learning the language of the host country in the context of the sociocultural situation of the migrant family.* Helsinki: Finnish National Commission for the United Nations Educational, Scientific, and Cultural Organization.

Slobin, D. (1985). *The crosslinguistic study of language acquisition:* Volume 1. The data. Hillsdale, NJ: Erlbaum.

Social dialects: A position paper. (1983). *ASHA, 25*(9) 23–24.

Spencer, G. (1986). *Projections of the Hispanic population: 1983–2080, current population reports, population estimates and projection.* Series P-25, No. 995. Washington, DC: Bureau of the Census, United States Department of Commerce.

Spinelli, F. M., & Ripich, D. N. (1985). Discourse and education. In D. N. Ripich & F. M. Spinelli (Eds.), *School discourse problems.* San Diego, CA: College-Hill.

Stewart, J. L. (1986). Hearing disorders among the indigenous peoples of North American and the Pacific Basin. In O. L. Taylor (ed.), *Nature of communication disorders in culturally and linguistically diverse populations.* San Diego, CA: College-Hill.

Taylor, O. L. (1993). Foreword. In D. E. Battle (ed.), *Communication disorders in multicultural populations.* Boston: Andover Medical Publishers.

Taylor, O. L. (Ed.). (1986). *Nature of communication disorders in culturally and linguistically diverse populations.* San Diego, CA: College-Hill.

Taylor, O. L., & Payne, K. T. (1983). Culturally valid testing: A proactive approach. *Topics in Language Disorders, 3,* 1–7.

Terrell, F., & Terrell, S. L. (1981). An inventory to measure cultural mistrust among blacks. *Western Journal Black Studies, 5,* 180–85.

Terrell, S. L., & Terrell, F. (1993). African-American cultures. In D. E. Battle (Ed.), *Communication disorders in multicultural populations.* Boston: Andover Medical Publishers.

Tikunoff, W. J. (1987). Providing instructional leadership: The key to effectiveness. In S. H. Frad & W. J. Tikunoff (eds.), *Bilingual education and bilingual special education: A guide for administrators.* Boston: Little Brown Co.

Trueba, H. T. (1987). *Success or failure? Learning and the language minority student.* Cambridge, MA: Newbury House Publishers.

Tucker, J. A. (1980). Ethnic proportions in classes for the learning disabled: Issues in non-biased assessment. *Journal of Special Education, 14*(1), 93–105.

United States Bureau of the Census. (1984). *Projections of the population of the U.S. by age, sex, race, 1983 to 2000. Series P-25-N0952.* Washington, DC: U.S. Government Printing Office.

United States Department of State/Department of Defense. (1985). *The Soviet-Cuban connection in Central America and the Carribbean.* Washington, DC: U.S. Government Printing Office.

United States Bureau of the Census. (1990a). *Current Population Reports. The Hispanic population in the United States: March 1990.* Washington, DC: U.S. Government Printing Office.

United States Bureau of the Census. (1990b). *Projections of the population of states by age, sex and race: 1989–2020.* Current Population Reports, Series D-25, no. 1055. Washington, DC: U.S. Government Printing Office.

United States Bureau of the Census. *Statistical Abstract of the U.S.* (1991). 111th ed., no. 1434. Washington, DC: U.S. Government Printing Office.

Valdez-Fallis, F. (1978). Code switching, and the classroom teacher. In F. Valdez-Fallis (Ed.), *Language in education: Theory and practice,* vol. 4. Arlington, VA: Center for Applied Linguistics.

Veltman, C. (1990). Status of the Spanish language in the United States. *International Migration Review, 24*(1), 108–23.

Waggoner, D. (1984). *Language minority children at risk in America: Concepts, definitions and estimates.* Washington, DC: National Council of La Raza. [ERIC Reproduction 110. ED 253-632]

Waggoner, D. (1984). The need for bilingual education: Estimates from the 1980 census. *Journal of the National Association for Bilingual Education, 8,* 1–14.

Ward, M. C. (1982). *Them children: A study in language learning.* New York: Irving Press.

Weddington, G. T. (1987). The assessment and treatment of communication disorders in culturally diverse populations. [Unpublished manuscript]

Westby, C. (1988). Assessing narrative competence. *Seminars in Speech and Language, 9,* 1–14.

Westby, C. (in press). Cultural variation in story telling. In L. Cole & V. Deal (eds.), *Communication disorders in multicultural populations. Rockville, MD: American Speech-Language Hearing Association.*

Westby, C., & Rouse, G. (1985). Culture in education and the instruction of language-learning disabled students. *Topics in Language Disorders, 5*(4), 15–28.

Wilkinson, C. Y., & Ortiz, A. A. (1986). *Characteristics of limited English proficient and English proficient learning disabled Hispanic students at initial assessment and at re-evaluation.* Austin: University of Texas, Handicapped Minority Research Institute on Language Proficiency.

STUDY GUIDE 6

1. According to the 1990 U.S. Census, what percentage of the national population is composed of people who identify with racial or ethnic minority groups?

2. What is the estimated population growth rate for each of the following groups?
   a. Asian/Pacific-Americans
   b. Hispanic-Americans
   c. Native Americans and Eskimos
   d. Americans of European descent (non-Hispanic)
3. What is the estimated proportion of the national population that will be composed of racial/ethnic minorities by the year 2010?
4. When is it predicted that the current majority will become the minority?
5. How do these demographic changes affect the profession of speech-language pathology?
6. Explain ASHA's commitment and position as it prepares to address the communication needs of minority people.
7. Describe Multicultural Agenda 2000 as it relates to each of the following.
   a. ASHA membership
   b. professional leadership
   c. ASHA national Office structure and staff
   d. policies and programs affecting professional services, education, and research
   e. governmental and legislative efforts
   f. public image
8. Define and differentiate between each of the following terms.
   a. race
   b. ethnicity
   c. culture
9. Describe how language and culture are dependent on each other.
10. Define each of the following terms, and give a personal example of each.
    a. ethnocentrism
    b. racism
    c. prejudice
    d. stereotype
    e. discrimination
11. Describe the cohesive and corrosive sides of ethnocentrism.
12. Define each of the following terms.
    a. cultural pluralism
    b. cultural relativism
13. How might you go beyond cultural relativism in order to effectively counter negative teachings and attitudes?
14. Define and differentiate between the following terms.
    a. language and dialect
    b. language difference and language disorder
15. How do we know if a language difference and language disorder occur concomitantly?

16. Describe and differentiate between the following levels of language proficiency in bilingual people. Which category is indicative of a disorder?
    a. bilingual English proficient
    b. limited English proficient (LEP)
    c. limited in both languages
17. Describe how language competency relates to language context.
18. Describe how language competency relates to language mastery.
19. Describe each of the four levels of language proficiency, and give an example of each.
20. How do the levels of language competency relate to assessment and intervention for children of minority background?
21. What are some of the reasons behind the pattern of overrepresentation for minorities who receive special education services?
22. How do stereotypes and misconceptions about minorities affect referral practices?
23. What are some common misconceptions about the process of learning a second language?
24. How can stereotyping be manifest in the classroom, and why are these patterns important for the speech-language pathologist to identify?
25. Why do so many people who identify with racial/ethnic minority groups receive services from speech-language pathologists who are not familiar with the minority language and culture?
26. What percentage of speech-language pathologists identifies with a racial/ethnic minority group? How does this compare to the overall population of people served by the profession? What are the likely consequences of this pattern?
27. How does the percentage of minority students in speech-language pathology compare to the national trend for minority representation? What are the likely consequences of this pattern? Are there any alternatives? If so, what are they?
28. Discuss the problems that have been noticed with using referral checklists for the purpose of identifying minority-language children who need speech-language services.
29. Discuss the problems that have been noticed with using academic performance observations for the purpose of identifying minority-language children who need speech-language services.
30. Describe some commonly used assessment procedures that are inappropriate for minority-language children.
31. Describe some commonly used intervention procedures that are inappropriate for minority-language children.
32. For how long has Spanish been spoken in what is now known as the southwestern part of the United States?
33. What is the racial heritage of Hispanic people?
34. What is the largest minority group in the United States?

35. What is the largest group of people with non-English background in the United States?
36. Where are the largest concentrations of Hispanic people in the United States?
37. What are the countries of origin for most Hispanic Americans?
38. Give some examples of Hispanic cultural characteristics?
39. What are the probable outcomes of being exposed to two languages simultaneously during language acquisition?
40. Describe some of the phonological and syntactic differences between Spanish and English. How might these influence the acquisition of English as a second language?
41. Describe some of the attitudes toward communication disorders (and other health-related problems) that might be found among Hispanic people.
42. Describe the process by which Black English and Standard American English came to evolve side-by-side but independently.
43. Who uses Black English?
44. Describe some of the phonological and syntactic differences between Black English and Standard American English.
45. How are communication disorders viewed among African-Americans?
46. Native Americans have a high prevalence of three conditions that are considered to be etiological factors related to communication disorders. What are they?
47. Where do the Native Americans reside?
48. What are some of the cultural and social characteristics of Native-American culture? How might these influence the way Native-Americans perform in school?
49. How does the pidginization of Native-American languages affect learning English as a second language?
50. Phonologically and syntactically, what are some of the differences between the Navajo language and English?
51. Describe how Native Americans generally view individuals with handicapping conditions.
52. Which is probably the most extremely diverse cultural minority in the United States? Why is this probably the case?
53. Which is the most rapidly growing cultural minority in the United States?
54. Where are the highest concentrations of Asian/Pacific-Americans?
55. Describe some of the cultural and social characteristics of Asian/Pacific groups.
56. Describe how some Asian languages are different from English phonologically and syntactically. How might these differences impact learning English as a second language?
57. How are communication disorders (and other health-related concerns) viewed by Asian/Pacific people?

58. Describe the groups of people who are likely to identify with deaf culture.

59. What is the native language of those who identify with deaf culture and how is it learned?

60. Why is third-party communication necessary for many deaf people? Describe the third-party communication options.

61. What is the only function that is served by an interpreter? How does this affect your responsibility as a communicator when you use one?

62. How is comprehension of spoken communication affected by deafness? How does this affect your responsibility as a communication partner?

63. How is written communication affected by deafness? What can you do to facilitate written communication when necessary?

64. What are some of the potential problems with using figurative spoken-language when communicating with a deaf person? Why are the same problems not apparent when using signs?

65. How might deafness affect eye contact and speaker-listener distance in conversation?

66. How is speech intelligibility affected by deafness? What can you do to facilitate your understanding of semi-intelligible and unintelligible speech?

67. How is access to news and events affected by deafness?

68. What variables influence language dominance and proficiency in deaf people? What language is likely to be dominant for the deaf person? Do all deaf people develop competency in a language? If not, why not?

69. Describe some family patterns that are common to deaf culture.

70. How do members of deaf culture relate to the mainstream culture?

71. What are the academic and clinical preparations that are necessary for delivering services to minority-language clients?

72. What are the characteristics of a culturally literate professional?

73. What percentage of ASHA professionals are bilingual?

74. What are the competencies required to consider oneself bilingual for the purpose of delivering services to minority-language clients? How are these competencies different for each of the following groups?
    a. bilingual English-proficient clients
    b. limited English-proficient clients (LEP)
    c. limited in minority language and English

75. Discuss each of the general guidelines that should be followed whenever serving individuals who identify with a cultural group other than your own.

76. Discuss the collaboration strategies that are recommended for professionals who are not adequately prepared to independently serve minority-language clients.

77. Discuss why knowledge of language acquisition milestones is central to appropriate language assessment for minority-language children.

78. Outline the eight-step preassessment process and discuss why it is used.

79. What is meant by determining language competency of the child?

80. Why is it necessary to determine language competency before beginning the assessment procedures?
81. Describe how each of the following procedures is used to determine language competency:
    a. language sampling
    b. observing and charting language behavior
    c. questionnaires
82. Why is testing in both languages critical to unbiased assessment of minority-language children?
83. Why are natural communication measures preferred to standardized testing when assessing minority-language children?
84. Discuss each of the following alternatives to standardized testing.
    a. systematic modification of a standardized procedure
    b. adapting a test
    c. language sampling
    d. criterion-referenced testing
85. Why is it important to document linguistic differences and socioeconomic status when assessing a minority-language child?
86. Differentiate between Type I, Type II, and Type III Learning Problems. Which type of learning problem requires intervention and why?
87. What is culturally valid intervention?
88. Discuss the following intervention considerations in terms of what is meant by them and in terms of how they are to be implemented.
    a. native-language instruction
    b. utilization of home-cultural information
    c. using comprehensible input
    d. employing nonlinguistic means for encouraging comprehension
    e. utilizing high-context and low-context activities
    f. giving consideration to academic level and social skills
    g. gradually reducing context and increasing cognitive demand

Appendices

APPENDIX 3–1.   PERMISSION TO SCREEN: SAMPLE

Date

Dear PARENT (OR INSERT NAME):

We are pleased to announce that a communication screening will be done at the (NAME OF SCHOOL) on (DATE OF SCREENING). The screening will be done to identify children who may have difficulties with speech/language or hearing. If you wish for your child to participate in the screening, sign the attached form and return it by (DEADLINE— MAY BE DATE OF SCREENING).

A certified speech-language pathologist from (NAME OF AGENCY) will conduct the screening. The results will be given to you, in writing when the screening is complete.

If you have any questions, please call. We hope that you and your child will be able to take advantage of this opportunity.

Sincerely,

(NAME, CREDENTIALS, AND AFFILIATION OF PERSON COORDINATING THE SCREENING—USUALLY SOMEONE FROM THE CHILD'S SCHOOL)

Date

I understand that a communication screening will take place on (DATE) at the (NAME OF SCHOOL), and I agree that my child will participate in the screening. I understand that the screening involves a hearing test and a speech-language test. I also understand that I will be informed of the screening results on (DATE).

_____

(Name of Child)

_____

(Name of Parent)

_____

(Signature of Parent)

_____

(Date)

APPENDIX 3–2.   SCREENING RESULTS: SAMPLE

<u>Date</u>

Dear (NAMES OF CHILD'S PARENTS):

With your permission, (NAME OF CHILD) participated in a communication screening today at the (NAME OF SCHOOL). As a result of the screening we recommend that your child

_____   receive no further testing at this time.

_____   receive a complete speech-language assessment in order to rule out or identify any problems that your child may have with speaking or listening to spoken language. This testing should be done by an ASHA-certified speech-language pathologist (list attached).

_____   receive a complete audiological assessment in order to rule out or identify any problems that your child may have with hearing. This testing should be done by an ASHA-certified audiologist (list attached).

If you have any questions about these results, or wish to discuss them, please contact me. I will be pleased to answer any questions about your child's performance on the screening.

Sincerely,

(NAME, CREDENTIALS AND AFFILIATION OF ASHA-CERTIFIED PERSON WHO SUPERVISED OR CONDUCTED THE SCREENING)

APPENDIX 3–3. AGREEMENT TO RECEIVE SERVICES: SAMPLE

Name of Client _____ ID # _____

I represent the above-named client and desire for that person to receive speech-language and/or audiology services at the (NAME OF CENTER). I agree to the terms, benefits, obligations, and potential risks of such services as they have been explained to me.

I understand that the center provides speech-language and audiology services with the intent to benefit the communication abilities of the client and that, in the event that the professionals at the center determine that services are not likely to benefit the client, the center will discontinue the services. Further, I understand that I may terminate the services at any time by informing the center of my plans to discontinue, and that the center may terminate services for any of the following reasons: completion of discharge objectives, lack of benefit received by client, professional judgment of the supervisor, and frequent absenteeism or tardiness.

I agree to attend sessions as scheduled, pay for services at the time that they are rendered, give one working-day's notice of cancellation, and pay for any sessions that are cancelled with less than one-working-day's notice. I have been issued a fee schedule and am aware of the cost of services and payment procedures.

I understand that the center is a part of an academic program at (NAME OF UNIVERSITY) and that the services will be provided by students who are appropriately supervised by professional university employees holding the appropriate Certificate of Clinical Competence from the American Speech-Language-Hearing Association (ASHA). I understand that the supervisory policies of the center meet the minimum standards of ASHA as defined by the standards of the Educational Standards Board and Professional Services Board of the Association.

I understand that the services that the client receives will be observed on a regular basis by the designated supervisor, and that they may be observed by students of speech-language pathology for educational purposes only. I also understand that family members of the above-named client are encouraged to observe the services by using the designated observation facility.

I understand that video and audio taping may be used for assessment and educational purposes only. I have been informed that in the event that video- or audiotaping is used for purposes other than assessment of client and education of students, that I will be informed in writing of the exact nature of the project and will be given the option to agree or disagree with participation in the project.

Although risks are not usually associated with speech-language and audiology services, in the event that the above-mentioned client is to receive services in a high-risk category, I understand that the risks will be explained to me, and that I will be given the opportunity to terminate services if I deem that the potential risks outweigh the potential benefits.

Signature _____ Date _____
Relationship to Client _____
Supervisor _____

APPENDIX 3–4. AUTHORIZATION TO SEEK AND RELEASE INFORMATION: SAMPLE

Name of Client _____ ID # _____

I represent the above-named client who receives speech-language and/or audiology services at the (NAME OF CENTER). I agree that the providing agency listed below will send information to the receiving agency listed below. I agree to this exchange with the understanding that all information received by the center is confidential and will not be shared further without my written consent.

Name and address of agency that will send information:

_____

_____

_____

_____

Name and address of agency that will receive information:

_____

_____

_____

_____

Signature _____ Date _____

Relationship to Client _____

Supervisor _____

APPENDIX 3–5.   CASE-HISTORY INTAKE FORM: SAMPLE

Date _____ ID # _____

<u>Identifying Information</u>

<u>Client's Name</u> _____

Address _____

_____

_____

Phone Number _____

Birth date _____Age _____

Language(s) spoken in the home _____

Mother's Name _____

Address _____

_____

_____

Phone Numbers: Home _____Work _____

Occupation _____

Education _____

_____

Age _____

Father's Name _____

Address _____

_____

Phone Numbers: Home _____Work _____

Occupation _____

_____

Age _____

Legal Guardian(s) _____

Address _____

_____

Phone Numbers: Home _____Work _____

Occupation _____

Education _____

_____

Age _____

How did you learn about the Speech and Hearing Center? _____

_____

Describe the problem. _____

_____

_____

_____

Exactly what would you like the staff at the Speech and Hearing Center to do for you? _____

_____

_____

_____

Speech-Language

At what age did the child begin to respond to speech? _____

At what age did the child respond to his/her own name? _____

Did the child coo and babble? _____

At what age did the child begin to interact socially? _____

At what age did the child begin to make a deliberate effort to make wants and needs known? _____

At what age did the child say first words? _____
What were the first words?

_____

When did the child begin to combine words to make short sentences? __

_____

Give an example of a first short sentence. _____

_____

_____

Does the child use language that is similar to that of other children at the same age? If not, please explain. _____

_____

_____

_____

Are family members able to understand the child's speech? If not, please explain. _____

_____

_____

_____

Are strangers able to understand the child's speech? If not, please explain.

_____

_____

_____

Describe the speech/language that child uses at this time. _____

_____

_____

_____

What language(s) does child use at school? _____

What language(s) does child use at home? _____

What language(s) is the child most comfortable using? _____

_____

Hearing

Has the child's hearing been tested? _____

Do you suspect a hearing problem? _____

Does the child respond to environmental noises (e.g., doorbell, telephone, radio, doors opening and closing, papers shuffling)? If not, please explain.

_____

_____

_____

Does the child wear a hearing aid? _____
If so, please describe. _____

_____

_____

_____

If so, at what age did the child begin wearing hearing aid(s)? _____

If so, at what times during the day and for what activities does the child wear the hearing aid(s)? _____

Does the child have a history of ear infections? Explain. _____

_____

_____

_____

When watching TV, does the child turn the volume up so that it is uncomfortable for other people in the same room? _____

<u>Physical</u>

Birth-length _____Birth-weight _____

Age when child first held head up _____

Age when child first rolled over _____

Age when child first sat up _____

Age when child first crawled _____

Age when child first stood alone _____

Age when child first walked _____

Age when child gained daytime bladder control _____

Age when child gained nighttime bladder control _____

Age when child gained control of bowels _____

Current height _____Current weight _____

Is the child's coordination similar to other children of the same age? ____
If not, please describe. _____

_____

_____

_____

Does the child wear glasses? _____

If so, since what age? _____

If so, is vision corrected to 20/20? _____

Cognitive

Have difficulties with learning been noticed? _____
If so, please explain. _____

_____

_____

_____

Is the child's knowledge of the world similar to other children at the same age? _____
If no, please explain _____

_____

_____

_____

Has the child been identified as mentally retarded? _____
If so, please explain. _____

_____

_____

_____

Has the child experienced problems in school? _____
If so, please explain. _____

_____

_____

_____

Health and Medical

Length of pregnancy _____

Complications during pregnancy _____

_____

_____

_____

Length of labor _____

Complications during delivery _____

_____

_____

_____

Health problems identified at birth _____
_____
_____
_____

Number of days in hospital at birth   _____

Serious illnesses, syndromes, diseases, chronic medical conditions _____
_____
_____
_____

Hospitalizations (reason and length of stay)   _____
_____
_____
_____

Social

Does the child use language for social purposes? _____

Does the child have friends? List first names/ages _____
_____
_____
_____

Does the child play well with other children? _____

Describe. _____
_____
_____
_____

How does the child react to meeting strangers?   _____
_____
_____
_____

How does the child respond to unfamiliar surroundings? _____
_____
_____
_____

What kinds of games and activities does the child enjoy? _____

_____

_____

_____

Family

Names and ages of all members of household

_____

_____

_____

_____

Is this a foster child? _____

Is the child adopted? _____

Describe how the child relates to other members of the household. ____

_____

_____

_____

Educational

Current grade in school _____

Have any grades been repeated? _____

If so, which grade(s)? _____

If so, what was the reason given?_____

_____

_____

_____

Name of the school at which the child is enrolled _____

_____

_____

_____

Do you have any questions that you would like us to answer? _____

If so, list your questions below.

_____
_____
_____
_____
_____
_____
_____

Exactly what would you like to accomplish by your visit to the speech and hearing center? _____

_____
_____
_____
_____
_____

APPENDIX 3–6. ASSESSMENT REPORT FORMAT: SAMPLE

I. Identifying Information
II. Statement of the Problem
III. Significant Background Information
IV. Testing Procedures and Results of Testing
    A. Detailed testing of expressive and receptive language, including all three dimensions
    B. Articulation or phonology testing
    C. Oral-mechanism examination
    D. Hearing screening
    E. Other testing
V. Behavioral Observations and Clinical Impressions
VI. Diagnosis
VII. Prognosis
VIII. Recommendations
IX. Signatures with Credentials and Dates

APPENDIX 4–1.   INTERVENTION PLAN FORMAT: SAMPLE 1

I.   Identifying Information
II.   Diagnosis
III.   Significant Background Information
IV.   Objectives and Procedures (see Appendix 4–3)
V.   Prognosis
VI.   Recommendations
VII. Signatures with Credentials and Dates

APPENDIX 4–2.   INTERVENTION PLAN FORMAT: SAMPLE 2

I.   Identifying Information
II.   Diagnosis
III.   Significant Background Information
IV.   Objectives (see Appendix 4–4)
V.   Procedures (see Appendix 4–4)
VI.   Prognosis
VII.   Recommendations
VIII.   Signatures with Credentials and Dates

APPENDIX 4–3   FORMAT OPTION FOR RECORDING OBJECTIVES AND PROCEDURES IN AN INTERVENTION PLAN

IV. Objectives and Procedures
  Long-Term Objective I.
      Short-Term Objective A. (Leads to accomplishing long-term objective I.)
          Procedure 1. (Addresses short-term objective I.A.)
          Procedure 2. (Addresses short-term objective I.A.)
      Short-Term Objective B. (Leads to accomplishing long-term objective I.)
          Procedure 1. (Addresses short-term objective I.B.)
          Procedure 2. (Addresses short-term objective I.B.)
  Long-Term Objective II.
      Short-Term Objective A. (Leads to accomplishing long-term objective II.)
          Procedure 1. (Addresses short-term objective II.A.)
          Procedure 2. (Addresses short-term objective II.A.)
      Short-Term Objective B. (Leads to accomplishing long-term objective II.)
          Procedure 1. (Addresses short-term objective II.B.)
          Procedure 2. (Addresses short-term objective II.B.)

APPENDIX 4–4   ALTERNATIVE FORMAT OPTION FOR RECORDING OBJECTIVES AND PROCEDURES IN AN INTERVENTION PLAN

IV. Objectives

Long-Term Objective I.

Short-Term Objective A. (Leads to accomplishing long-term objective I.)

Short-Term Objective B. (Leads to accomplishing long-term objective I.)

Short-Term Objective C. (Leads to accomplishing long-term objective I.)

Long-Term Objective II.

Short-Term Objective A. (Leads to accomplishing long-term objective II.)

Short-Term Objective B. (Leads to accomplishing long-term objective II.)

V. Procedures

Procedure 1. (Addresses short-term objective I.A. and B.)

Procedure 2. (Addresses short-term objective I.A. and C.)

Procedure 3. (Addresses short-term objective II.A. and B.)

APPENDIX 4–5   PROGRESS REPORT FORMAT: SAMPLE

I.   Identifying Information
II.   Diagnosis
III.   Significant Background Information
IV.   Objectives and Progress
    A. Long-term Objective 1
        1.   Short-term Objective 1a
        2.   Short-term Objective 1b
    B. Long-term Objective 2
        1.   Short-term Objective 2a
        2.   Short-term Objective 2b
V.   Clinical Impressions
VI.   Prognosis
VII.   Recommendations
VIII. Signatures with Credentials and Dates

APPENDIX 4–6 MAINTAINING AND MONITORING A HEARING AID

Speech-language pathologists should check each of the following at the beginning of every assessment or intervention session. Parents and/or clients should be taught to make the same check at the end of each day. Checking at the end of the day is better than checking at the beginning of the day because weak batteries recharge overnight but are not apt to last throughout the day.

1. Check to make sure that batteries have sufficient power.
   a. Use a volt meter to check batteries.
   b. Discard and replace batteries as soon as voltage drops below the level prescribed in that particular hearing aid's handbook.
2. For body hearing aids, check cords. They should be in good condition.
   a. Replace broken cords.
   b. Replace fractured cords. To identify fractured cords, place the receiver against microphone and shake the cord. Fractured cords will cause intermittent feedback.
3. Check receivers for body aids. There should be no evidence of damage.
   a. Examine casing for cracks.
   b. Check washer between earmold and receiver for snug fit. Loose fit may result in feedback.
   c. If hearing aid does not work and cords and batteries are known to be in good condition, a new receiver should be tried. If aid still does not function, internal damage to the hearing aid may be assumed.
4. Hearing aids (both body aids and behind-the-ear aids) should be checked to make sure that they reproduce speech clearly. Use a custom earmold, stethoscope, or plug with tubing and listen through the hearing aid to the five sounds ([u], [a], [e], [ʃ], and [s]). Any distortion of sound may indicate internal malfunction (Johnson & Paterson, 1991).

APPENDIX 4–7   TROUBLESHOOTING A HEARING AID

1. Complaint: The hearing aid is not working properly.
    a. Check "M-T-O" position. Switch should be set to "M."
    b. Check battery for leakage. If leaking, wipe compartment with a soft cloth, discard battery, and replace it.
    c. Check battery for voltage using a volt meter. If voltage is below recommended level, discard battery and replace. If a volt meter is not handy, turn aid to full volume. If feedback does not occur, battery is weak or dead.
    d. If sound distortion or intermittent signal occurs, send hearing aid for repairs. It may have internal problems.
    e. Check for plugged tube. If tube is plugged, remove blockage or replace tube.
    f. Check for clogged hook. If hook is clogged, remove blockage or replace hook.
    g. Check for clogged filter. If filter is clogged, wash or replace.
    h. Check tubing for evidence of a tear or perforation. If torn or perforated, replace tubing.
2. Complaint: The hearing aid is not working at all. With the hearing aid system intact, turn the aid on full volume and listen for feedback.
    a. If there is no feedback, check the battery.
    b. If the battery has sufficient voltage, leave the volume on and remove the ear mold and ear hook. If feedback occurs, the problem is external to the aid (ear mold, tube or hook). Check the following:
        i. Attach the ear hook. If no feedback occurs, the hook may be blocked. Clear blockage or replace hook. If the hook appears to be clear, check the screw threads. If screw threads are damaged, make arrangements for service.
        ii. If feedback continues when you attach the hook, attach the earmold and tubing to the hook. If feedback stops, the earmold bore or tubing may be blocked. Clear blockage or replace the blocked part.
    c. If no feedback occurs when you turn the aid to full volume the problem is internal to the aid. Check the following:
        i. on/off switch
        ii. volume control
        iii. battery compartment
        iv. microphone port
3. Complaint: The hearing aid is "feeding back." With the hearing aid system intact, turn the aid to full volume and listen for feedback. Then:
    a. Cover the tip of the ear mold with your finger. If the feedback stops, the cause may be a poor-fitting ear mold. Make arrangements to adjust the ear mold fitting.

b. If the feedback continues, remove the ear mold and cover the tip of the hook with your finger. If the feedback stops, the cause may be a hole or tear in the tubing. Replace the tubing.

c. If feedback continues, remove the hook and cover the tip of the microphone port with your finger. If feedback stops, the cause may be due to a broken hook. Replace the hook.

d. If feedback continues, look for a crack in the case. If the case is intact, the problem is probably internal to the hearing aid. In either event, the hearing aid is in need of repair.

APPENDIX 6–1.   DEFINITION OF A BILINGUAL
SPEECH-LANGUAGE PATHOLOGIST

Speech-language pathologists or audiologists who present themselves as bilingual for the purposes of providing clinical services must be able to speak their primary language *and* speak (or sign) at least one other language with native or near-native proficiency in lexicon (vocabulary), semantics (meaning), phonology (pronunciation), morphology/syntax (grammar), and pragmatics (use) during clinical management.

To provide bilingual assessment and remediation services in the client's language, the bilingual speech-language pathologist or audiologist should possess (1) ability to describe the process of normal speech and language acquisition for both bilingual and monolingual individuals and how those processes are manifested in oral (or manually coded) and written language; (2) ability to administer and interpret formal and informal assessment procedures to distinguish between communication differences and communication disorders in oral (or manually coded) and written language; (3) ability to apply intervention strategies for treatment of communicative disorders in the client's language; and (4) ability to recognize cultural factors which affect the delivery of speech-language pathology and audiology services to the client's language community (Payne, 1986).

Glossary

Adventitious—acquired after the time when the individual has command of a first language.

Anatomy—physical or biological structure.

Antecedent—an event that precedes and elicits a response or target behavior.

Antecedent stimulus—See Antecedent.

Apraxia of speech—a sensorimotor speech disorder that impairs one's ability to voluntarily produce phonemes and words.

Assessment—an in-depth evaluation for the purposes of diagnosing and making recommendations.

Authorization—permission.

Behavioral audiometry—engaging a child in play activities that are specifically designed to prepare him or her for accurately responding to a hearing screening or audiological assessment.

Bicultural—having a background that includes significant firsthand experience with two distinct cultural groups.

Bilateral—on two sides.

Bilingual—having fluency in two languages.

Canonical babbling—See Reduplicated babbling.

Carryover—transfer, as in transfer of intervention accomplishments for spontaneous use in activities of daily living.

Chromosome—an x-shaped body contained in the cell nuclei of plants and animals, which is responsible for transmitting genetic characteristics from one generation to the next.

Code—a system whereby one thing (or symbol) is used to represent another.

Code switching—the alternating use of two languages at the word, phrase, and sentence levels, with a complete phonological break between languages.

Cognition—knowledge and the ability to use knowledge.

Cohesive markers—words that serve to link the parts of a conversation.

Communication breakdown—a misunderstanding resulting from failure to adequately send or receive the intended message.

Communication code—a variation in communication that reflects one's political, social, or religious orientation and thus characteristically communicates something about identity in relation to the groups; not necessarily situation-dependent.

Communication register—a situation-dependent variation in communication, including changes in word selection, pronunciation, and inflectional and pragmatic characteristics.

Communication style—See Communication register.

Comprehensible—understandable.

Confidentiality—honoring of a person's right to privacy.

Congenital—apparent at birth.

Consequence—event that occurs immediately after the response to an antecedent and can be used to increase, maintain, decrease, or extinguish a response.

Consequent stimulus—See Consequence.

Constriction—pre-consonant; approximation of a consonant sound.

Content-form interaction—the dependent relationship between language form and language content that occurs whenever content obligates the use of a particular form.

Content words—major building blocks of a language, including nouns, verbs, adjectives, and adverbs.

Contingent—logically related.

Conversational cohesion—the degree to which the words and sentences of a conversation are logically connected.

Conversational repair—identification of the source of a communication breakdown and the provision of needed information in order to clear up the misunderstanding or confusion.

Conversational speech sample—a taped conversation that is taken for the purposes of informally judging intelligibility, language performance level, voice, fluency, prosody, and pragmatics.

Copula—verb *(to be)* that links the subject with the predicate to describe a state of being (e.g., "The cat *is* big"; "We *are* hungry").

Cryptophasia—private language.

Cultural chauvinism—the attitude which presumes that people of one's own group are superior to members of other groups and thus that members of other cultural groups are not only different, but wrong and inferior.

Cultural degradation—the act of giving a cultural group the impression that its culture is believed to be inadequate, backward or inferior, and thus debasing the self-esteem of group members.

Cultural literacy—familiarity with cultural groups other than one's own as well as having the understanding that culture involves much more than characteristics of language and dialect, that one's culture permeates every dimension of communication, and that each person views the world in a way that can only be completely understood through the eyes of the culture with which that person identifies.

Culturally salient—meaningful and familiar to individuals who belong to a particular cultural group.

Culturally valid—See Culturally salient.

Cultural pluralism—the coexistence of a number of diverse and mutually supportive cultural groups within the boundaries of one nation.

Cultural pride—universal attitude of self-respect and satisfaction based on one's heritage within a particular cultural group, enhancing self-esteem within the group.

Cultural relativism—the position that each culture is different, but not necessarily inferior or superior; perceiving each culture from its own perspective and not from the perspective of the individual's own culture.

Culture—a term used to describe behaviors, beliefs, and values of a group of people who are brought together by commonalities.

Data—organized set of information.

Decibel (dB)—unit used to measure amplitude of sound.

Deictic term—word whose meaning depends on the speaker's perspective as a point of reference.

Deixis—use of a deictic term. See Deictic term.

Deviant language—See Language disorder.

Diagnosis—identification of a problem by formal examination or assessment.

Dialect—a subset of language referring to the phonemic, lexical, and semantic variations that occur within a language and are common to a particular group of people from the same region, of the same socioeconomic group, or of a similar ethnic heritage.

Discharge—release, dismissal.

Discharge objective—See Long-term objective.

Discrimination—differentiating between things based on an awareness of identified characteristic properties; consists of direct or indirect acts of exclusion, distinction, differentiation, or preference on account of group membership.

Disfluent—choppy; not flowing smoothly.

Dismissal—See Discharge.

Dominant gene type—gene whose characteristics are capable of being manifest whether paired with a similar or dissimilar gene type.

Dyad—a pair of individuals conversing.

Dysarthrias—a heterogeneous group of communication disorders generally resulting in difficulties with coordinating and performing acts of respiration for speech, phonation, articulation, resonance, and prosody.

Echolalia—the repetition of an utterance that was just spoken by another person, with no apparent intent to convey, emphasize, or elaborate on the information communicated by the previous speaker.

Ethics—rules or standards governing the conduct of members of a profession; principles of right or good conduct.

Ethnicity—heritage and group membership, based on race, origin, characteristics, and institutions.

Ethnocentrism—the attitude of focusing on one's own heritage, which can be used as a cohesive or corrosive force depending on how it is applied; includes cultural pride, cultural degradation, and cultural chauvinism.

Etiology—cause as determined by diagnosis.

Expressive jargon—See Variegated babbling.

Figurative—meaning does not correspond to the exact meanings of the words in the text.

Fluency—flow, smoothness.

Follow-up—action taken to inquire about the outcome of a recommendation or action taken after discharge.

Functional gain—difference between the weakest sounds a person is able to hear with (as opposed to without) hearing aids.

Function words—words whose exact meaning depends significantly on the content words that they connect, including prepositions, articles, conjunctions, and pronouns.

Gene—structure that codes specific genetic information as it is passed down from one generation to the next; genes are located on chromosomes.

Generalization—See Carryover.

Genetic—inherited, as genes carrying a particular trait are passed down from one generation to the next.

Hertz (Hz)—unit used to measure sound frequency.

Identification—recognizing or demonstrating awareness of a target's characteristic properties; the act of recognizing a deficit in performance; also, the act of recognizing individuals who require assessment and/or intervention services.

Idioglossia—See Cryptophasia.

Illocution—conventional, socially recognized, nonverbal signals that are intended to convey requests and guide attention.

Inherited—resulting from a gene being passed from one generation to the next.

Interdisciplinary team—a group of professionals, representing a variety of disciplines, who meet to address the needs of individuals receiving services from the group.

Interpersonal communication—communication between people.

Intervention—the act of doing something to or for someone in order to initiate change.

Intrapersonal communication—communication with one's self.

Jargon—unintelligible strings of syllables.

Language—a code whereby ideas about the world are expressed through a conventional system of arbitrary signals for communication.

Language competence—the successful integration of the three dimensions of language: form, content, and use.

Language content—the meaning, or semantics, of language.

Language delay—See Language disorder.

Language difference—a variation in a symbol system used by an entire group of individuals; this unique symbol system reflects shared regional, social, cultural, or ethnic factors and is typically characterized by variations in vocabulary, pronunciation, grammar, and pragmatics.

Language disability—See Language disorder.

Language disorder—a term used to describe a heterogeneous group of children whose language behaviors are different from, and not superior to, the language behaviors of their same-age counterparts.

Language form—the shape of the language, including all aspects that contribute to the surface features of the language (how it is perceived auditorily and/or visually).

Language impairment—See Language disorder.

Language sample—part of formal language testing; a carefully planned conversation that is taped and subsequently evaluated for the purpose of in-depth analysis.

Language use—the dimension of language that considers the function of the utterance and its context, also called pragmatics.

Lesion—injury, wound.

Lexical item—word.

Locative—a word designating location.

Locution—meaningful words that are used purposefully.

Long-term objective—a general goal that defines the expected communication status at discharge.

Marginal babbling—long series of syllabic segments that resemble adult syllables only in that they are composed of both consonants and vowels. Sounds and sound patterns; duration of syllables; frequency and duration of pauses between syllables; and pitch, inflection, and stress patterns differ from adult language.

Mental retardation—a condition that occurs when an individual's cognitive, intellectual, and behavioral skills are below those of same-age peers.

Metalinguistics—language (talking) about language; instructions pertaining to language.

Metaphoric—See Figurative.

Misdiagnosis—failure to identify a problem through assessment, inaccurate identification of a problem through assessment, or identification of a problem through assessment when, in fact, a problem does not exist.

Monolingual—having fluency in one language only.

Monologue—a long speech.

Morpheme—the smallest unit of language that carries meaning.

Morphology—study of morphemes; includes the words and morphemes of a language.

Morphophonemic rules—rules that govern the changes in pronunciation of words as morphemes are added.

Motherese—linguistic adaptations made by an adult caretaker in order to accommodate a child socially, linguistically, and contextually.

Narration—uninterrupted monologue that is generated for the purpose of entertaining or informing a listener.

Neologism—invented word.

Neonate—newborn.

Neurological—having to do with the brain or nervous system.

Nonfluent—choppy; not flowing smoothly.

Nonverbal—without spoken words.

Obligatory—compulsory, required by context.

Orthographic—written.

Otitis media—middle ear infection; fluid in the middle ear.

Overreferral—the act of recommending assessment and/or intervention for individuals who are not in need of services.

Paralinguistics—aspects of language apart from phonology, morphology, and syntax; includes prosody, voice, fluency, and some aspects of pragmatics.

Parallel play—the act of playing side-by-side and independently.

Parallel-talk—making comments about the actions of the child and objects that appear to hold the child's attention without an attempt to obtain a response.

Perception—achieving understanding.

Perinatal—at birth, during the birth process.

Perlocution—actions that unintentionally communicate a need and thereby result in a change in caretaker behavior such that the need is met.

Perseveration—meaningless repetition of a behavior, which may or may not have been useful, meaningful, or contextually appropriate at an earlier time.

Phoneme—the smallest pronounceable unit of a language.

Phonetically consistent form (PCF)—See Vocable.

Phonological process—simplification pattern used in the attempted pronunciation of words, phrases, and phoneme sequences.

Phonology—the system of sounds and sound patterns that characterize the language, including phonemes and syllables.

Physiology—function of anatomical structures.

Pidginization—modifications of a language that evolve for the purpose of communicating with people from dissimilar linguistic backgrounds.

Pidginized language—a language that evolves as a result of communication between individuals from dissimilar linguistic backgrounds and characterized by features of both languages, composed of short, simple utterances that contain only substantive words, and often resembling telegraphic speech.

Polyocular view—appreciating a circumstance from the perspective of many individuals.

Practicum—the experience of engaging in supervised clinical practice.

Pragmatics—See Language use.

Pre-consonant—See Constriction.

Prejudice—a negative a priori judgment about a group or about a group's individual members.

Prelingual—before the time when the individual has command of a first language.

Preverbal—before the time when an individual begins to use words for communication.

Prevowel—See Resonant.

Process—a natural phenomenon marked by gradual changes that lead toward a particular result.

Prognosis—a statement of one's professional opinion regarding whether a client is likely to benefit from intervention.

Prosody—the suprasegmental aspects of a language, comprising vocal inflection, stress, intonation, pausing, and all other variables that contribute to the rhythmic contour of the spoken segments or syllables.

Protocol—plan.

Pseudo-deficit—difference in performance that is based on gaps in the mastery of English, not to be used as evidence of a language disorder.

Quantify—measure numerically.

Race—a term describing one's biological and anatomical attributes as determined by heredity, including skin color, facial features, and hair texture.

Racism—the attitude that one's racial group is inherently superior to another group, corresponding to cultural degradation and cultural chauvinism.

Rapport—relationship of mutual trust.

Rationale—evidence on which a decision is based.

Recessive gene type—a gene whose characteristics are incapable of being manifested when paired with a dominant gene type.

Recommendation—advice based on findings.

Reduplicated babbling—series of repeated consonant-vowel syllables; syllable duration, duration and frequency of pauses, and pitch, inflection and stress patterns somewhat resemble adult language patterns.

Referral—a recommendation to consult an outside source.

Reflexive vocalization—vocalizations that are automatic in nature and occur in response to stimuli.

Reinforcement—See Consequence.

Reinforcer—See Consequence.

Resonance—tone as determined by vibrations within a hollow chamber.

Resonant—pre-vowel; approximation of a vowel.

Response—target behavior, or what the client does immediately after an antecedent.

Screening—brief evaluation to determine whether an assessment is necessary.

Segment—See Syllable.

Self-play—the act of entertaining one's self in the absence of interaction with other people.

Self-talk—long, audible, self-directed private monologue characterized by behaviors such as verbal play, songs, rhymes, accounts of imaginative stories and events, and expressions of emotions; the act of verbalizing whatever one is seeing, hearing, doing or feeling.

Semantic category—classifications used to sort words according to identified aspects of language content.

Semantics—refers to the meaning conveyed by words, phrases, utterances, gestures, and body language.

Short-term objective—a specific goal that clearly defines the immediate steps to be achieved while working toward a particular long-term objective.

Simultaneous communication—the act of speaking and signing at the same time for the purpose of communication.

Single-word utterance—expression that is similar in form to an adult word or phrase and is consistently used by the child in reference to a particular object or situation.

Specific language disability—See Language disorder.

Specific language impairment—See Language disorder.

Speech-language pathologist—a person who is certified by the American Speech-Language-Hearing Association in speech-language pathology and therefore is qualified to diagnose and treat individuals with speech-language disorders.

Stereotype—an oversimplified, often negative, concept about members of a particular group.

Stimulus—See Antecedent, Consequence.

Style switching—changes of linguistic form within a language in order to accommodate situational demands, including changing from one dialect to another as well as situation-dependent changes that occur within a dialect.

Suprasegmental—See Prosody.

Syllable—smallest possible combinations of two or more phonemes, comprising the segments of the language.

Syntax—system of rules for combining linguistic units, such as morphemes and words.

Target behavior—See Response.

Terminal objective—See Long-term objective.

Third-party payer—an agency that pays on behalf of a private individual for services rendered.

Time out—temporary removal from stimulation and opportunity.

Triad—a group of three; specifically, three individuals conversing.

Trisomy—a disorder of human chromosome number in which one of the 23 chromosome pairs has three members instead of the normal two.

Twin talk—See Cryptophasia.

Unilateral—on one side.

Variegated babbling—syllable series that resembles the adult language in all respects expect comprehensibility.

Vascular lesion—a lesion caused by interrupted blood supply.

Vocable—utterance that does not resemble the form of an adult word but is used repeatedly and consistently by the child to represent the same object, event, or relation.

Vocal play—experimentation with pitch and volume extremes.

Index